Achieving Child Health Equity

Editors

ROBERT S. KAHN
MONICA J. MITCHELL
TINA L. CHENG

PEDIATRIC CLINICS
OF NORTH AMERICA

www.pediatric.theclinics.com

Consulting Editor
TINA L. CHENG

August 2023 • Volume 70 • Number 4

ELSEVIER

1600 John F. Kennedy Boulevard • Suite 1800 • Philadelphia, Pennsylvania, 19103-2899

http://www.theclinics.com

THE PEDIATRIC CLINICS OF NORTH AMERICA Volume 70, Number 4
August 2023 ISSN 0031-3955, ISBN-13: 978-0-323-93907-2

Editor: Kerry Holland
Developmental Editor: Axell Ivan Jade M. Purificacion

The Pediatric Clinics of North America (ISSN 0031-3955) is published bimonthly by Elsevier Inc., 360 Park Avenue South, New York, NY 10010-1710. Months of issue are February, April, June, August, October, and December. Periodicals postage paid at New York, NY and additional mailing offices. Subscription prices are $279.00 per year (US individuals), $827.00 per year (US institutions), $351.00 per year (Canadian individuals), $1100.00 per year (Canadian institutions), $419.00 per year (international individuals), $1100.00 per year (international institutions), $100.00 per year (US students and residents), $100.00 per year (Canadian students and residents), and $165.00 per year (international residents and students). To receive students/resident rare, orders must be accompanied by name of affiliated institution, date of term, and the signature of program/residency coordinator on institution letterhead. Orders will be billed at individual rate until proof of status is received. Foreign air speed delivery is included in all *Clinics* subscription prices. All prices are subject to change without notice. **POSTMASTER:** Send address changes to *The Pediatric Clinics of North America*, Elsevier Health Sciences Division, Subscription Customer Service, 3251 Riverport Lane, Maryland Heights, MO 63043. **Customer Service: 1-800-654-2452 (US and Canada). From outside of the US and Canada: 1-314-447-8871. Fax: 1-314-447-8029. For print support, E-mail: JournalsCustomerService-usa@elsevier. com. For online support, E-mail: JournalsOnlineSupport-usa@elsevier.com.**

Reprints. For copies of 100 or more, of articles in this publication, please contact the Commercial Reprints Department, Elsevier Inc., 360 Park Avenue South, New York, NY 10010-1710. Tel.: 212-633-3874; Fax: 212-633-3820; E-mail: reprints@elsevier.com.

The Pediatric Clinics of North America is also published in Spanish by McGraw-Hill Inter-americana Editores S.A., Mexico City, Mexico; in Portuguese by Riechmann and Affonso Editores, Rua Comandante Coelho 1085, CEP 21250, Rio de Janeiro, Brazil; and in Greek by Althayia SA, Athens, Greece.

The Pediatric Clinics of North America is covered in *MEDLINE/PubMed (Index Medicus), Excerpta Medica, Current Contents, Current Contents/Clinical Medicine, Science Citation Index, ASCA, ISI/BIOMED,* and *BIOSIS.*

PROGRAM OBJECTIVE

The goal of the *Pediatric Clinics of North America* is to keep practicing physicians and residents up to date with current clinical practice in pediatrics by providing timely articles reviewing the state-of-the-art in patient care.

TARGET AUDIENCE

All practicing pediatricians, physicians, and healthcare professionals who provide patient care to pediatric patients.

LEARNING OBJECTIVES

Upon completion of this activity, participants will be able to:

1. Review challenges, barriers, and underlying causes adversely impacting optimal health for every child.
2. Discuss effective partnerships that address health care access and promote child health equity.
3. Recognize efficient modalities Pediatricians and other health care providers can take to improve child health outcomes and advance progress towards health equity.

ACCREDITATIONS

Physician Credit

The Elsevier Office of Continuing Medical Education (EOCME) is accredited by the Accreditation Council for Continuing Medical Education (ACCME) to provide continuing medical education for physicians.

The EOCME designates this journal-based activity for a maximum of 16 *AMA PRA Category 1 Credit*(s)™.- Physicians should claim only the credit commensurate with the extent of their participation in the activity.

All other healthcare professionals requesting continuing education credit for this journal-based activity will be issued a certificate of participation.

ABP Maintenance of Certification Credit

Successful completion of this CME activity, which includes participation in the activity and individual assessment of and feedback to the learner, enables the learner to earn up to 16 MOC points in the American Board of Pediatrics' (ABP) Maintenance of Certification (MOC) program. It is the CME activity provider's responsibility to submit learner completion information to ACCME for the purpose of granting ABP MOC credit.

DISCLOSURE OF CONFLICTS OF INTEREST

The EOCME assesses conflict of interest with its instructors, faculty, planners, and other individuals who are in a position to control the content of CME activities. All relevant conflicts of interest that are identified are thoroughly vetted by EOCME for fair balance, scientific objectivity, and patient care recommendations. EOCME is committed to providing its learners with CME activities that promote improvements or quality in healthcare and not a specific proprietary business or a commercial interest.

The planning committee, staff, authors, and editors listed below have identified no financial relationships or relationships to products or devices they or their spouse/life partner have with commercial interest related to the content of this CME activity:

Maria J. Arrojo, MA; Andrew F. Beck, MD, MPH; Jonas Bromberg, PsyD; Katherine C. Budolfson, MD, MPH; Tina L. Cheng, MD, MPH; Alexandra M. S. Corley, MD, MPH; Lori Crosby, PsyD; R. Neal Davis, MD, MSc; Lisa Ross DeCamp, MD, MSPH; Elena Dicus, JD, MBA; Benard P. Dreyer, MD; Ashley Durkin, MPH, PMP; Ruth A. Etzel, MD, PhD; Errol L. Fields, MD, PhD, MPH, FAAP; Arvin Garg, MD, MPH; Angelo P. Giardino, MD, PhD; Daniella Gratale, MA; Adrienne W. Henize, JD; Robert S. Kahn, MD, MPH; Melissa D. Klein, MD, MEd; Daniel Kozman, MD, MPH; Marciana Laster, MD, MSCR; Michelle Littlejohn, Melissa R. Lutz, MD, MHS; Keith J. Martin, DO, MS; Rajkumar Mayakrishnan, BSc, MBA; Kamila B. Mistry, PhD, MPH; Monica J. Mitchell, PhD, MBA; Monica Johnson Mitchell, PhD, MBA; David Nichols, MD, MBA; Eliana M. Perrin, MD, MPH; Sarah Polk, MD, ScM; Carolyn Reynolds, APRN, MS; Carley Riley, MD; Barry S. Solomon, MD, MPH; Tiffany A. Stewart, MD; Rachel L.J. Thornton, MD, PhD; Alicia Tieder, MSW, LICSW; Ndidi I. Unaka, MD, MEd; Louis Vernacchio, MD, MSc; Kara O. Walker, MD, MPH, MSHS; Leslie R. Walker-Harding, MD, FAAP, FSAHM; Heather J. Walter, MD, MPH; Karen M. Wilding, MHA; Desiree Yeboah, MD, FAAP; H. Shonna Yin, MD, MS; Janine Young, MD.

The planning committee, staff, authors, and editors listed below have identified financial relationships or relationships to products or devices they or their spouse/life partner have with commercial interest related to the content of this CME activity:

Keith C. Norris, MD, PhD: Consultant: Atlantis Health.

UNAPPROVED/OFF-LABEL USE DISCLOSURE

The EOCME requires CME faculty to disclose to the participants:

1. When products or procedures being discussed are off-label, unlabelled, experimental, and/or investigational (not US Food and Drug Administration [FDA] approved); and
2. Any limitations on the information presented, such as data that are preliminary or that represent ongoing research, interim analyses, and/or unsupported opinions. Faculty may discuss information about pharmaceutical agents that is outside of FDA-approved labelling. This information is intended solely for CME and is not intended to promote off-label use of these medications. If you have any questions, contact the medical affairs department of the manufacturer for the most recent prescribing information.

TO ENROLL

To enroll in the *Pediatric Clinics of North America* Continuing Medical Education program, call customer service at 1-800-654-2452 or sign up online at http://www.theclinics.com/home/cme. The CME program is available to subscribers for an additional annual fee of USD 214.00.

METHOD OF PARTICIPATION

In order to claim credit, participants must complete the following:

1. Complete enrolment as indicated above.
2. Read the activity.
3. Complete the CME Test and Evaluation. Participants must achieve a score of 70% on the test. All CME Tests and Evaluations must be completed online.

In order to claim MOC points, participants must complete the following:

1. Complete steps listed above for claiming CME credit
2. Provide your specialty board ID#, birth date (MM/DD), and attestation.
3. Online MOC submission is only available for the American Board of pediatrics' (ABP) Maintenance of Certification (MOC) program

CME INQUIRIES/SPECIAL NEEDS

For all CME inquiries or special needs, please contact elsevierCME@elsevier.com.

Contributors

CONSULTING EDITOR

TINA L. CHENG, MD, MPH
BK Rachford Professor and Chair of Pediatrics, University of Cincinnati, University of Cincinnati College of Medicine, Director, Cincinnati Children's Research Foundation, Chief Medical Officer, Cincinnati Children's Hospital Medical Center, Cincinnati, Ohio

EDITORS

ROBERT S. KAHN, MD, MPH
Professor of Pediatrics, University of Cincinnati, Vice President, Health Equity Strategy and Lead, Michael Fisher Child Health Equity Center, Cincinnati Children's Hospital Medical Center, Cincinnati, Ohio

MONICA J. MITCHELL, PhD, MBA
Professor, Division of Behavioral Medicine and Clinical Psychology, University of Cincinnati, Senior Director, Community Relations, Co-Director, Center for Clinical and Translational Science and Training, Community Engagement, Michael Fisher Child Health Equity Center, Cincinnati Children's Hospital Medical Center, Department of Pediatrics, University of Cincinnati College of Medicine, Cincinnati, Ohio

TINA L. CHENG, MD, MPH
BK Rachford Professor and Chair of Pediatrics, University of Cincinnati, University of Cincinnati College of Medicine, Director, Cincinnati Children's Research Foundation, Chief Medical Officer, Cincinnati Children's Hospital Medical Center, Cincinnati, Ohio

AUTHORS

MARIA J. ARROJO, MA
Pediatric Physicians' Organization at Children's, Wellesley, Massachusetts; Boston Children's Hospital, Boston, Massachusetts

ANDREW F. BECK, MD, MPH
Associate Professor, Department of Pediatrics, University of Cincinnati College of Medicine, Divisions of General and Community Pediatrics, and Hospital Medicine, Cincinnati Children's Hospital Medical Center, Cincinnati, Ohio

JONAS BROMBERG, PsyD
Pediatric Physicians' Organization at Children's, Wellesley, Massachusetts; Boston Children's Hospital, Harvard Medical School, Boston, Massachusetts

KATHERINE C. BUDOLFSON, MD, MPH
Academic General Pediatrics Fellow, Baylor College of Medicine, Texas Children's Hospital, Houston, Texas

TINA L. CHENG, MD, MPH
BK Rachford Professor and Chair of Pediatrics, University of Cincinnati, University of Cincinnati College of Medicine, Director, Cincinnati Children's Research Foundation, Chief Medical Officer, Cincinnati Children's Hospital Medical Center, Cincinnati, Ohio

ALEXANDRA M.S. CORLEY, MD, MPH
Assistant Professor, Department of Pediatrics, University of Cincinnati College of Medicine, Division of General and Community Pediatrics, Cincinnati Children's Hospital Medical Center, Cincinnati, Ohio

LORI E. CROSBY, PsyD
Professor, Division of Behavioral Medicine, Cincinnati Children's Hospital Medical Center, Department of Pediatrics, University of Cincinnati College of Medicine, Cincinnati, Ohio

R. NEAL DAVIS, MD, MSc
Intermountain Health, Senior Medical Director, Intermountain Children's Health, Murray, Utah

ELENA DICUS, JD, MBA
Executive Network Director, Intermountain Health, Intermountain Children's Health, Salt Lake City, Utah

LISA ROSS DeCAMP, MD, MSPH
Children's Hospital Colorado, Department of Pediatrics, University of Colorado School of Medicine, Adult and Child Center for Outcomes Research and Delivery Science, Aurora, Colorado; Latino Research and Policy Center, Denver, Colorado

BENARD P. DREYER, MD
Professor and Vice Chair for Diversity, Equity and Inclusion, Department of Pediatrics, NYU Grossman School of Medicine, New York, New York

ASHLEY DURKIN, MPH, PMP
Seattle Children's Center for Diversity and Health Equity, Seattle, Washington

RUTH A. ETZEL, MD, PhD
Adjunct Professor, Milken Institute School of Public Health, The George Washington University, Washington, DC

ERROL L. FIELDS, MD, PhD, MPH, FAAP
Division of Adolescent/Young Adult Medicine, Department of Pediatrics, Johns Hopkins School of Medicine, Baltimore, Maryland

ARVIN GARG, MD, MPH
Professor, Department of Pediatrics, Child Health Equity Center, UMass Chan Medical School, UMass Memorial Children's Medical Center, Worcester, Massachusetts

ANGELO P. GIARDINO, MD, PhD
Wilma T. Gibson Presidential Professor, Chair, Department of Pediatrics, University of Utah School of Medicine, Chief Medical Officer, Intermountain Primary Children's Hospital, Salt Lake City, Utah

DANIELLA GRATALE, MA
Associate Vice President, Federal Affairs, Nemours Children's Health, National Office of Policy and Prevention, Washington, DC

ADRIENNE W. HENIZE, JD
Program Manager, Child HeLP and Community Partnerships, Division of General and Community Pediatrics, Cincinnati Children's Hospital Medical Center, Cincinnati, Ohio

ROBERT S. KAHN, MD, MPH
Professor of Pediatrics, University of Cincinnati, Vice President, Health Equity Strategy and Lead, Michael Fisher Child Health Equity Center, Cincinnati Children's Hospital Medical Center, Cincinnati, Ohio

MELISSA D. KLEIN, MD, MEd
Professor, Department of Pediatrics, University of Cincinnati College of Medicine, Divisions of General and Community Pediatrics, and Hospital Medicine, Cincinnati Children's Hospital Medical Center, Cincinnati, Ohio

DANIEL KOZMAN, MD, MPH
David Geffen School of Medicine, UCLA Department of Medicine, Section of Medicine-Pediatrics and Preventive Medicine, University of California, Los Angeles, Los Angeles, California

MARCIANA LASTER, MD, MSCR
David Geffen School of Medicine, University of California, Los Angeles, Division of Pediatric Nephrology, UCLA Department of Pediatrics, Los Angeles, California

MELISSA R. LUTZ, MD, MHS
General Academic Pediatrics Fellow, Department of Pediatrics, Johns Hopkins School of Medicine, Baltimore, Maryland

KEITH J. MARTIN, DO, MS
Department of Pediatrics, Johns Hopkins School of Medicine, Centro SOL-Center for Salud/Health and Opportunity for Latinos, Baltimore, Maryland

KAMILA B. MISTRY, PhD, MPH
Associate Director, Office of Extramural Research, Education and Priority Populations, Sr Advisor Health Equity and Child Health and Quality Improvement, US Department of Health and Human Services, Agency for Healthcare Research and Quality, Rockville, Maryland; Department of Pediatrics, Johns Hopkins School of Medicine, Baltimore, Maryland

MONICA J. MITCHELL, PhD, MBA
Professor, Division of Behavioral Medicine and Clinical Psychology, University of Cincinnati, Senior Director, Community Relations, Co-Director, Center for Clinical and Translational Science and Training, Community Engagement, Michael Fisher Child Health Equity Center, Cincinnati Children's Hospital Medical Center, Department of Pediatrics, University of Cincinnati College of Medicine, Cincinnati, Ohio

DAVID NICHOLS, MD, MBA
President and CEO, Emeritus, The American Board of Pediatrics, Chapel Hill, North Carolina

KEITH C. NORRIS, MD, PhD
David Geffen School of Medicine, University of California, Los Angeles, Division of General Internal Medicine and Health Services Research, UCLA Department of Medicine, Los Angeles, California

ELIANA M. PERRIN, MD, MPH
Bloomberg Distinguished Professor, Department of Pediatrics, Johns Hopkins School of Medicine/School of Nursing, Baltimore, Maryland

SARAH POLK, MD, SCM
Department of Pediatrics, Johns Hopkins School of Medicine, Centro SOL-Center for Salud/Health and Opportunity for Latinos, Baltimore, Maryland

CAROLYN REYNOLDS, APRN, MS
Intermountain Health, Executive Clinical Director, Intermountain Children's Health, Murray, Utah

CARLEY L. RILEY, MD
Associate Professor, Department of Pediatrics, University of Cincinnati College of Medicine, Division of Critical Care, Cincinnati Children's Hospital Medical Center, Cincinnati, Ohio

BARRY S. SOLOMON, MD, MPH
Professor, Department of Pediatrics, Johns Hopkins School of Medicine, Baltimore, Maryland

TIFFANY A. STEWART, MD
Department of Pediatrics, NYU Grossman School of Medicine, Bellevue Hospital, New York, New York

RACHEL L.J. THORNTON, MD, PhD
Vice President, Chief Health Equity Officer, Nemours Children's Health, Wilmington, Delaware

ALICIA TIEDER, MSW, LICSW
Seattle Children's Center for Diversity and Health Equity, Seattle, Washington

NDIDI I. UNAKA, MD, MEd
Professor, Department of Pediatrics, University of Cincinnati College of Medicine, Cincinnati Children's Hospital Medical Center, Cincinnati, Ohio

LOUIS VERNACCHIO, MD, MSc
Pediatric Physicians' Organization at Children's, Wellesley, Massachusetts; Boston Children's Hospital, Harvard Medical School, Boston, Massachusetts

KARA O. WALKER, MD, MPH, MSHS
Executive Vice President, Chief Population Health Officer, Nemours Children's Health, Washington, DC

LESLIE R. WALKER-HARDING, MD, FAAP, FSAHM
University of Washington/Seattle Children's Hospital, Seattle, Washington

HEATHER J. WALTER, MD, MPH
Harvard Medical School, Boston Children's Hospital, Boston, Massachusetts; Pediatric Physicians' Organization at Children's, Wellesley, Massachusetts

KAREN M. WILDING, MHA
Vice President, Chief Value Officer, Nemours Children's Health, Wilmington, Delaware

DESIREE YEBOAH, MD, FAAP
University of Washington/Seattle Children's Hospital, Seattle, Washington

HSIANG SHONNA YIN, MD, MS
Department of Pediatrics, NYU Grossman School of Medicine, Bellevue Hospital, Population Health, New York, New York

JANINE YOUNG, MD
Department of Pediatrics, University of California, San Diego School of Medicine, Rady Children's Hospital San Diego

Contents

Preface: Achieving Child Health Equity   xvii

Robert S. Kahn, Monica J. Mitchell, and Tina L. Cheng

A Framework for Pursuing Child Health Equity in Pediatric Practice   629

Robert S. Kahn, Tina L. Cheng, and Monica J. Mitchell

> This article brings together several disparate frameworks to help outline a
> needed shift in pediatric practice to ensure child health equity. That shift
> involves moving from a commitment to equal care delivery to an explicit
> commitment to equitable health outcomes. The frameworks describe (1)
> the distinct domains of child health where inequity can be expressed, (2)
> the shortfalls of equal care delivery in meeting that promise, (3) a coherent
> typology of the barriers that drive health inequity and (4) a characterization
> of interventions as downstream, midstream, and upstream in nature.

Clarity on Disparity: Who, What, When, Where, Why, and How   639

Tina L. Cheng and Kamila B. Mistry

> This article offers a framework of *who, what, when, where, why, and how* of
> health disparities that can serve as a systematic approach to move from
> description to understanding causes and taking action to ensure health
> equity.

Population Healthcare Practice Management

**Population Health in Pediatric Primary Care as a Means to Achieving Child Health
Equity**   651

R. Neal Davis, Carolyn Reynolds, Elena Dicus, and Angelo P. Giardino

> We propose population health as a model of care to advance efforts to
> achieve child health equity. We use the structure-process-outcome frame-
> work to highlight key structures of pediatric population health necessary to
> catalyze what has been slow progress to date. Using specific ongoing ex-
> amples, we then show how different models of integrated health care de-
> livery systems align population health structures to enable processes
> aimed to achieve child health equity. We conclude by highlighting the crit-
> ical role of committed leadership to drive progress.

**Alternative Payment Models and Working with Payers–Key Considerations for
Advancing Population Health Goals and Achieving Child Health Equity**   667

Rachel L.J. Thornton, Karen M. Wilding, Daniella Gratale, and Kara O. Walker

> This article summarizes approaches to achieving value-based care in Pe-
> diatrics, providing a framework for understanding the continuum of models
> from fee-for-service to advanced alternative payment models. We present
> key examples of how alternative payment models have been developed
> and applied at the federal level within Medicare through the work of
> the Centers for Medicare and Medicaid Services (CMS) and the Center

for Medicaid and Medicaid Innovation (CMMI). We further describe key lessons learned and opportunities to adapt value-based payment models to promote whole child health and equity. Finally, we summarize policy considerations and challenges in achieving accountability and aligning financial incentives for children's health within a complex payer landscape.

Moving Beyond Health Care to Achieve Health Equity

Partnering with Families and Communities to Improve Child Health and Health Equity   683

Monica J. Mitchell, Carley L. Riley, and Lori E. Crosby

Pediatricians and other pediatric health providers collaborate with families and communities, including schools, health departments, and other partners to advance pediatric health challenges and health equity. This article will discuss best practices and guiding principles to support engagement and effective partnership with families and communities. Models for engaging families and communities while promoting health equity will also be discussed. Case studies and examples will be shared, as well as how they may be applied by pediatric health providers to promote child health.

Addressing Social Determinants of Health in Practice   695

Melissa R. Lutz, Arvin Garg, and Barry S. Solomon

This review summarizes the current pediatric literature related to social determinants of health, including strengths and weaknesses of screening practices and intervention strategies, common concerns and potential unintended consequences, opportunities for further research, and provides evidence-informed practical strategies for clinicians.

Pursuing a Cross-Sector Approach to Advance Child Health Equity   709

Alexandra M.S. Corley, Adrienne W. Henize, Melissa D. Klein, and Andrew F. Beck

Cross-sector partnerships are essential to ensure a safe and effective system of care for children, their caregivers, and communities. A "system of care" should have a well-defined population, vision, and measures shared by health care and community stakeholders, and an efficient modality for tracking progress toward better, more equitable outcomes. Effective partnerships could be clinically integrated, built atop coordinated awareness and assistance, and community-connected opportunities for networked learning. As opportunities for partnership continue to be uncovered, it will be vital to broadly assess their impact, using clinical and nonclinical metrics.

Addressing Structural Racism in Pediatric Clinical Practice   725

Marciana Laster, Daniel Kozman, and Keith C. Norris

Structural racism is the inequitable allocation of various social determinants of health to different communities. Exposure to this and other discrimination levied from intersectional identities is the primary driver of disproportionately adverse health outcomes for minoritized children and their families. Pediatric clinicians must vigilantly identify and mitigate racism in health care systems and delivery, assess for any impact of patient and family exposure to racism and direct them to appropriate health resources, foster an environment of inclusion and respect, and ensure that all care is delivered through a race-conscious lens with the utmost cultural humility and shared decision-making

Addressing Health Literacy in Pediatric Practice: A Health Equity Lens   745

Tiffany A. Stewart, Eliana M. Perrin, and Hsiang Shonna Yin

Low health literacy has been linked to worse child health-related knowledge, behaviors, and outcomes across multiple health domains. As low health literacy is highly prevalent and an important mediator of income- and race/ethnicity-associated disparities, provider adoption of health literacy best practices advances health equity. A multidisciplinary effort involving all providers engaged in communication with families should include a universal precautions approach, with clear communication strategies employed with all patients, and advocacy for health system change.

Health Care Anchors' Responsibilities and Approaches to Achieving Child Health Equity   761

Desiree Yeboah, Alicia Tieder, Ashley Durkin, and Leslie R. Walker-Harding

This article provides an overview of the anchor institution concept, recommended strategies for embracing an anchor mission, and the challenges that can arise in the process. An anchor mission centers on advocacy, social justice, and health equity. Hospitals and health systems are anchor institutions that are uniquely positioned to utilize their economic and intellectual resources in partnership with communities to mutually benefit the long-term well-being of both. Anchor institutions have a responsibility to invest in the education and development of their leaders, staff, and clinicians in health equity, diversity, inclusion, and anti-racism.

Special Topics

Pediatric Primary-Care Integrated Behavioral Health: A Framework for Reducing Inequities in Behavioral Health Care and Outcomes for Children   775

Maria J. Arrojo, Jonas Bromberg, Heather J. Walter, and Louis Vernacchio

Nearly half of US children and adolescents will suffer a behavioral health (BH) disorder, with substantially higher rates among more disadvantaged children such as racial/ethnic minorities, LGBTQ + youth, and poor children. The current specialty pediatric BH workforce is inadequate to meet the need and the uneven distribution of specialists as well as other barriers to care, such as insurance coverage and systemic racism/bias, further exacerbate disparities in BH care and outcomes. Integrating BH care into the pediatric primary care medical home has the potential to expand access to BH care and reduce the disparities inherent in the current system.

Health Care for Children in Immigrant Families: Key Considerations and Addressing Barriers   791

Keith J. Martin, Sarah Polk, Janine Young, and Lisa Ross DeCamp

One in four US children is a child in an immigrant family. Children in immigrant families (CIF) have distinct health and health care needs that vary by documentation status, countries of origin, and health care and community experience caring for immigrant populations. Health insurance access and language services are fundamental to providing health care to CIF. Promoting health equity for CIF requires a comprehensive approach to both the health and social determinants of health needs of CIF. Child health providers can promote health equity for this population through tailored primary care services and partnerships with immigrant-serving community organizations.

Achieving Health Equity for Sexual and Gender-Diverse Youth   813

Errol L. Fields

Compared to their heterosexual and cisgender peers, sexual and gender diverse (SGD) youth, especially those from minoritized racial/ethnic groups, experience significant disparities in health, health care, and social conditions that can threaten their health and well-being. This article describes the disparities impacting SGD youth, their differential exposure to the stigma and discrimination that foster these disparities, and the protective factors that can mitigate or disrupt the impact of these exposures. On the final point, the article specifically focuses on pediatric providers and inclusive, affirming, medical homes as critical protective factors for SGD youth and their families.

Climate Change and Child Health Equity   837

Katherine C. Budolfson and Ruth A. Etzel

The climate crisis is a major public health threat for children, disproportionately affecting the most vulnerable populations. Climate change causes a myriad of health issues for children, including respiratory illness, heat stress, infectious disease, the effects of weather-related disasters, and psychological sequelae. Pediatric clinicians must identify and address these issues in the clinical setting. Strong advocacy from pediatric clinicians is needed to help prevent the worst effects of the climate crisis and to support the elimination of use of fossil fuels and enactment of climate-friendly policies.

Practice and Policy Change

Crossing the Quality Chasm and the Ignored Pillar of Health Care Equity   855

Tina L. Cheng, Ndidi I. Unaka, and David Nichols

Although there has been tremendous progress toward the aspiration of delivering quality health care, among the National Academy of Medicine's (previously Institute of Medicine) six pillars of quality (health care should be safe, effective, timely, patient-centered, efficient, and equitable), the last pillar, equity, has been largely ignored. Examples of how the quality improvement (QI) process leads to improvements are numerous and must be applied to the pillar of equity related to race/ethnicity and socio-economic status. This article describes how equity should be addressed using the QI process.

Achieving Child Health Equity: Policy Solutions 863

Benard P. Dreyer

Policy solutions to address child health equity, with evidence to support the policies, are presented. Policies address health care, direct financial support to families, nutrition, support for early childhood and brain development, ending family homelessness, making housing and neighborhoods environmentally safe, gun violence prevention, LGBTQ + health equity, and protecting immigrant children and families. Federal, state, and local policies are addressed. Recommendations of the National Academy of Science, Engineering, and Medicine and the American Academy of Pediatrics are highlighted when appropriate.

PEDIATRIC CLINICS OF NORTH AMERICA

FORTHCOMING ISSUES

October 2023
Pediatric Genetics
Anne Slavotinek, *Editor*

December 2023
Everyday Ethics in the Clinical Practice of Pediatrics and Young Adult Medicine
Margaret R. Moon, *Editor*

February 2024
Addressing Violence in Pediatric Practice
Joel A. Fein and Megan H. Bair-Merritt, *Editors*

RECENT ISSUES

June 2023
Pediatric Rehabilitation
Mary McMahon and Amy Houtrow, *Editors*

April 2023
Vaccine Hesitancy
Peter G. Szilagyi, Sharon G. Humiston, and Tamera Coyne-Beasley, *Editors*

February 2023
Child Advocacy in Action
Lisa J. Chamberlain, Tina L. Cheng, David M. Keller, *Editors*

THE CLINICS ARE AVAILABLE ONLINE!
Access your subscription at:
www.theclinics.com

Preface

Achieving Child Health Equity

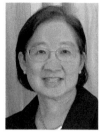
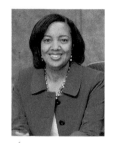
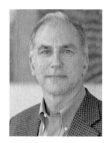

Tina L. Cheng, MD, MPH   Monica J. Mitchell, PhD, MBA   Robert S. Kahn, MD, MPH
Editors

Injustice anywhere is a threat to justice everywhere. We are caught in an inescapable network of mutuality, tied in a single garment of destiny. Whatever affects one directly, affects all indirectly.
—*Martin Luther King Jr, Letter from Birmingham, Alabama jail, April 16, 1963.*

As pediatric professionals, we must ensure that every child is healthy, ready to learn, and on their optimal trajectory to healthy adulthood. Excellent and equitable health outcomes are our goal. This issue of Pediatric Clinics of North America does not simply describe health disparities across different populations but also delves deeper into causes and how to take action to achieve equity. As pediatric clinicians, we have focused on actions that can be implemented in practice and advocacy on the system level. This issue's authors make a compelling argument that to achieve health equity, the scope of what is formally "in practice" must be broadened.

This issue recognizes that a child's well-being is inextricably tied to the well-being of their family and community. Achieving health equity acknowledges the importance of the family and community context and requires multilevel intervention, including the practice, health institution, community, and policy levels (**Fig. 1**). Recognizing this, each article includes practical tips for extending clinical practice into these spheres.

The first articles in this issue, by Kahn and colleagues and Cheng and Mistry, offer frameworks for addressing child health equity with an emphasis on clarity in language when discussing health disparities. With a shift in focus from individual care to population care (**Fig. 2**), the next section focuses on population health care practice management with articles on population health management in practice and working with payers on population health. Population health improvement involves work on the community level addressing social determinants and structural drivers. The articles by Mitchell and colleagues, Lutz and colleagues, Beck and colleagues, Norris, Williams and colleagues, and Walker-Harding and colleagues discuss working with families and

Pediatr Clin N Am 70 (2023) xvii–xix
https://doi.org/10.1016/j.pcl.2023.05.002
0031-3955/23/© 2023 Published by Elsevier Inc.

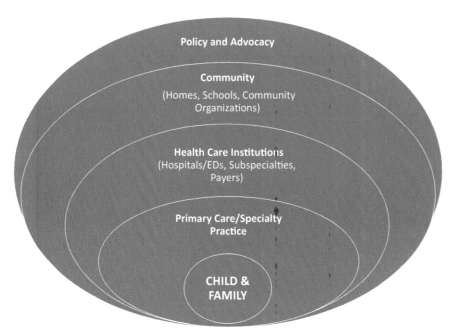

Fig. 1. Levels of intervention to achieve health equity.

communities, screening for social determinants, integrating work across sectors, addressing structural racism and health literacy in practice, and taking responsibility as anchor institutions.

Four "hot-topic" areas are discussed in the articles by Vernacchio, Polk and colleagues, Fields, and Etzel and Budolfson, including health equity related to mental

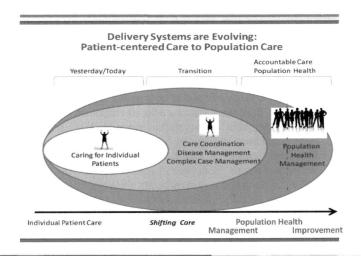

Fig. 2. Delivery systems are evolving: patient-centered care to population care. (*Adapted from* Linda Dunbar, with permission.)

health and climate change and to two populations of focus: immigrants and LGBTQ health. Finally, quality improvement and policy interventions to achieve health equity are highlighted in the final articles, written by Cheng and colleagues and Dreyer.

The COVID-19 pandemic and the murder of George Floyd have yet again laid bare the longstanding health disparities that exist by race/ethnicity, language, and socio-economic status. That evidence is clear. This issue of *Pediatric Clinics of North America* focuses on drivers of inequity and specific actions to achieve health equity and justice. It is time for pediatric clinicians to heed Dr King's call—to lean into the inescapable network and co-create the equitable, caring system that all children and families deserve.

Tina L. Cheng, MD, MPH
University of Cincinnati
Cincinnati Children's Research Foundation
Cincinnati Children's Hospital Medical Center
Michael Fisher Child Health Equity Center
3333 Burnet Avenue MLC 3016
Cincinnati, OH 45229-3026, USA

Monica J. Mitchell, PhD, MBA
Division of Behavioral Medicine and
Clinical Psychology
Center for Clinical and Translational Science
and Training, Community Engagement
Cincinnati Children's Hospital Medical Center
Michael Fisher Child Health Equity Center
3333 Burnet Avenue MLC 3015
Cincinnati, OH 45229-3026, USA

Robert S. Kahn, MD, MPH
University of Cincinnati
Cincinnati Children's Hospital Medical Center
Michael Fisher Child Health Equity Center
3333 Burnet Avenue
Cincinnati, OH 45229-3026, USA

E-mail addresses:
Tina.cheng@cchmc.org (T.L. Cheng)
Monica.Mitchell@cchmc.org (M.J. Mitchell)
Robert.kahn@cchmc.org (R.S. Kahn)

A Framework for Pursuing Child Health Equity in Pediatric Practice

Robert S. Kahn, MD, MPH[a],*, Tina L. Cheng, MD, MPH[b], Monica J. Mitchell, PhD, MBA[c,d]

KEYWORDS

- Child health equity • Pediatric practice • Community partnerships
- Social determinants of health

KEY POINTS

- Rather than seeking equal delivery of pediatric clinical services, the goal should be equitable child health outcomes.
- To achieve equitable health outcomes, one needs to appreciate that 80% of the variation in outcomes is explained by factors outside of medical care.
- Pediatric practice change to address those factors outside of clinical care will require we address both family-level social needs and community-level structural factors.

THE COMPLEXITY OF HEALTH DISPARITIES

Health disparities remain pervasive across conditions in children and youth. Preterm birth, infant mortality, asthma, diabetes, and depression all show evidence for variation in outcomes.[1] That variation is driven by social, environmental, and physical conditions.[2] These disparities occur not just in health conditions but also in well-being outcomes for children, such as kindergarten readiness and high school graduation. Racism and poverty are two of the foundational drivers of these inequities but, as papers throughout this issue demonstrate, inequities emerge wherever there are differentials in power and status that lead to discrimination and differentials in access to needed supports.

[a] University of Cincinnati, Michael Fisher Child Health Equity Center, Cincinnati Children's Hospital Medical Center, 3333 Burnet Avenue, Cincinnati, OH 45229-3026, USA; [b] University of Cincinnati, Cincinnati Children's Research Foundation, Cincinnati Children's Hospital Medical Center, Michael Fisher Child Health Equity Center, 3333 Burnet Avenue MLC 3106, Cincinnati, OH 45229-3026, USA; [c] Division of Behavioral Medicine and Clinical Psychology, University of Cincinnati; [d] Community Relations, Center for Clinical and Translational Science and Training, Community Engagement, Michael Fisher Child Health Equity Center, Cincinnati Children's Hospital Medical Center, 3333 Burnet Avenue MLC 3015, Cincinnati, OH 45229-3026, USA
* Corresponding author.
E-mail address: Robert.kahn@cchmc.org

Pediatr Clin N Am 70 (2023) 629–638
https://doi.org/10.1016/j.pcl.2023.03.002
0031-3955/23/© 2023 Elsevier Inc. All rights reserved.

Increasingly medical leaders have drawn attention to these disparities. The National Academy of Science, Engineering, and Medicine, American Academy of Pediatrics, Academic Pediatric Association, Society for Pediatric Research, and American Pediatric Society have all focused attention on the issue.[3,4] Pediatric professionals, across all disciplines and subspecialties, are uniquely positioned to see the impact of these social forces and highlight preventable and unjust morbidity. Further, through our research insights, the field is positioned to characterize how these social forces 'get under the skin' of children to cause and to perpetuate worse outcomes.

But the pathways or mechanisms that lead from these foundational drivers to inequitable outcomes are complex. The pathways can cross over one or more than one generation, they can act directly on individuals, families, communities, or at a population level, and they can interact in ways that are hard to discern. Many pathways can lead to the same adverse outcome and a single pathway can have multiple adverse impacts.[5] The pathways can have many modifiable upstream and downstream points or they can be short with a limited window for intervention. Further, the pathways, when fully laid out, offer many arenas for action—from political and social advocacy to food and housing policy to school and early education supports to health care access and treatment.

Given the complexity of the causal pathways, pediatric professionals are not nearly as well positioned to address disparities as they are to document them. This article seeks to offer an approach to this challenge. The goal of pediatric professionals should be equitable child outcomes among those that come to care and among all children in our community. The goal must be achieved through a logical and disciplined set of upstream interventions. To guide the needed pediatric practice changes amid this complexity the article brings together and briefly describes four frameworks: the first framework describes the multiple domains of child health in which inequity can emerge, the second highlights the needed shift from pursuing equal care delivery to pursuing equity in child health, the third framework offers a coherent depiction of causes of inequities (and hence a rationale and logic for change efforts), and the final framework characterizes strategies for intervention. These existing frameworks, familiar to some, have not previously been brought together to inform pediatric practice change. Further, the four frameworks provide logic for many of the topics included in this issue, as outlined below.

To achieve equitable child health outcomes

- Shift mindset from pursuing equal care to achieving equitable outcomes
- Adopt a coherent framework of non-medical causes of inequity
- Partner to pursue midstream and upstream interventions to address those causes

FRAMEWORK FOR CHILD HEALTH OUTCOMES: MORE THAN DISEASE

Child health disparities often focus on inequities in health conditions or diseases, but a broader frame is needed. The National Research Council and Institute of Medicine report on "Children's Health, The Nation's Wealth" outlined three domains of health fundamental to the assessment of children's health: health conditions, functioning, and health potential (**Table 1**). Health conditions include alterations in health status by disease, injuries, impairments, or pathophysiological manifestations of disorders (signs and symptoms) and are critical to assess in addition to the length of life. Disparities are evident across almost every pediatric health condition.[1] Health functioning includes all aspects of physical, psychological, cognitive, and social functioning in daily life as a child develops. Health potential involves a child's competency and capacity in

Table 1		
Domains of child health		
Health Conditions	**Functioning**	**Health Potential**
Alternations in health status due to disease, disability, or injury	Physical, cognitive, emotional, and social functioning and deficits	Competency and capacity in physical, cognitive, emotional, social well-being, and development potential
Symptoms	Functional deficit, disability (disability days, bed days)	Resilience
	Restrictions in activity, morbidity burden	
	Flourishing	

Institute of Medicine. 2004. Children's Health, the Nation's Wealth: Assessing and Improving Child Health. Washington, DC: The National Academies Press. https://doi.org/10.17226/10886.

physical, cognitive, emotional, social well-being, and their developmental potential. It also includes health assets or resilience, a child's ability to respond to future health challenges. Pediatric clinicians must broaden their attention to disparities in functioning and health potential which may be more visible in other settings, such as home and school. As a corollary, clinicians will have to broaden their strategies to assess and address these domains.

FRAMEWORK FOR CHILD EQUITABLE HEALTH OUTCOMES VERSUS EQUAL HEALTH CARE SERVICES

The next framework highlights that excellence in equal delivery of care is not enough. Equity in outcomes should be the goal of pediatric practice. Equality in care delivery means every child is offered the same access to phone triage, the same set of immunizations, and the same treatment protocols. Yet as the other papers will highlight across their case studies, treating all equally with standard care will lead to differential outcomes. The message in **Fig. 1** will be familiar to most. A prior version shows individuals of different heights trying to watch a baseball game from behind a tall fence. In the first panel, they all stand on equal boxes. The one who is tall can see the game and the one who is short cannot. The second panel shows that the box height has been tailored to the individual and now all can see the game. The Robert Wood Johnson Foundation recently updated the graphic to align the concept more closely to health equity (see **Fig. 1**).[6] Pursuing Equality, in panel 1, everyone gets the same, regardless of whether it is needed, right, or sufficient for the desired outcome. When Pursuing Equity, panel 2, everyone gets what is needed to overcome their foundational barriers and conditions. Of note, the solutions in panel 2 are structural ones, rather than ones that expect each individual to adapt to circumstances.

Alexandra M.S. Corley and colleagues' article, "Pursuing a Cross-Sector Approach to Advance Child Health Equity," note in their paper, for some children with asthma, there are barriers and conditions, such as poor quality housing, that lead to worse outcomes. In their paper on health literacy, Tiffany A. Stewart and colleagues' article, "Addressing Health Literacy in Pediatric Practice: A Health Equity Lens," in this issue point out that low literacy is an important mediator of poverty and racism-related conditions. Both give practical advice on how standard pediatric care can be adapted or tailored to meet the unique needs of some families to ensure children achieve

EQUALITY:
Everyone gets the same – regardless if it's needed or right for them.

EQUITY:
Everyone gets what they need – understanding the barriers, circumstances, and conditions.

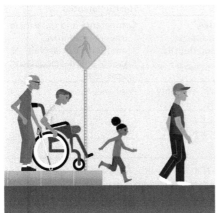 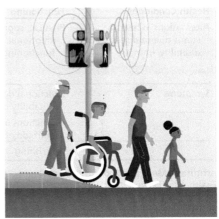

Fig. 1. A framework to differentiate the delivery of equal care from the adaptations needs to achieve equitable outcomes. Copyright 2022 Robert Wood Johnson Foundation.

equitable outcomes. The American Academy of Pediatrics and others[7] have proposed updated models of the Medical Home and offer guidance and resources to help ensure health equity. In summary, the first framework highlights the difference between equal health care delivery and the needed adaptations in pediatric practice to ensure equitable child health outcomes.

However, there are so many potential adaptations. The next framework offers a simple and coherent way to think about the causes of inequitable outcomes before moving to interventions.

FRAMEWORK FOR THE CAUSES OF CHILD HEALTH EQUITY

Given the complexity of the pathways that lead to health disparities, the third framework offers a simple, coherent depiction of causes. There are many graphical representations of the social, economic, and environmental factors that cause health inequities. **Fig. 2** shows one of the most common representations, constructed by the University of Wisconsin Population Health Institute for the County Health Rankings and Roadmap initiative.[8] This figure is chosen here because its implications for clinical practice are clearest. Importantly, the antecedents to these outcomes begin during infancy and childhood and possibly in utero and preconception.

The model draws on research literature[9] that indicates that medical care accounts only for 5% to 15% of the variation in premature death. In this figure, health behaviors account for an estimated 30%, social and economic factors 40%, and physical environment 10%. Further characterization of social and economic factors highlights the roles of education, income, and community safety, among others. These primary and secondary drivers offer a simple, coherent way to think about the cause of child health inequities. It is important to note that this model does not include some foundational causes identified in this volume, such as current and historical racism, as noted by Norris and colleagues, and discrimination against sexual and gender diverse youth and families or immigrants, as highlighted by Fields and #. Although pediatric practice's central objective is the delivery of clinical care, the figure illustrates that even

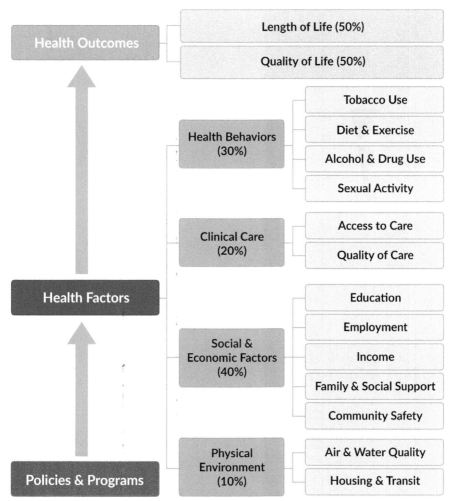

Fig. 2. A framework around the causes of variation in health outcomes with the estimated percentage of effect of each cause. County health rankings model ©2014 UWPHI.

the best clinical care will miss 80% of the factors driving variation in the child's long-term health. There are many potential opportunities for intervention.

FRAMEWORK FOR STRATEGIC EQUITY INTERVENTIONS

As noted above, there are many causes of health inequities and therefore many possible interventions. **Fig. 2** offered a simple frame for bucketing the causes. With those causes in mind, **Fig. 3** offers a frame for disciplined, strategic discussions around interventions. Originally developed by Castrucci and Auerbach and adapted in a recent Federal report,[10] the Figure highlights the notion of upstream and downstream work. Furthest downstream is the standard, daily work of clinicians providing medical care. Midstream efforts reflect much of our current work to screen for and address family-level social needs. This level of intervention would include providing community health workers or referrals to food banks. Finally, upstream efforts focus

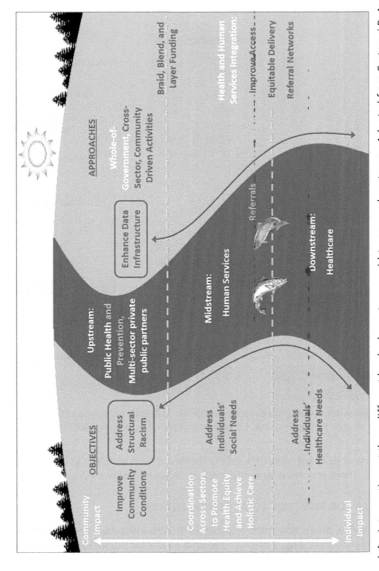

Fig. 3. A framework for interventions at three different levels: downstream, midstream, and upstream. *Adapted from* Castrucci B, Auerbach J, Meeting individual social needs falls short of addressing social determinants of health. Health affairs blog. January 16, 2019.

Table 2
Examples of interventions (framework 3) addressing select causes (framework 2) of child health inequity

	Social	Economic	Physical Environment
Downstream (equal health care)	Easy front desk appointment-making for all families	Free drug samples in the practice	Stronger asthma medicines when current regimen fails
Midstream (meeting family levels needs)	Refer to a community health worker to assist with coordinating appointments and transportation	Local community organization staff available to assist with Earned Income Tax Credit filing	Refer to city housing authority for home inspection and remediation
Upstream (addressing population-level structural barriers)	Health system pursuit of mission as an Anchor Institution, eg, fair wages, supplier diversity, community engagement	Join advocacy effort for renewal of the Child Tax Credit	Support City effort to hold the landlord accountable by testifying on health effects of poor-quality housing

on community level impact with more structural change. These include working on laws and policies like the Child Tax credit to reduce family poverty or addressing the legacy of structural racism by working on residential segregation and home ownership. Pediatric practices can start at either level and intentionally choose which pathways to address. **Table 2** lays out a range of potential actions at each level for some common risk domains. This issue is replete with practical advice on how to get started.

CHALLENGES TO PURSUING OUTCOMES EQUITY IN PRACTICES: POPULATIONS, PARTNERSHIPS, PAYMENT

Moving from equal care to equitable outcomes, using a disciplined approach to downstream, midstream, and upstream interventions is the aspiration. To achieve that aspiration, though, there are at least three important challenges to address as part of an overall framework: populations, partnerships, and payment.

Populations

The term population is used so loosely that it can be problematic. A population, when used clinically, can refer to those currently with active medical records in one's practice or a subset of those with a specific medical condition listed. For payers or Accountable Care Organizations, a population might be that with a specific type of health insurance. More typically through a public health lens, the population will refer to those within a geographic boundary, or a subset of those within a geographic boundary.

Inequities in health outcomes, however, are often driven by those children who cannot routinely access and benefit from medical care. They may not appear on any practice's medical panel as "active". Further, families may have frequent changes in their health insurance. Payers then have no long-term accountability for improved outcomes. Finally, individual practices rarely care for most children in a geographic area. In summary, no single health care entity has the accountability and leverage to drive child health equity for all children. Future progress on child health equity will require more collaborative approaches across health systems and practices, and across payers, to ensure strong support for all vulnerable children and families. Significant improvements in disease outcomes across competitive health systems are emerging from new approaches such as Learning Networks.[11,12] These networks are now beginning to focus on health equity. By bringing multiple systems together to achieve a shared goal, they offer an important strategy for improving equity at the level of geographic populations.

Partnerships

Pediatric practices are well positioned to screen for and identify the social, economic, and environmental factors influencing child health, but practices are rarely positioned to prevent or mitigate those risks directly. As Corley and colleagues and Mitchell and colleagues discuss in detail in this issue, effective multi-sector partnerships are critical. An important additional question to highlight here is who, in an equitable outcomes-focused medical home, is accountable for developing and managing the partnerships. Traditional physician, nursing, care management, and community health worker roles are not scoped for the focus and skills to maintain these partnerships. Further, quality improvement, as outlined by Cheng and colleagues, is difficult enough when applied within the medical practice. Applying those methods to improve outcomes of a health care–community partnership is even more complex. To achieve child health equity at the population level, through high-quality community partnerships, pediatric practices will need to re-envision and rewrite traditional clinical roles and build new capabilities and capacities.

Payment

A final major consideration is payment and how to ensure it aligns with and adequately supports the pursuit of equitable health outcomes. Thornton and colleagues lay out the opportunities and the challenges for value-based payment to align with child health equity goals. In value-based payment, as opposed to payment for care utilization, the incentive is to keep children healthy. Federal and state agencies are exploring new ways to incentivize prevention and the needed multi-sector collaborations.

What, more precisely, must be supported by these changes in payment? As noted above, the frameworks suggest several areas that will require investment. Building practice roles and capabilities for equity will require financial support. Who will take on practice accountability for equitable outcomes and for building community collaborations? Who will bring the quality improvement skills to bear on those partnerships to ensure they are optimized? And what resources will be needed for practices to join in new cross-system and cross-sector learning networks to ensure child health equity across geographic populations? Further, as the number of health care-community partnerships grow, and the flow of referrals to community agencies increase, what financial resources will be available to support those community agencies, and how should that support be structured?

SUMMARY

A pediatric commitment to *equal* care delivery is a commitment to *inequitable* child health outcomes. A vision in which all children thrive requires us to begin adapting clinical practice to meet children and families where they are and to help them to overcome the family-level and structural barriers to health. That can feel like trying to boil the ocean or solve world hunger. The frameworks described here offer distinct domains of child health, a coherent typology of the barriers that drive health inequity, and a way to think about downstream, midstream, and upstream interventions. The midstream and upstream approaches naturally lead to community allies—partnerships to achieve the desired outcomes to address causes that lie beyond medical care. There remain challenges, such as reaching all children and aligning payment to support these practice changes. Yet, as other papers in this issue reveal, the field is more than ready to move forward. The papers capture many examples of practice changes that lead to more equitable child and youth outcomes, including across a range of special populations, and they offer practical steps forward. It is time for pediatric practice to achieve its great aspiration for every child.

CLINICS CARE POINTS

- Pause to consider the outcomes you wish every child in your practice could achieve.
- Identify a few children less likely to reach those outcomes because of family hardships, system barriers, or other hurdles.
- Identify one or two professionals from other disciplines that are critically important for those particular children to reach the outcomes – e.g., a teacher, a pharmacist, an adult mental health provider.
- To begin to put this framework into practice, carve out 15 minutes and, with one family's consent, reach out to the relevant professionals to brainstorm how, together, you might more effectively support the family and the child.

DISCLOSURE

The authors have no relevant disclosures to report.

REFERENCES

1. Beck AF, Riley CL, Taylor SC, et al. pervasive income-based disparities in inpatient bed-day rates across conditions and subspecialties. Health Aff 2018; 37(4):551–9.
2. Beck AF, Cohen AJ, Colvin JD, et al. Perspectives from the society for pediatric research: interventions targeting social needs in pediatric clinical care. Pediatr Res 2018;84(1):10–21.
3. Council On Community Pediatrics. Poverty and child health in the United States. Pediatrics 2016;137(4). https://doi.org/10.1542/peds.2016-0339.
4. Beck AF, Marcil LE, Klein MD, et al. Pediatricians contributing to poverty reduction through clinical-community partnership and collective action: a narrative review. Acad Pediatr 2021;21(8S):S200–6.
5. Cicchetti D, Rogosch FA. Equifinality and multifinality in developmental psychopathology. Dev Psychopathol 1996;8(4):597–600.
6. Robert Wood Johnson Foundation. Equality Equity Curb Graphic. 2022. Available at: https://www.rwjf.org/en/insights/our-research/infographics/visualizing-health-equity.html. Accessed January 10, 2023.
7. Garg A, Sandel M, Dworkin PH, et al. From medical home to health neighborhood: transforming the medical home into a community-based health neighborhood. J Pediatr 2012;160(4):535–536 e1.

8. The University of Wisconsin Population Health Institute. County Health Rankings & Roadmaps. 2023. www.countyhealthrankings.org. Accessed January 10, 2023.

9. Kaplan RM, Milstein A. Contributions of Health Care to Longevity: A Review of 4 Estimation Methods. Ann Fam Med 2019;17(3):267–72.

10. Whitman A., De Lew N., Chappel A., et al., Addressing Social Determinants of Health: Examples of Successful Evidence-Based Strategies and Current Federal Efforts, *ASPE Office of Health Policy*, HP-2022-12., 2022. https://aspe.hhs.gov/reports/sdoh-evidence-review.

11. Britto MT, Fuller SC, Kaplan HC, et al. Using a network organisational architecture to support the development of Learning Healthcare Systems. BMJ Qual Saf 2018; 27(11):937–46.

12. Seid M, Hartley DM, Margolis PA. A science of collaborative learning health systems. Learn Health Syst 2021;5(3):e10278.

Clarity on Disparity
Who, What, When, Where, Why, and How

Tina L. Cheng, MD, MPH[a,b,*], Kamila B. Mistry, PhD MPH[c,d]

KEYWORDS

- Disparities • Equity • Child • Racism • Stress • Access to care • Allostatic load

KEY POINTS

- To achieve health equity, the field must move beyond describing health disparities to understanding underlying causes and taking action to eliminate disparities.
- Clarity and explicit language are important in discussing and eliminating health disparities.
- Addressing the *who, what, when, where, why, and how* of health disparities is vital to advancing equitable health outcomes.

INTRODUCTION

Identifying and addressing disparities early in the life course offer an opportunity to improve overall population health and well-being. Although the Coronavirus Disease 2019 (COVID-19) pandemic and murder of George Floyd have exposed longstanding health disparities, many aspects of investigating and defining health disparities lack the clarity required to facilitate meaningful efforts toward advancing equity in health and health care delivery. This article offers a framework of *who, what, when, where, why, and how* that can serve as a systematic approach to move beyond cursory or proforma descriptions of health equity initiatives or research studies. Clarity in language and approach has the potential for deeper insights into scientific rationale, working hypotheses, analytical definitions, appropriate interventions, and other elements that cannot and should not be assumed. The framework focuses deliberately on the goal of questioning, a central aspect of scientific inquiry, and encourages sharing of thoughts and ideas based on the current level of understanding—with intent of driving further investigation and action to address inequities.

[a] Department of Pediatrics, University of Cincinnati College of Medicine, Cincinnati, OH, USA; [b] Cincinnati Children's Hospital Medical Center, 3333 Burnet Avenue. MLC 3016, Cincinnati, OH, USA; [c] US Department of Health and Human Services, Agency for Healthcare Research and Quality, 5600 Fishers Lane, Room 06N03, Rockville, MD, USA; [d] Department of Pediatrics, Johns Hopkins School of Medicine, Baltimore, MD, USA
* Corresponding author.
E-mail address: Tina.Cheng@cchmc.org

Pediatr Clin N Am 70 (2023) 639–650
https://doi.org/10.1016/j.pcl.2023.03.003
0031-3955/23/© 2023 Elsevier Inc. All rights reserved.

Previously, we have highlighted a set of unique considerations on health disparities in children, that are distinct from the underlying mechanisms for disparities among adults (**Table 1**).[1–3] The "5 Ds", as they are termed, offer a guide for researchers, practitioners, and policymakers in examining children's unique characteristics with regard to their demographics, development, disease/differential epidemiology, dependency, and dollars. The 5 Ds deepen our understanding and distinguish between factors that influence disparities in health care delivery and outcome for children compared with adults: *Demographic patterns* for US children continue to indicate higher rates of poverty and growing racial/ethnic diversity. Children, uniquely, have a *dependency* on parents or other caregivers for basic needs including health care requiring family input and family health. Children are predominantly healthy and have *differential epidemiology* with regard to chronic conditions, with many being relatively rare and requiring specialized care. *Development* in childhood and adolescence is characterized by continuous growth and transitions thereby setting a trajectory upon which adult health builds. Finally, costs or *dollars* spent on child health are relatively small compared to adults and the return on investment is not immediate but realized over the life course. In addition, almost half of all US children are enrolled in Medicaid or the Children's Health Insurance Program. Ultimately, these distinctions are important to inform the need, design, and implementation of approaches to eliminate disparities in children that decrease reliance on adult-focused solutions that are adapted or retrofit.

Perhaps a sixth D is "Do Now and Disseminate". The literature is rife with descriptions of disparities. However, there is a dearth of literature and evidence on

Table 1
The 5 Ds highlighting unique differences between the adult vs child/adolescent medical home

The 5 Ds	Adults	Children/Adolescents
Developmental Change	• Health maintenance • Prevention of adverse sequelae • Rehabilitative	• Enhance developmental progress • Habilitative
Dependency	• Independent and autonomous • Patient-centered Medical Home (PCMH)	• Dependent on adults • Parents are essential partners • Team members: family, child care providers, teachers, others • Family-centered Medical Home (FCMH)
Differential Epidemiology	• Large number of common chronic conditions (eg, heart disease, diabetes, hypertension) • Subspecialists in the community	• Predominantly healthy • Large number of relatively rare chronic conditions • Subspecialists based in academic medical centers
Demographic Patterns	• Poverty among elderly has declined in part due to Medicare	• Disproportionate rates of poverty • Disproportionate racial and ethnic diversity
Dollars	• Higher health care costs • Private insurers and Medicare • Focus on return on investment on secondary and tertiary prevention	• Overall costs are small • Private insurers, state Medicaid, CHIP • Return on investment over long-term life course

From Stille C, Turchi RM, Antonelli R, Cabana MD, Cheng TL, Laraque D, et al. The family-centered medical home: specific considerations for child health research and policy. Academic Pediatrics 2010; 10:211-7, copyright Elsevier. With copyright permission Elsevier.[3]

interventions to achieve health equity.[4] The future health and well-being of US children are linked to how successfully we manage, not just describe or report on the health and well-being of today's children. The persistence of disparities highlights a need to "disseminate" and apply what we know and "do" and "do now" rather than treat adult morbidities. In the path forward, translation of research to practice and policy and greater investment in dissemination and implementation research will allow us to "do" what is needed to improve population health and reduce disparities.

The Ds are vital, yet unless there is a deliberate focus on deconstructing and explicitly clarifying the *who, what, when/where, why, and how* of children's health disparities, progress will be slow. Addressing these questions can further target research and successful intervention.

CLARITY ON DISPARITY

To eliminate disparities and promote equity, focusing on a set of key questions can help to provide clarity regarding the current evidence base and how it can be used to pinpoint the "do" (and even the don't). Below, using racial/ethnic disparities in infant mortality (IM) as an example, we operationalize the *who, what, when/where, why, and how of children's disparities* to illustrate a systematic approach to using data and evidence to clarify current status and direct action.

WHO has the Disparity?

Too often, the term "disparity" is used generally without specificity to the population of focus. There are many dimensions that may relate to a population at risk. Healthy People 2030 defines a health disparity as, "a particular type of health difference that is closely linked with social, economic, and/or environmental disadvantage" and notes that disparities, "adversely affect groups of people who have systematically experienced greater obstacles to health based on their racial or ethnic group; religion; socioeconomic status; gender; age; mental health; cognitive, sensory, or physical disability; sexual orientation or gender identity; geographic location; or other characteristics historically linked to discrimination or exclusion."[5] Clarity on which population or dimension is the focus seems obvious but is often not specified with the term "disparities" used generically.

The concept of intersectionality further highlights the ways in which inequities based on gender, race, disability, and other factors related to discrimination can "intersect" to create unique and dynamic effects. With intersectionality and interactions among multiple dimensions, clarity on population or dimension of focus and understanding the contributions of the different dimensions are critical. Without necessary grounding and explicit information, incorrect assumptions can be made which then limits the overall value of the research and how it can be leveraged. This article focuses on disparities related to race/ethnicity and socioeconomic status though concepts presented may apply to other disparity dimensions.

The source of any population classification, such as self-reported or investigator observed may also be important in clarifying the "who". Additionally, who is selected as the reference population in a study and the underlying reasoning for the selection requires critical thought. Utilizing a different reference group could produce different results.

In the United States there are clear differences in infant mortality by race. The preterm birth rate is nearly 50% higher for Black compared to White infants[6] and there are nearly four times more deaths among Black infants related to short gestation and low birth weight. To disentangle and clarify "who" has the disparity, it is important to ascertain the contribution of race/ethnicity, socioeconomic status, or other factors to guide intervention.

WHAT is a Disparity?

Terms such as difference, disparity, inequality are often used interchangeably, yet each is distinct. Not all differences are health disparities.[7] As noted above, the US Department of Health and Human Services defines disparities as "a particular type of health difference that is closely linked with social, economic, and/or environmental disadvantage."[5] This definition purports that a disparity is not merely a difference but a difference due to greater obstacles. The World Health Organization has defined disparities as "differences in health which are not only unnecessary and avoidable but, in addition, are considered unfair and unjust."[8] Definitions are important and should be clearly articulated, as they have implications for both research and action. The definitions noted here move beyond describing the difference and making comparisons among subgroups. Rather, they signal a deeper focus on showing and addressing unfair treatment that warrant investigation and correction. Disparities should and do imply areas of disadvantage that often occur systematically and cause obstacles to health and fewer opportunities based on demographic, social, economic, and environmental factors.

In the case of infant mortality, the magnitude and severity of the disparity by race/ethnicity in infant mortality are staggering. Defining it as a disparity indicates that the differences are unfair and unjust, and avoidable. It delineates a path forward in defining both the aim and scope of investigation and intervention. Although some may consider differences unavoidable or rooted in conditions beyond control, assessing the notion of "avoidability" is critical. The Centers for Disease Control and Prevention (CDC) recently reported that more than 80% of pregnancy-related deaths were preventable.[9] Maternal morbidity and mortality correlate with infant survival and share risk factors.[10]

WHAT Kind of Disparity?

Health and health care disparities are often co-mingled. **Fig. 1** displays the levels at which disparities may occur differentiating health care disparities from health

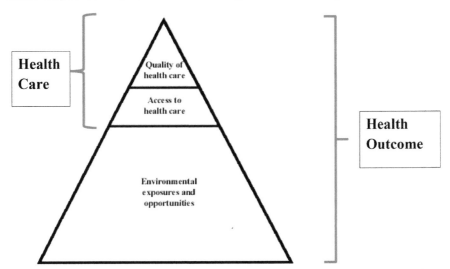

Fig. 1. Health or health care disparities: levels at which health disparities are produced. Camara Phyllis Jones. "Confronting Institutionalized Racism." Phylon (1960-) 50, no. 1/2 (2002): 7–22. https://doi.org/10.2307/4149999.

disparities. Health disparity refers to differences in burden of illness, disability or mortality experienced by one population compared to another. A health care disparity refers to differences in health care coverage, access, and quality of care. Although health and health care disparities are related, it is necessary to distinguish between the two as the potential sources and solutions are distinct.[11] Health care disparities often involve poor access and quality of care requiring health system solutions. **Fig. 2** demonstrates potential sources of disparities related to health care which may involve the patient, the clinician, the patient–clinician interaction, and/or the health system. Disparities in health outcomes may be produced from health care disparities and/or other levels and may require broader solutions.

As children are acquiring skills and developing their health potential, discussions of health and health care disparities must consider a broad range of outcomes such as well-being, life chances, opportunity, risk and resilience, and quality of life as well as the more traditional health status and the provision of health care.[12,13] Interventions to address IM have largely focused on delivery and quality of prenatal care. However, growing research demonstrates that health care-focused interventions are necessary but not sufficient to eliminate the health disparity in IM.[14]

WHEN/WHERE did the Exposure Underlying the Disparity Occur?

A key concept underlying life course population health is the critical and sensitive periods of exposures and their effects on children and even future generations. **Fig. 3** shows how children's health is affected by multiple influences and is changing across the life course starting in utero.[13] The timing of an exposure in childhood is critical to understanding mechanisms and exploring solutions. Risk factors associated with disparities will vary depending on the timing or developmental age and magnitude of exposure. In addition, there may be sensitive periods when exposures, positive or negative, are most detrimental or protective in relation to disparate health outcomes.[15] For instance, several studies have now shown cumulative life course exposure to low socioeconomic status conditions, starting in childhood, is associated with increases in cardiovascular disease outcomes in adulthood.[16]

Fig. 4 illustrates a life course view of health risk emphasizing developmental origins of health and disease and underlying epigenetic and other mechanisms involved in both disruptive and nondisruptive pathways to disease including evidence for transgenerational passage of risk from both maternal and paternal lines.[17] Adverse childhood experiences have been linked to chronic health problems, mental illness, and substance use problems in adolescence and adulthood.[18] There are growing examples of how exposures in utero can have effects across generations. For example, diethylstibestrol (DES) exposure during pregnancy has had multigenerational

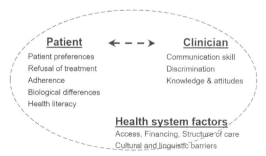

Fig. 2. Health care disparities: Potential sources involving the patient, clinician, interaction between the patient and clinician, and health system factors.

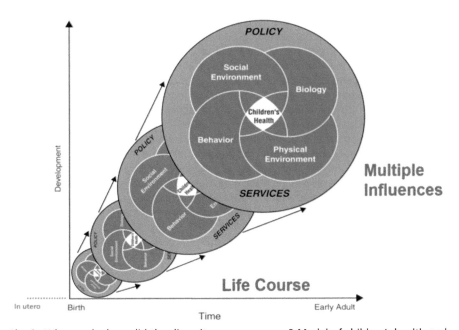

Fig. 3. When and where did the disparity exposure occur? Model of children's health and influences. (National Research Council and Institute of Medicine. 2004. Children's Health, the Nation's Wealth: Assessing and Improving Child Health. https://doi.org/10.17226/10886. Reproduced with permission from the National Academy of Sciences, Courtesy of the National Academies Press, Washington, D.C.)

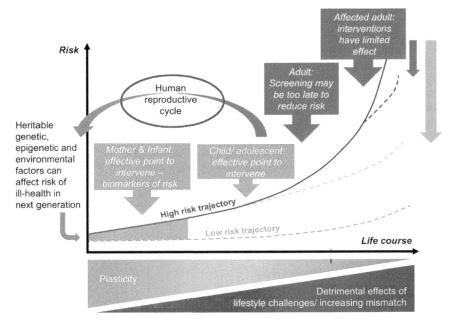

Fig. 4. When and where did the disparity exposure occur? Life course view of health risk. (*From* Hanson MA, Gluckman PD. Early Developmental Conditioning of Later Health and Disease: Physiology or Pathophysiology? Physiol Rev 2014; 94(4): 1027-1076. © The American Physiological Society (APS). All rights reserved.)

neurodevelopment effects.[19] A pregnant woman would be the first generation with her fetus representing the second generation. Exposure of the fetus' reproductive cells are the third generation and the potential mechanism for disruption.[20] Understanding mechanisms for transgenerational effects requires a three-generation approach and may guide intervention.[21]

Place-based approaches to address disparities in health and health care have been a growing focus.[22] These approaches highlight the importance of understanding and accounting for the context in which disparities occur. Investigation of the "where" can provide vital information on the cultural, social, and other specific local circumstances that need to be evaluated to address the disparity. However, while there are various terms and models that are considered in placed-based approaches, the emerging evidence continues to suggest that participatory and inclusive methods, working directly with communities, and grounded understanding are key elements for addressing contextual factors that influence health and health care disparities.

For infant mortality, there is growing research demonstrating that it is not only prenatal but also preconception influences that affect outcomes.[14,23] This requires a universal approach to ensuring all women of childbearing age are healthy. One pediatric-specific approach is to address the interconception care needs of mothers in pediatric practice. Studies of a preconception women's health screener used in pediatric practice increased positive maternal health behaviors including smoking cessation, folate use, and health knowledge around healthy interconception interval.[24–26]

Examples of placed-based approaches to IM reduction offer keen insights into interrelated contextual factors contributing to IM and emphasize the potential of intergenerational strategies addressing maternal and child health needs.[27] Evidence-based home visiting programs have shown promise in mitigating disparities by using culturally responsive and community driven approaches that carefully assess and meet the needs of at-risk families.[28]

WHY/HOW did the Disparity Occur?

Health and health care disparities are complex and multifactorial. Social, economic, and physical exposures (eg, poverty, racial discrimination, stress, housing instability) including those specific to the health care system (eg, access to services, quality of care) contribute to disparities, as well as their interactions. Research must go beyond describing disparities to ascertaining the "why" and "how" of health and health care disparities. A conceptual map or model incorporating the "why and how" is vital as it describes the underlying assumptions regarding how various factors may contribute to a specified disparity. This allows the field to grow as it openly invites challenge and evaluation of new theories and mechanisms which is critical to guide appropriate intervention. Emerging research on a range of factors from allostatic load (AL), racial discrimination, and access to care, among others, enhance our understanding of how exposures get "under the skin" leading to racial disparities in infant mortality.[14,29,30]

To reduce racial and ethnic disparities in infant mortality, the focus must turn to root causes and potential underlying mechanisms. Low birthweight (LBW) is the second leading cause, after birth defects, of infant mortality in the United States with Black infants being almost twice as likely to have LBW than White infants. Accumulating evidence shows chronic maternal stress among Black women to be one likely cause of infant LBW.[31] Chronic stress is shown to produce hormones which wear down the body over time and impact blood pressure and cholesterol. The cumulative impacts of stress are measured on a multi-system AL index of physiological function, with higher scores being associated with LBW and other pregnancy complications.[32] Recent studies looking carefully at the racial/ethnic disparities and their link to AL, have shown that differences in AL index scores are not explained by differences in socioeconomic factors, including education level and income among Black women. Thus, the findings suggest the role of racism in affecting AL and may underlie LBW deliveries.[33]

A framework by Camera Jones explores race-associated differences and how racism may operate at three levels: institutionalized, personally mediated, and internalized in affecting health outcomes.[34,35] Institutional racism is the structural differential access to goods, services, and opportunities of society by race while personally mediated racism involves prejudice and discrimination. Internalized racism is defined as the acceptance of negative messages about their own abilities and intrinsic worth among those stigmatized. The framework suggests that internalized racism may influence health outcomes through health behaviors. Institutionalized racism may operate through socioeconomic status or access to health care while personally mediated racism may operate through stress and differential treatment.[34] Using an allegory about a gardener, Jones describes flower boxes (rich and poor soil and red and pink flowers) to illustrate how racism affects growth.[35] The allegory is intended to guide explicit thinking about the multiple impacts of racism and can serve as a tool to understand and mitigate effects on maternal health and subsequently infant outcomes.

All three types of racism likely contribute to maternal morbidity and mortality. Recent studies have explored provider discrimination during pregnancy and delivery, particularly the role of implicit bias in influencing provider behavior.[36] Maternal mortality case reviews have highlighted a number of maternal deaths and near misses among minority women where providers did not or were slow to listen to patients. Additionally, study findings have also indicated significantly higher rates of disrespect and mistreatment (ie, shouting, ignoring, or refusing requests for help) during pregnancy and birth among Black, Latino, and Indigenous women.[37] Stress and AL related to racism may be another mechanism and target for intervention to drive improvements in maternal and infant morbidity and mortality.

Access to high-quality maternal care during pregnancy, birth, and postpartum is vital for optimal development and can influence IM and birth outcomes. Eisenberg and Power have outlined "voltage drops" or steps from the potential to receive high-quality health care to quality care received.[38] The steps include the availability of insurance, enrollment in insurance, coverage of services and providers, availability of informed choice, availability of a consistent source of primary care, accessibility of referral services, and delivery of high-quality care. Access to care may be an obstacle at one or more of these steps and may relate to the three types of racism. Understanding and addressing barriers are key.

For maternal access to care particularly in rural areas, the literature suggests that two key factors, insurance coverage and availability of providers and services, underlie existing racial/ethnic and geographic disparities. Medicaid is the largest payer for maternity care in the United States covering approximately 42% of all births with the largest share among Latino, Black, American Indian, and Alaska Native individuals and those who live in rural areas.[39,40] Many pregnant women enrolled in Medicaid experience a coverage gap during both the prenatal and postpartum periods, times that are critical to assuring both maternal and infant health. States have the option to extend postpartum Medicaid eligibility so mothers can stay insured for a full year after giving birth rather than losing coverage at 6 weeks. However, expansions continue to be uneven across the United States perpetuating disparities.[41] Beyond coverage, limited access to providers and obstetric/birthing facilities continue to drive disparities. Data suggest that a rise in both rural and medically underserved areas disproportionately impact communities with larger percentages of minority patients. Beyond describing disparities, digging deeper into the contribution of multiple potential mechanisms is critical to the design of appropriate and successful interventions.

SUMMARY

Eliminating disparities and ensuring equity must start early in the life course with an understanding of the unique considerations for child disparities related to demographics, development, dependency, disease/differential epidemiology, dollars, and dissemination. To further health equity research, programs, and policies, it is critical to clarify the *who, what, when/where, and why/how of disparities*. Clarity on the description of the population and disparity to be addressed are the first step (who/what). Delving deeper to understand when and where the disparity manifests and the mechanisms and processes (why/how) that underlie disparities in partnership with communities must guide intervention. Although descriptive statistics and studies of child health disparities are important for monitoring progress, it is incumbent that we systematically address the *who, what, when, where, how, and why* of disparities to enable more rapid and targeted action. Explicit language to address these questions, commitment to dissemination and implementation of best practices, and rooting out unfair, entrenched policies that have perpetuated structural inequities, are urgently needed to achieve health equity for children and their families.

CLINICS CARE POINTS

- Identifying and understanding disparities in health by race/ethnicity, socioeconomic status, and language are important in clinical care as a step toward health equity.
- Using the who, what, when, where, and how framework can assist in designing interventions in practice and policy.

DISCLOSURE

No financial assistance was received to support this article. This work is original, not previously published, and not submitted for publication or consideration elsewhere. The authors are solely responsible for this document's contents, findings, and conclusions, which do not necessarily represent the views or serve as an official position of AHRQ or HHS.

REFERENCES

1. Cheng TL, Mistry KB. The uniqueness and importance of children in addressing health disparities across the life course: implications for research. Epidemiology 2019;30(2):S60–4.
2. Forrest CB, Simpson L, Clancy C. Child health services research. Challenges and opportunities. JAMA 1997;277:1787–93.
3. Stille C, Turchi RM, Antonelli R, et al. The family-centered medical home: specific considerations for child health research and policy. Academic Pediatrics 2010; 10:211–7, copyright Elsevier.

4. Flores G, American Academy of Pediatrics Committee on Pediatric Research. Technical report: Racial and Ethnic Disparities in the Health and Health Care of Children. Pediatrics 2010;125:e979–1020.

5. Healthy People 2030. Health Equity in Healthy People 2030. Available at: https://health.gov/healthypeople/priority-areas/health-equity-healthy-people-2030#:~:text=Healthy%20People%202030%20defines%20a,%2C%20and%2For%20environmental%20disadvantage. Accessed October 23, 2022.

6. Riddell CA, Harper S, Kaufman JS. Trends in Differences in US Mortality Rates Between Black and White Infants. JAMA Pediatr 2017;171:911–3.

7. Braveman P. Health disparities and health equity: concepts and measurement. Annu Rev Public Health 2006;27:167–94.

8. Whitehead M. The concepts and principles of equity and health. Copenhagen, Denmark: World Health Organization Regional Office for Europe; 1990. Contract No.: EUR/ICP/RPD 414 7734r ORIGINAL: ENGLISH.

9. Trost SL, Beauregard J, Njie F, et al. Pregnancy-related deaths: data from maternal mortality review committees in 36 US states, 2017–2019. Atlanta, GA: Centers for Disease Control and Prevention, US Department of Health and Human Services; 2022.

10. Moucheraud C, Worku A, Molla M, et al. Consequences of maternal mortality on infant and child survival: a 25-year longitudinal analysis in Butajira Ethiopia (1987-2011). Reprod Health 2015;12(Suppl 1):S4.

11. Jones CP. National Center for Chronic Disease Prevention and Health Promotion (U.S.). Division of Adult and Community Health. Emerging Investigations and Analytic Methods Branch. Confronting institutionalized racism. Phylon 2002;50: 7–22. Available at: https://stacks.cdc.gov/view/cdc/104986. Accessed August 9, 2022.

12. Horn I, Cheng TL. Jenkins R and the DC Baltimore Research Center on Child Health Disparities Writing Group. Starting Early: A life-course perspective on child health disparities: Research Recommendations. Pediatrics 2009;124: S257–61.

13. National Research Council (US); Institute of Medicine (US). Children's Health. The Nation's Wealth: assessing and improving child health. Washington (DC): National Academies Press (US); 2004.

14. Lu MC, Kotelchuck M, Hogan V, et al. Closing the Black-White Gap in Birth Outcomes: A Life-course Approach. Ethn Dis 2010;20(1 0 2):S62–76.

15. Halfon N, Hochstein M. Life course health development: an integrated framework for developing health, policy and research. Milbank Q 2002;80:433–79.

16. Pollitt RA, Rose KM, Kaufman JS. Evaluating the evidence for models of life course socioeconomic factors and cardiovascular outcomes: a systematic review. BMC Publ Health 2005;5:7.

17. Hanson MA, Gluckman PD. Early developmental conditioning of later health and disease: physiology or pathophysiology? Physiol Rev 2014 Oct;94(4):1027–76.

18. Centers for Disease Control and Prevention. Fast Facts: Adverse Childhood Experiences (ACEs). 2022. Available at: https://www.cdc.gov/violenceprevention/aces/fastfact.html. Accessed October 23, 2022.

19. Kioumourtzoglou MA, Coull BA, O'Reilly ÉJ, et al. Association of Exposure to Diethylstilbestrol During Pregnancy With Multigenerational Neurodevelopmental Deficits. JAMA Pediatr 2018;172(7):670–7.

20. Cheng TL, Miranda ML, Child Enrollment Scientific Vision Working Group of the NIH All of Us Research Program. https://allofus.nih.gov/sites/default/files/cesvwg_1-18-18.pdf. Accessed October 23, 2022.

21. Cheng TL, Johnson SB, Goodman E. Breaking the Intergenerational Cycle of Disadvantage: The Three Generation Approach. Pediatrics 2016;137:1–12.

22. Dankwa-Mullan I, Pérez-Stable EJ. Addressing Health Disparities Is a Place-Based Issue. Am J Public Health 2016;106(4):637–9.

23. Centers for Disease Control and Prevention. Recommendations to improve pre-conception health and health care—United States: a report of the CDC/ATSDR Preconception Care Work Group and the Select Panel on Preconception Care. MMWR (Morb Mortal Wkly Rep) 2006;55(RR06):1–23.

24. Chilukuri N, Cheng TL, Psoter K, et al. Effectiveness of a Pediatric Primary Care Intervention to Increase Maternal Folate Use: Results from a Cluster Randomized Control Trial. J Pediatr 2018;192:247–52.

25. Upadhya KK, Psoter KJ, Connor KA, et al. Cluster randomized trial of a precon-ception health intervention for mothers in pediatric visits. Acad Pediatr 2020 Jul; 20(5):660–9.

26. Gregory EF, Upadhya KK, Cheng TL, et al. Enabling factors associated with receipt of interconception health care. Matern Child Health J 2020;24(3):275–82.

27. J. Taylor, C. Novoa, K. Hamm, S. Phadke. "Eliminating Racial Disparities in Maternal and Infant Mortality: A Comprehensive Policy Blueprint." Center for American Progress. May 2019. Available at: https://www.americanprogress.org/issues/women/reports/2019/05/02/469186/eliminating-racial-disparities-maternal-infant-mortality/. Accessed April 23, 2023.

28. Michalopoulos C, Faucetta K, Hill C.J, et al. "Impacts on Family Outcomes of Ev-idence-Based Early Childhood Home Visiting: Results from the Mother and Infant Home Visiting Program Evaluation." OPRE Report 2019-07. January 2019. Avail-able at: https://www.acf.hhs.gov/sites/default/files/documents/opre/mihope_impact_report_final20_508_0.pdf. Accessed April 23, 2023.

29. Wallace M, Harville E, Theall K, et al. Preconception Biomarkers of Allostatic Load and Racial Disparities in Adverse Birth Outcomes: the Bogalusa Heart Study. Paediatr Perinat Epidemiol 2013;27(6):587–97.

30. Witt WP, Cheng ER, Wisk LE, et al. Maternal Stressful Life Events Prior to Concep-tion and the Impact on Infant Birth Weight in the United States. Am J Public Health 2014;104(Suppl 1):S81–9.

31. Centers for Disease Control and Prevention. Infant Mortality. Available at: https://www.cdc.gov/reproductivehealth/maternalinfanthealth/infantmortality.htm#causes. Accessed October 23, 2022.

32. Beckie TM. A systematic review of allostatic load, health, and health disparities. Biol Res Nurs 2012;14(4):311–46.

33. Mays VM, Cochran SD, Barnes NW. Race, race-based discrimination, and health outcomes among African Americans. Annu Rev Psychol 2007;58:201–25.

34. Jones CP. Levels of racism: a theoretic framework and a gardener's tale. Am J Public Health 2000;90(8):1212–5.

35. Jones CP. Invited commentary: "race," racism, and the practice of epidemiology. Am J Epidemiol 2001;154(4):299–304 [discussion: 305-6].

36. Saluja B, Bryant Z. How Implicit Bias Contributes to Racial Disparities in Maternal Morbidity and Mortality in the United States. J Womens Health (Larchmt) 2021; 30(2):270–3.

37. Vedam S, Stoll K, Taiwo TK, et al. The Giving Voice to Mothers study: inequity and mistreatment during pregnancy and childbirth in the United States. Reprod Health 2019;16:77.

38. Eisenberg JM, Power EJ. Transforming insurance coverage into quality health care: voltage drops from potential to delivered quality. JAMA 2000;284(16): 2100–7.
39. Medicaid and CHIP Payment and Access Commission. Medicaid's Role in Financing Maternity Care. January 2020 Fact Sheet. Available at: https://www.macpac.gov/wp-content/uploads/2020/01/Medicaid's-Role-in-Financing-Maternity-Care.pdf. Accessed April 23, 2023.
40. Centers for Disease Control and Prevention National Center for Health Statistics. Key Birth Statistics. 2018 data. Available at: https://www.cdc.gov/nchs/nvss/births.htm. Accessed 23 October, 2022.
41. Admon LK, Daw JR, Winkelman TN, et al. Insurance Coverage and Perinatal Health Care Use Among Low-Income Women in the US, 2015-2017. JAMA Netw Open 2021;4(1):e2034549.

Population Healthcare Practice Management

Population Health in Pediatric Primary Care as a Means to Achieving Child Health Equity

R. Neal Davis, MD, MSc[a,*], Carolyn Reynolds, APRN, MS[a],
Elena Dicus, JD, MBA[b], Angelo P. Giardino, MD, PhD[c]

KEYWORDS

- Population health • Pediatric primary care • Financial integration
- Clinical integration • Clinically integrated networks • Social determinants of health
- Child health equity

KEY POINTS

- Progress on achieving child health equity has been slow despite being a critical priority.
- High-quality pediatric primary care is designed to advance child health equity within a population health model.
- Current structures of health care delivery, still largely supported by fee-for-service payments, are not designed to advance the practice transformation required to implement high-quality pediatric primary care.
- Integrated health care delivery systems, innovative structures with financial and clinical integration, may catalyze progress to achieve child health equity.
- Pediatric clinically integrated networks supported by children's hospitals offer a structure currently innovating to achieve child health equity within a population health model.

CASE STUDY

Sarah is a 5-year-old with asthma. She and her family are part of a refugee community in a large, urban US city. Her asthma is uncontrolled, and she has been to the emergency department (ED) several times for exacerbations as it is close to her home and

---

The authors have no financial disclosures or financial conflicts of interest.

[a] Intermountain Health, Intermountain Children's Health, 5026 South State Street, Murray, UT 84107, USA; [b] Intermountain Health, Intermountain Children's Health, 80 North Mario Capecchi Drive, Salt Lake City, UT 84102, USA; [c] Department of Pediatrics, University of Utah School of Medicine, Intermountain Primary Children's Hospital, 295 Chipeta Way, Salt Lake City, UT 84108, USA
* Corresponding author.
E-mail address: Neal.Davis@imail.org

her family has limited means of transportation. She has insurance through Medicaid and has been attributed (assigned administratively by Medicaid) to a local pediatric clinician. The local pediatrician, part of a productive fee-for-service office, is not aware of Sarah and her health or transportation challenges. Sarah is not the only child in her community with unmet needs, but there are no data resources devoted to understanding her communities' health. (Continued-end of the article.)

ACHIEVING CHILD HEALTH EQUITY

Equitable care was defined as one of six domains of quality in health care in 2001 in the Institute of Medicine's (IOM) seminal publication, Crossing the Quality Chasm.[1] Despite that prominent recognition of equity being a domain of health care quality, attention to incorporating equity in quality-improvement work has lagged behind in terms of effort and achievement.[2] This is especially true when compared to the effort devoted to patient safety, another of the six domains. For example, among a convenience sample of pediatric quality leaders, the Children's Hospital Association estimated that in 2019, while over 40% of their effort was directed toward patient safety, less than 10% of their effort was directed at health equity.[2]

Not long after the release of the Crossing Chasm, the IOM in 2003 released another report, Unequal Treatment, focused on the definition and measurement of inequitable care.[3] Overarching findings in this report included (1) racial and ethnic disparities in health care exist and, because they are associated with worse outcomes in many cases, are unacceptable, and (2) racial and ethnic disparities in health care occur in the context of broader historic and contemporary social and economic inequality and evidence of persistent racial and ethnic discrimination in many sectors of American life. Of note, pediatric care was included in the literature review and analysis that underpin the findings and recommendations from Unequal Treatment.[3] In 2010, the IOM empaneled a workgroup to determine if progress had occurred in the preceding decade. The findings were indeed disappointing, and among the key themes that emerged during the workgroup's deliberations was the persistence of health disparities: "Health disparities are not going away. Many participants agreed that health disparities have persisted over time and across the life course. Furthermore, people of color experience an earlier onset and a greater severity of negative health outcomes."[4] Despite equitable care being an IOM-designated domain of quality, and in the context of having an entire report focused on the striking disparities in care affecting large segments of the US population, equity in health care has remained elusive.

In this section, we propose population health as a model of care to advance efforts to achieve child health equity. We use the structure-process-outcome framework to highlight key structures of pediatric population health necessary to catalyze what has been slow progress to date. Using specific ongoing examples, we then show how different models of integrated health care delivery systems (IDSs) align population health structures to enable processes aimed to achieve child health equity. We conclude by highlighting the critical role of committed leadership to drive progress.

POPULATION HEALTH: CONCEPT, APPROACH, AND OUTCOME

In 2003, health service researchers, Drs David Kindig and Greg Stoddart proposed the definition of population health as "the health outcomes of a group of individuals, including the distribution of such outcomes within the group." They went on to declare that the practice of population health should include attention to not only health outcomes but also to patterns of health determinants, health policies, and health interventions.[5] The mention of health determinants presaged the eventual connection of the population health model to address what are now called the social determinants of health or social drivers of health (SDOHs) and the policies and actions necessary to promote optimal health. Kindig and Stoddart described determinants of health as including (1) social, economic, and physical environments; (2) personal health practices; (3) individual capacity and coping skills; (4) one's biology; (5) early developmental trajectory; and (6) access to health services. Within a population health approach, the focus is on the interrelationship of conditions and factors that affect defined groups, longitudinally over the life course. Ideally, this focus then leads to the identification of systematic variation in patterns of occurrence within and among different groups and correspondingly to a deeper understanding of these patterns along with implications on policies and actions aimed at improving the health of those groups in need.[5] Conceptually, population health connects the study of the distribution of various health outcomes (i.e., dependent variable) within a specified group of patients with the measured patterns of observable determinants of health (i.e., independent variable) along with the policies that influence those determinants (**Fig. 1**).

PRIMARY CARE, POPULATION HEALTH, AND ACHIEVING HEALTH EQUITY

In 2019, Silberberg and colleagues adopted the definition of population health described above and applied it specifically to primary care. "What PCPs do every day is designed to improve the health of their patients. However, taking a population

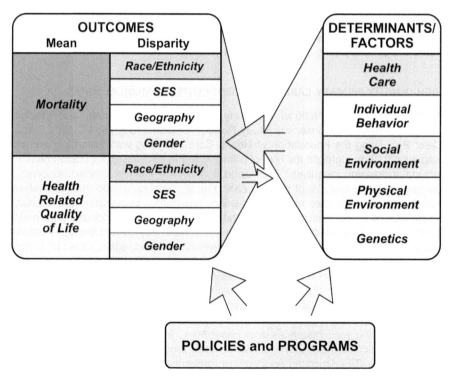

Fig. 1. Population health model. David Kindig PhD, Department of Population Health Sciences, University of Wisconsin, and Greg Stoddart, Department of Clinical Epidemiology and Biostatistics, McMaster University. (Used with permission and available at https://www.improvingpopulationhealth.org/blog/what-is-population-health.html.)

health perspective can lead providers to think differently about health problems and solutions and to use their time and resources in very different ways than when they consider the needs of patients one at a time."[6] They further prioritized the impact of SDOH on the distribution of health outcomes within a population. They argued that the practice of primary care is ideally suited to influence policies and interventions to eventually affect outcomes in a population specifically calling out the importance of attending to the influence of SDOH:

> Put simply, social determinants often confound the efforts of primary care to improve their patients' health. Despite the great gains in knowledge surrounding the science and methods of medicine and prevention, unhealthy environments and social inequalities result in unhealthy lifestyles, deficiencies in medical care and self-management, and health disparities. To make a significant change in population health, primary care professionals will have to collaborate with each other and with other sectors of society to address social and environmental determinants.[6]

Using a socio-ecological lens, Silberberg and colleagues advocated for primary care providers (PCPs) to embrace a population health approach to primary care at several levels, namely, individual, practice, institutional, and community:

> PCPs have several assets for engaging in population health. Patient data can be used to identify patterns of health outcomes that indicate the need to explore social determinants (e.g., a pattern of uncontrolled pediatric asthma in one area of town). The stories of individual patients are powerful tools for increasing the visibility of an issue. PCPs can leverage the respect afforded to their profession and their expertise about health and illness to increase the awareness of policymakers and the general public about the impact of social conditions on health.

HIGH-QUALITY PRIMARY CARE AND PATIENT-CENTERED MEDICAL HOME

In May of 2021, the National Academy of Science, Engineering, and Medicine (NASEM) issued the Consensus Study Report, "Implementing High-Quality Primary Care: Rebuilding the Foundation of Health Care", aligning with Silverberg and colleagues (2019) to highlight the role of primary care in advancing population health to include addressing inequities.[7] The report built on the well-established concepts of primary care, the four C's of primary care (**Fig. 2**),[8] and expanded them by defining high-quality primary care as "whole-person, integrated, accessible, and equitable health care by interprofessional teams who are accountable for addressing the majority of an individual's health and wellness needs across settings and through sustained relationships with patients, families, and communities." This, again, called on primary care to extend their focus not only to include children and families regularly engaging with their care but also to include all children and families attributed to their care, considering how these children interface with other health care institutions, their communities, and even the policy environment (**Fig. 3**).

However, achieving this expanded view of primary care requires practice transformation including new resources and capabilities. In recent decades, the patient-centered medical home (PCMH) has been widely promoted as the model for practice transformation. The American Academy of Pediatrics (AAP) defined a medical home as "an approach to providing comprehensive primary care that facilitates partnerships between patients, clinicians, medical staff, and families ... extend[ing] beyond the four walls of a clinical practice."[9] The National Committee for Quality Assurance (NCQA) outlined six concept areas for PCMH recognition: team-based care and practice

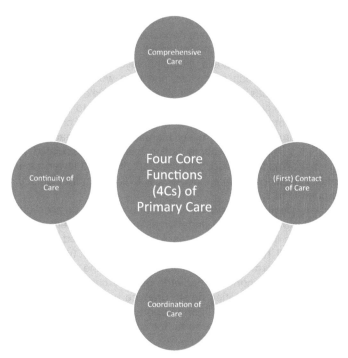

Fig. 2. The 4Cs of primary care.

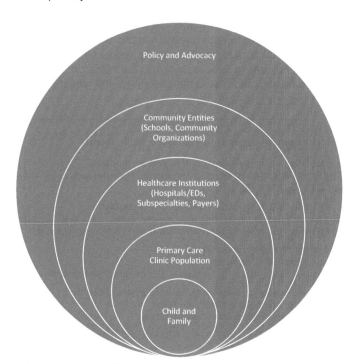

Fig. 3. Pediatric Population Health Socio-ecological Lens based on Silverberg and colleagues (2019) and NASEM Report on High-Quality Primary Care (2021).

organization, knowing and managing your patients, patient-centered access and continuity, care management support, care coordination and care transitions, and performance measurement and quality improvement.[10] Ideally, pediatric clinicians would regularly review their patient panels, including validated and meaningfully stratified data on quality and utilization outcomes, and then work with their care teams on outreach, needed services, and coordination of complex medical and social care (**Box 1**). Pediatric practices that have engaged in work to become PCMHs have achieved significant practice transformation in areas such as chronic condition management, care coordination, community outreach, data management, and quality improvement.[11] Notably, PCMH accreditation has been associated with improved quality outcomes, including reduced health disparities and lower costs.[12] As such, professional organizations, such as the AAP, actively promote PCMH for all primary care offices caring for children.[8]

However, many primary care clinicians do not practice in an accredited PCMH. In May of 2022, the Kaiser Family Foundation estimated that there were 441,439 primary care clinicians in the United States[13] with an estimated 67,000 practicing in an NCQA-accredited medical home,[14] or around 15%. (While there are other PCMH accreditation organizations, NCQA remains the major accreditor.)[9] As such, it is likely that a minority of pediatric primary care clinicians practice in an accredited PCMH with population health practice transformation capabilities. Understanding this discrepancy may inform opportunities for change that could potentially improve population health efforts for children including progress toward achieving child health equity.

INTEGRATED HEALTH CARE DELIVERY SYSTEMS

Dr Avedis Donabedian proposed structure, process, and outcome as a conceptual framework for advancing health care quality.[15] In this framework, structure includes the context in which care is delivered including physical facilities, payment models, data infrastructure, and staffing; process includes the interactions between the health care team and patients; and outcomes refers to the effects on patients and

---

Box 1
How pediatric clinicians can practice in a population health model

1. Define a population at the pediatric clinician and/or clinic level
   - Full attributed patient panel or condition-specific registries such as asthma, depression, children with medical complexity

2. Define meaningful and actionable measures for the population
   - Quality measures such as well-child visits, immunizations, asthma action plan
   - Utilization measures such as emergency department visits, inpatient visits

3. Stratify measures for equity focus such as:
   - Payer level: commercial, Medicaid
   - Community level: race, ethnicity, language, and geography/neighborhood

4. Universally screen/respond to social determinants/drivers of health
   - Evidence-based screening and clinic workflows
   - Partnerships with community-based organizations

5. Care team collaboration for outreach, gap closures, and community connections
   - Care management and care coordination
   - Parent and adolescent advisory groups
   - Partnerships with community groups

populations. Donabedian suggested generally that structure leads to processes, which lead to outcomes (**Fig. 4**), or in other words, meaningful change often starts with structure.

Importantly, the NASEM report on high-quality primary care suggested structural challenges that primary care practices face to achieve population health practice transformation.[7] Many of these can be organized generally in areas of value-based financial alignment, expanded care teams, and data capabilities. For example, the NASEM report calls for a shift from fee-for-service payment to value-based payments, from physician-centric care delivery models to team-based care enabled by robust care management and care coordination, and from fragmented data reporting to comprehensive population health data tools. These three areas are interdependent (**Fig. 5**). Success in value-based payments may finance expanded care teams or improved data capabilities. However, success in value-based payments depend on both expanded care teams and improved data capabilities. It is, therefore, daunting for primary care practices to take on value-based contracts without those capabilities in place. It is similarly difficult to invest in expanded care teams or data capabilities without the assurance of sustained value-based payment structures. As such, the default path for many primary care offices may be stagnation, lack of practice transformation, and inability to embrace a population health model. On the other hand, if there are structures that can aid primary care practices in overcoming these fundamental barriers, they may catalyze a cycle of continued progress in population health. For example, if practices can be a part of structures aligning financial support with practice transformation capabilities, they may gain confidence in their capabilities to practice in a population health model and be willing to take on further innovative initiatives necessary to achieve child health equity.

INTEGRATED HEALTH CARE DELIVERY SYSTEMS AS A POTENTIAL CATALYTIC STRUCTURE

In recent years, various forms of IDSs have emerged to support primary care practices with population health practice transformation (**Table 1**). Dr Stephen Shortell defined an IDS as "[a] network of organizations that provides or arranges to provide a coordinated continuum of services to a defined population and is *clinically and fiscally accountable* for the costs, outcomes, and (working with others) the health status of the population served."[16] Given the focus on accountability for quality outcomes and cost, an IDS structure may be well suited to overcome some of the challenges practices face in PCMH practice transformation and overcome stagnation in achieving child health equity.

CLINICALLY AND FINANCIALLY INTEGRATED HEALTH SYSTEMS

Since the 1990s, there has been growth of financial and clinical integration attributed to changes in the payment environment, including the passage of the Affordable Care

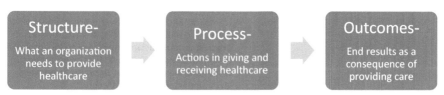

Fig. 4. Donabedian structure-process-outcome framework.

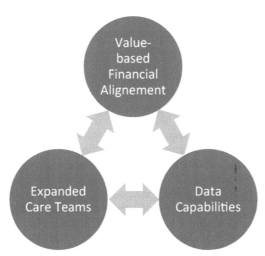

Fig. 5. Interdependence of financial alignment and practice transformation capabilities—intractable barrier or virtuous cycle for population health?

Act in 2010, as well as local market dynamics, rising technology costs, and local market forces.[17] These integration strategies have been undertaken for economic and quality rationales, particularly as recognition of the link between quality and efficiency has grown.[18] In one model, health care systems can integrate through ownership

Table 1
Population health definitions

Concept	Definition
Population health	The health outcomes of a group of individuals, including the distribution of such outcomes within the group[5]
Patient-centered medical home (PCMH)	An approach to providing comprehensive primary care that facilitates partnerships between patients, clinicians, medical staff, and families … extend[ing] beyond the four walls of a clinical practice[8]
Value-based payments/contracts	Arrangement where payment for health care services is based on health outcomes and/or health care utilization of a defined population, ranging from pay-for-performance to full capitation
Integrated health care systems	Network of organizations that provides or arranges to provide a coordinated continuum of services to a defined population and is *clinically and fiscally accountable* for the costs, outcomes, and the health status of the population served[14]
Pediatric clinically integrated networks	A formal organization or governance arrangement, with a focus on pediatric health care, among physicians or physicians and one or more hospitals to facilitate quality improvement, coordination of care, data sharing, and, at the most integrated level, undertake joint contracting[16,20]

arrangements that consolidate providers of similar types of services, such as multiple physician groups or hospitals, or consolidate providers of different types of services, such as primary care, acute care, and post-acute care. Some integrated health care systems have created further financial alignment through ownership of health plans. Commonly cited examples of this IDS model include Intermountain Healthcare (Intermountain hospitals and medical facilities, Intermountain Medical Groups, and Select Health insurance) and Kaiser Permanente (Kaiser Hospitals and medical facilities and Permanente Medical Groups, Kaiser Foundation Health Plan). With clinical and financial alignment and similarity in their not-for-profit missions, Intermountain Healthcare and Kaiser Permanente have both advanced population health models with significant investment in primary care practice transformation including innovations to address SDOH.[19,20] As such, IDS, particularly when connected to payers and holding full financial risk for a population, may be a structure to catalyze population health innovation (see **Fig. 5**).

An example of this occurred in Utah from 2017 to 2021. Intermountain Healthcare's structure includes Select Health, a wholly owned subsidiary health plan. Select Health administers an Accountable Care Organization for the state of Utah's Medicaid population, called Community Care. In 2017, Intermountain Healthcare executive leadership asked if they, as an IDS, could positively impact SDOH for the Community Care population. Sharing the idea with community partners led to the formation of a community collaboration to align goals, processes, data, resources, and outcomes to provide a continuum of care for community members. This demonstration project was called the Alliance for Determinants of Health.[21]

Two communities in Utah, Weber and Washington counties, were chosen for the Alliance as they exhibited higher-than-average SDOH factors including lower education and income as well as high ED use, substance use disorder, and mental health needs. In addition, each community had a strong culture of collaboration on public health issues like intergenerational poverty.

The Alliance methodology was based on the Accountable Health Communities model of awareness, assistance, and alignment. Awareness included screening individuals for social needs; assistance included navigation to resources to address needs; and alignment was supporting the readiness and capability of the social services providers to meet the community needs. Alignment also was improved by utilization of a closed-loop digital referral system, Unite Us, which was implemented both in the health care system and in community-based organizations (CBOs).

SDOH screening was completed in primary care offices, the EDs, and through outreach from care coordinators. Although screening was a well-known mechanism for understanding needs, two fundamental barriers had to be overcome, namely primary care provider hesitance to screen/respond appropriately to identified needs, and ED workflows to screen. Primary care providers were provided expanded care teams to support screening and response and, over time, became more willing and adept at SDOH processes. In addition, social work resources were hired to perform screening in the ED.

Once a need was identified and understood, the client was offered connection to a community health worker (CHW) who could visit their home or connect virtually. Funded by Intermountain, CHWs were members of the Alliance communities and employees of CBOs and were critical to understanding needs more completely. Subsequent referrals were routed through Unite Us. CHWs also had access to discretionary funds that they could use for needs not readily filled by CBOs; needs such as a blanket, a taxi ride home from an appointment, or a phone charger.

While formal evaluation is pending, preliminary results of the Alliance include 20,697 social needs screenings (about one in four were screenings of families in pediatric clinics); 1811 CHW cases; 31.6% CHW clients that completed their program goals; 4912 Unite Us unique service episodes; 47% Unite Us service episodes resolved; and possible reduction in nonemergent ED use. Few of the pediatric screens resulted in a referral for CHW services because pediatric care teams worked directly to connect families with pre-existing community resources such as early childhood home visitation programs that played a similar role to CHWs. Notably, screening families in pediatric clinics may have been associated with increased subsequent well-child visits and connection to subspecialty appointments. Results of the full pediatric analysis are still in process.

Intermountain is actively preparing for graduated expansion of the Alliance to all service areas. In this example, Intermountain, as an IDS with a clinically and financially aligned structure as well as close community alignment, innovated processes of awareness and assistance and ultimately improved outcomes for a population, including the pediatric population that has a long-term return on this investment.

PEDIATRIC CLINICALLY INTEGRATED NETWORKS

While an ownership structure of IDS may catalyze population health advancement, many primary care practices want to remain independent and have little interest in an ownership model. Are there, then, other options among independently owned entities capable of achieving the financial and clinical alignment necessary for population health innovation? Clinical integration, often referred to as clinically integrated networks (CINs), is another form of delivery system integration that can coexist with financial integration, although not requiring ownership.[16,22] Through clinical integration, members of a health care market work together to facilitate quality improvement, coordination of care, data sharing, and, at the most integrated level, are permitted to undertake joint contracting including value-based contracts (see **Table 1**). This requires "a high degree of interdependence and cooperation among the physicians to control costs and ensure quality."[22]

In pediatrics, clinical and financial integration has been growing. Pediatric CINs have often taken the form of a free-standing children's hospital as an anchoring partner or founder. The other network partners typically include hospital-owned pediatric practices, both general pediatrics and subspecialty, as well as affiliation with independently owned pediatric practices. These networks may have joint contracts including value-based payments with government payers, such as Medicaid, commercial payers, or both, which facilitates new ways of coordinating and supporting pediatric systems of care. This structure often empowers pediatric primary care offices with value-based financial alignment, expanded care teams, and data capabilities (see **Fig. 5**) to achieve practice transformation consistent with the PCMH model. The network structure also creates a community of primary care practices focused on similar population health goals and best-practice sharing within a quality-improvement model. In addition, the alignment with children's hospitals enables connections to the other components of the pediatric population health socio-ecological lens including health care institutions such as EDs and specialty care teams, as well as community entities as part of a children's hospital community health and advocacy responsibility (**Fig. 6**).

In 2016, the Children's Hospital Association (CHA) organized an Accountable Healthcare Learning Collaborative (AHLC) to support the growth in pediatric CINs.

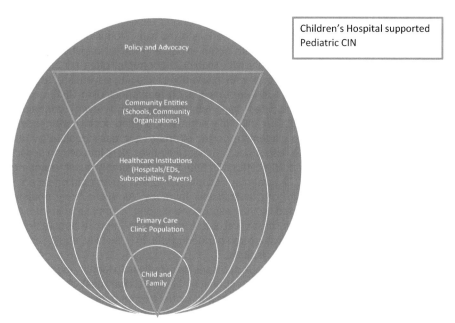

Fig. 6. Pediatric population health socio-ecological lens with facilitated connections via a children's hospital–supported pediatric clinically integrated network.

Starting with 16 networks, the AHLC grew to include 30 participants in 2022 (data from CHA to authors). As members of the AHLC and in light of this article, we collaborated with AHLC leadership to find out at a descriptive level how pediatric CINs across the United States are approaching work aiming to achieve child health equity. We asked which areas of population health equity pediatric CINs are focused on, specifically in the areas of SDOH, race and ethnicity, Medicaid, language services, and sexual orientation and gender identity. We also asked for a general text description of efforts. We received information from 20 of the 30 members, with basic descriptive information of networks provided in **Table 2**. As this was aimed at a general overview and not for research purposes, research should be caried out to further elucidate findings and themes mentioned below.

All AHLC pediatric CIN respondents reported value-based contracts with a mix of Medicaid, commercial, and even direct-to-employer arrangements. Nineteen percent of contracts were full or partial capitation, 50% shared risk or shared savings, and 31% pay for performance.

Table 2		
Descriptive information of networks from AHLC respondents		
Statistic	**Pediatric Clinicians (19 CIN Responses)**	**Patient Lives (20 CIN Responses)**
Sum	15,568	3,102,000
Average	819	155,100
Median	600	130,000
Min/Max	118/2860	14,000/470,000

Abbreviations: AHLC, Accountable Healthcare Learning Collaborative; CIN, clinically integrated network.

Nearly 90% of respondents reported specific efforts related to SDOH (**Fig. 7**). We noted in the text responses that most networks started with a focus on nutrition insecurity and/or transportation needs, with some expanding out as capabilities developed over time. In general, networks with Medicaid contracts, often full capitation, were most progressive in SDOH work with innovations including advanced data analysis of community needs, extended care navigation teams including CHWs sometimes resourced by sophisticated risk stratification, and even contractual connections/payments to CBOs to efficiently address identified social care needs.

Seventy-five percent of respondents reported efforts to address inequities by race and ethnicity. We noted in text responses that most initiatives were focused on collecting valid, self-reported data as a first step with future plans to stratify quality outcomes based on race and ethnicity. Several respondents noted that payer data on race and ethnicity were incomplete and of questionable accuracy. As such, many pediatric CINs were pairing data collected by their associated children's hospital or in their pediatric CINs using more standardized, validated methods to improve accuracy and completeness. These networks were often partnering with the diversity, equity, and inclusion leaders at the children's hospitals.

Seventy percent of respondents reported specific initiatives to identify inequities for their Medicaid population. In the text responses, we noted that most of these were related to addressing SDOH needs and were connected to contracts with higher levels of risk. While children's hospitals had a clear focus on language services, we found that a minority of networks reported extending this focus to their primary care networks. In addition, work related to sexual orientation and gender identity was often reported to be in planning phases. Finally, many networks commented on work to understand child health inequities by geography, either by focusing on certain urban neighborhoods or, more generally, urban versus rural.

While it was not possible to reflect all the work being done by AHLC pediatric CINs via a brief survey, we did reach out to leaders of five of the networks to understand more details of their initiatives (see acknowledgments). These discussions helped us understand and frame key concepts of how pediatric CINs are working on child health equity particularly in the areas of SDOH, Medicaid, and race and ethnicity (**Table 3**).

In addition, each of these five networks highlighted the critical role of leadership to advance efforts to achieve child health equity. This included synergy in leadership

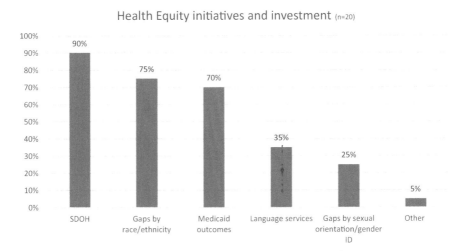

Fig. 7. AHLC respondents on children's health equity initiatives and investment.

Table 3
Key concepts from AHLC pediatric CINs work to achieve child health equity

Equity Area	Structures	Processes	Outcomes	Insights
Social determinants/drivers of health and Medicaid population	• Pediatric CINs with value-based contracts involving higher financial risk sharing (e.g., full or partial capitation Medicaid contracts) • Pediatric CINs supported by children's hospitals	• Enhanced data analytics to identify children and families with greatest need both medically and socially • Increased care team resources such as care coordination and CHWs • Primary care networks connected to community-based organizations and community partnerships historically developed by children's hospitals	• Improved access to medical and social care • Improved quality measures • Improved workflows in primary care to address identified social needs via community partners	• Value-based contracts with increased financial accountability for the pediatric CIN correlate with level of resources devoted to addressing SDOH • Relationships developed by children's hospitals with community partners can be extended to primary care networks
Race, ethnicity, and language (REaL)	• Pediatric CINs supported by children's hospitals	• Pediatric CINs supported by DEI leadership at children's hospitals • Improved efforts to collect valid and standardized data	• Meaningful quality outcome data stratified by REaL • Continuous quality improvement (CQI) initiatives in primary care focused on closing child health equity gaps by REaL	• Accurate race, ethnicity, and language data are complex to organize and act on; partnering with children's hospital's infrastructure can empower primary care teams to understand gaps and have the support to act

Abbreviations: AHLC, Accountable Healthcare Learning Collaborative; CHW, community health worker; CIN, clinically integrated network; DEI, diversity, equity, inclusion; SDOH, social drivers of health.

within the children's hospital, the pediatric CIN, and the communities served. This also involved focused efforts to prioritize equity in children's health, devote resources to it, and to influence primary care teams on the front lines to understand equity data and engage in change initiatives.

In 2021, Doherty and colleagues reported qualitative research to identify the central principles for advancing equity outcomes in health systems.[23] They found six themes: (1) committed and engaged leadership, (2) integrated organization structure, (3) commitment to quality improvement and safety, (4) ongoing training and education, (5) effective data collection and analytics, and (6) stakeholder communication, engagement, and collaboration. Notably, the key concepts from our brief AHLC overview of pediatric CINs, while not research, aligned with these findings suggesting that children's hospital–supported pediatric CINs may be an existing structure to catalyze population health processes in primary care to achieve child health equity.

ACHIEVING CHILD HEALTH EQUITY

In conclusion, we assert that a population health model, with a broadened socio-ecological lens, is fundamental to the future of primary care and is necessary to push past historical stagnation in achieving child health equity. While the PCMH model is a well-known framework for primary care practice transformation to population health, historical structures of health care delivery do not adequately support comprehensive adoption. IDS, whether in ownership models or children's hospital–supported pediatric CINs, may provide improved structural alignment for population health and, as such, support practice transformation processes necessary to achieve meaningful outcomes. Primary care pediatric practices, when appropriately structured and resourced, are ideally suited to implement a population health strategy aimed at reducing and ultimately eliminating inequitable care.

CASE STUDY (CONTINUED)

Sarah's pediatric office recently joined a children's hospital–supported pediatric CIN. The pediatric CIN has a population health value-based contract with Medicaid. With the support of the children's hospital's data analytics, the pediatric CIN created a disparity index of several key quality measures stratified by race, ethnicity, and geography and noted significant differences in asthma outcomes for children in Sarah's refugee community. The pediatric CIN shared these data with Sarah's pediatric clinician as part of regular data review. The pediatric office's expanded care team, now an accredited medical home with support and resources from the pediatric CIN, was tasked with contacting Sarah's family but was unsuccessful. Fortunately, the children's hospital had developed meaningful relationships with the refugee community, funding a CHW initiative. The pediatric care team worked with a CHW who connected to Sarah's family. The CHW identified the transportation challenges and arranged transportation options for Sarah to be able to access her medical home. Over time, as trust developed, Sarah received improved care for her asthma and has not returned to the ED. On a population level, the pediatric CIN team noted improvement in the asthma outcomes of the disparity index over time as they continued connecting children to high-quality primary care.

ACKNOWLEDGMENTS

The authors thank Emily Eresuma MBA from Primary Children's Hospital; Nancy Hanson and Stephanie Krogh from Children's Hospital Association; Mike Weiss, DO, Megan Beckerle, Karen Pugh, Erika Jewell, LCSW, and Sara Marchese, MD, from Children's

Hospital of Orange County; Jeffrey Simmons, MD, MSc, and Adriene Thornton, RN, MA, CIC, from Children's Minnesota; Sheryl Morelli, MD, from Seattle Children's Care Network; Snehal Shah, MD, MPH, and Sara Donahue from Boston Children's Hospital; Elizabeth Hogan and Brad Weselman, MD, from Children's Healthcare of Atlanta.

REFERENCES

1. Institute of Medicine. Crossing the quality chasm: a new health system for the 21st century. Washington, DC: National Academy Press; 2002.
2. Keren R, Pursuing Quality, Beyond Safety. Next Generation of Quality in Children's Healthcare Design Workshop. February 4, 2020. Children's Hospital Association, Dallas, TX.
3. Smedley BD, Nelson AR, Stith AY, editors. Unequal treatment confronting racial and ethnic disparities in healthcare. Washington: National Academies Press; 2002.
4. Anderson KM. How far have we come in reducing health disparities?: progress since 2000: workshop summary. Washington DC: National Academies Press; 2012.
5. Kindig D, Stoddart G. What is population health? Am J Public Health (N Y) 2003; 93:380–3.
6. Silberberg M, Martinez-Bianchi V, Lyn MJ. What is population health? Prim Care 2019;46:475–84.
7. McCauley L, Phillips RL, Meisnere M, et al. Implementing high-quality primary care: rebuilding the foundation of health care. Washington, DC: The National Academies Press; 2021.
8. Jimenez G, Matchar D, Choon Huat Koh G, et al. Revisiting the four core functions (4Cs) of primary care: operational definitions and complexities. Prim Health Care Res Dev 2021;22:e68.
9. American Academy of Pediatrics. Medical home. Available at: https://www.aap.org/en/practice-management/medical-home . Accessed September 29, 2022.
10. Philip S, Pantely S, Fovier D. Milliman white paper patient-centered medical home. Available at: https://www.ncqa.org/wp-content/uploads/2019/06/06142019_WhitePaper_Milliman_BusinessCasePCMH.pdf . Accessed September 29, 2022.
11. Agency for Healthcare Research and Quality (AHRQ). The National Evaluation of the CHIPRA Quality Demonstration Grant Program. Available at: https://www.ahrq.gov/sites/default/files/wysiwyg/policymakers/chipra/statesummaries/chipra-750-utah-state-snapshot.pdf . Published January 2018. Accessed September 29, 2022.
12. National Committee for Quality Assurance (NCQA). Latest evidence: benefits of NCQA patient-centered medical home recognition. Available at: https://www.ncqa.org/wp-content/uploads/2019/09/20190926_PCMH_Evidence_Report.pdf . Accessed September 29, 2022.
13. Kaiser Family Foundation. Professionally active primary care physicians by field. Available at: https://www.kff.org/other/state-indicator/primary-care-physicians-by-field/?currentTimeframe=0&sortModel=%7B%22colId%22%3A%22Location%22%2C%22sort%22%3A%22asc%22%7D . Published September 29, 2022. Accessed September 29, 2022.
14. O'Neill A. FAQs: Patient-centered medical home recognition program. National Committee for Quality Assurance (NCQA). Available at: https://www.ncqa.org/programs/health-care-providers-practices/patient-centered-medical-home-pcmh/faqs/. Published March 21, 2022. Accessed September 29, 2022.

15. Donabedian A. An introduction to quality assurance in health care. New York: Oxford University Press; 2003.

16. Shortell S. Integrated care: policy and evidence. HRSN/SDO Conference. June 2009. Available at: https://www.slideshare.net/NuffieldTrust/steve-shortell-integrated-care-policy-and-evidence . Accessed September 29, 2022.

17. RAND Corporation. What have we learned about the economic effects of vertical integration? Available at: https://www.rand.org/health-care/centers/health-system-performance/what-have-we-learned/vertical-integration.html . Accessed September 29, 2022.

18. Evans JM, Baker RG, Berta W. The evolution of integrated health care strategies. Adv Health Care Manag 2013;125–61. https://doi.org/10.1108/s1474-8231(2013) 0000015011.

19. Ross M. Understanding the value of the Kaiser Permanente model. Kaiser Permanente Institute for Health Policy. Available at: https://www.kpihp.org/blog/understanding-the-value-of-the-kaiser-permanente-model-integrated-care-stories/. Published August 23, 2022. Accessed September 29, 2022.

20. Reiss-Brennan B, Brunisholz KD, Dredge C, et al. Association of integrated team-based care with health care quality, utilization, and cost. JAMA 2016;316:826. https://doi.org/10.1001/jama.2016.11232.

21. Wu K, Strane D, Kellom K, et al. Implementation of social determinants screening for referral to a community health worker program: iterative evaluation and expert feedback. AcademyHealth. Available at: https://academyhealth.confex.com/academyhealth/2021arm/meetingapp.cgi/Paper/46050. Published June 16, 2021. Accessed September 28, 2022.

22. Jones Harbour P. American Hospital Association Annual Membership Meeting, In: *Clinical integration: the changing policy climate and what it means for care coordination*. In: Federal Trade Commission. 2009. p. 5–17. Washington, DC.

23. Doherty JA, Johnson M, McPheron H. Advancing health equity through organizational change: perspectives from health care leaders. Health Care Manage Rev 2021;47:263–70.

Alternative Payment Models and Working with Payers– Key Considerations for Advancing Population Health Goals and Achieving Child Health Equity

Rachel L.J. Thornton, MD, PhD[a],*, Karen M. Wilding, MHA[b],
Daniella Gratale, MA[c], Kara O. Walker, MD, MPH, MSHS[c]

KEYWORDS

- Whole child health • Value-based payment • Pediatric pay-for-performance
- Social determinants of health

KEY POINTS

- The transition from fee-for-service models to value-based care in the US has been predominantly focused on adult populations, and there is a need for concentrated attention to develop and adopt value-based payment in pediatric populations.
- Support for value-based payment innovation requires flexibility and accountability for results to advance child health equity, but this depends on the payer and provider incentives, data availability, performance metrics, and overall adoption within the model.
- We recommend a whole child health model as the foundation for value-based payment innovation and accountability with child health equity as the ultimate accountability metric because it recognizes the interdependence of health care, social services, education, community, and family supports in achieving optimal child health and well-being.

CASE EXAMPLE: In keeping with achieving improved outcomes for patients, providers in one of Nemours geographic markets were working under a new value-based contract with a larger commercial insurance company. In keeping with continued efforts to provide high-quality care while also meeting expectations under the contract, Nemours children's providers and clinical teams redoubled their efforts to optimize preventive care services for primary care patients and increase their focus on dispensing generic version of medications indicated for chronic disease

[a] Nemours Children's Health, 1201 15th Street Northwest, Suite 520, Wilmington, DE, USA;
[b] Nemours Children's Health, 1600 Rockland Road, Wilmington, DE 19803, USA; [c] Nemours Children's Health, 1201 15th Street Northwest, Suite 520, Washington, DC 20005, USA
* Corresponding author. 2200 Concord Pike, 8th Floor, Wilmington, DE 19803.
E-mail address: Rachel.thornton@nemours.org

Pediatr Clin N Am 70 (2023) 667–682
https://doi.org/10.1016/j.pcl.2023.03.005
0031-3955/23/© 2023 Elsevier Inc. All rights reserved.
pediatric.theclinics.com

management. Through these efforts, Nemours providers improved primary care and wellness outcomes while also reducing overall costs of care. In addition, because a new valued-based payment agreement provided flexible funding and incentives for managing hospitalizations and improving chronic disease management, providers were able to rely on an enhanced cadre of care managers to support the comprehensive care needs of many patients after hospital discharge. Through access to comprehensive care managers and part of the multidisciplinary care team, Nemours decreased hospital readmissions by 24% (compared with a 5.6% reduction among other similar providers). This meant that the organization improved patient outcomes in a cost-effective way, in keeping with the contract. As a result, they also received financial incentives from the insurer that could be used to reward teams and enhance services in keeping with the triple aim of patient-centered, high-quality, cost-effective care.

INTRODUCTION

Since the passage of the Affordable Care Act (ACA) more than a decade ago, the health care sector is increasingly focused on evolving from a "sick care" system organized around isolated transactions for medical services delivered in a fee-for-service model into a value-based system organized around patient and population-level health outcomes where the framework for financing prioritizes results instead of discrete services. As such, value-based payment models focus on achieving, sustaining, and incentivizing optimal health outcomes for patients. This "volume to value" transition was informed by the "triple aim"[8] model that became widely popularized during the ACA policy development and implementation process. Focused on optimizing experience of care, health outcomes of populations, and per capita costs in US health care, the triple aim has since expanded to include a fourth focus on well-being within the health care workforce (quadruple aim).[9] More recently, some have suggested expanding to include a fifth aim specifically focused on equity within health care delivery.[9–11]

Yet, as the SARS-CoV2 disease (COVID-19) pandemic vividly illustrated in real-time, the fragmented nature of US health care today, and the disconnect between some financial payment models and population-level health outcomes, the "volume to value" transition remains an aspirational goal. In fact, in their recent viewpoint, Nundy and colleagues[10] argue for an expanded focus on health equity above and beyond the inclusion of equity as one of six pillars of quality as articulated in the historic NASEM report, *Crossing the Quality Chasm*.[6] In fact, there is an inherent risk in value-based payment models that the focus on quality improvement and optimization may neglect to support the transformative efforts within health systems that are required to prioritize equitable outcomes at a population level. This is further evidenced by the lack of focus through regulatory and accreditation efforts to institutionalize equity within value-based models in prior decades, which have only taken hold as a mainstream imperatives within the last 4 to 6 years.[12,13]

A recent update to the Center for Medicaid and Medicaid Innovation (CMMI) strategy recognized the need to pause continued development of new models and instead accelerate the dissemination and evaluation of the models within its portfolio already, with a focus on summarizing and building the evidence about which models are producing results in keeping with triple aim.[12] One such example is the Accountable Care Organization (ACO) Investment Model (AIM) which showed $526 million in gross Medicare spending reductions in the first 3 years (2016–2018), which were associated with improvements in areas such as hospital utilization and long-term care.[14] Despite some promising examples, value-based alternative payment models are not reflected in most health care payments across the United States This is particularly true for pediatric populations. Even farther behind the general "volume to value" transition in the US health care system is the prioritization of equity in population health and health care delivery. Decades-old consensus that racial bias and racism contribute to racial/ethnic disparities in health care,[15] effective solutions to address systemic and structural drivers of health care disparities remain elusive, even in the face of payment innovation spurred by the ACA and the Centers for Medicare and Medicaid Services (CMS) Innovation Center (CMMI).[12]

Within the context of payment transformation, there is growing attention to identifying and reducing disparities and inappropriate variation in care, consistent with the pillars of health care quality. Equitable health care means providing care that does not vary in quality because of patients' sociodemographic characteristics such as gender, race/ethnicity, geography, or socioeconomic status.[6] Relatedly, health equity is achieved when everyone has the resources needed to achieve their full health potential or optimal health.[3,16] Measuring meaningful and unjust differences in outcomes across patient sociodemographic subgroups (ie, health disparities) is an important barometer for determining whether efforts are advancing health equity (**Box 1** for key concepts and definitions).[3]

Such a focus on identifying health disparities and implementing initiatives and programs to reduce disparities are still in a fledgling phase across much of the value-based care landscape. And current approaches to implementing value-based care models run the risk of further concentrating health care resources among advantaged populations thus worsening disparities in access to care and associated health outcomes for historically marginalized groups.[17] New coalitions, regulatory requirements,

---

Box 1
Key definitions

- Population Health—Health outcomes and their distribution in a population.[1] These outcomes are achieved by patterns of health determinants (eg, medical care, public health, socioeconomic status, physical environment, individual behavior, and genetics) over the life course produced by policies and interventions at the individual and population levels.[2]

- Health Disparities—Meaningful and unjust differences in health outcomes across patient sociodemographic subgroups (ie, health disparities), which can be used to measure progress in achieving health equity.[3]

- Health Equity—The state in which everyone has the opportunity to attain their full health potential and no one is disadvantaged from achieving this potential because of social position or other socially determined circumstances.[4]

- Value-Based Care—A framework for restructuring health care systems with the overarching goal of achieving *value*, which is the produce of quality plus patient experience at a given cost. Value is largely defined in terms of achieving the triple aim,[1] keeping additional aims (eg, workforce well-being, equity) in mind as implementation of value-based care matures.[5]

- Equitable Health Care—Care that does not vary in quality because of patients' sociodemographic characteristics such as gender, race/ethnicity, geography, or socioeconomic status.[6]

- Whole child health—A model that engages multi-sector partners to support the developmental, physical, mental, behavioral, and social needs of children and youth, and to help foster healthy relationships with caregivers, through individual, family-based, and community-level approaches and interventions.[7]

proposed rules, and accreditation initiatives across health care are directing attention toward establishing baseline performance, and driving accountability for reducing disparities as a core component of value-based care transformation.[12,18]

For example, guidance to state Medicaid directors on how to advance the adoption of value-based models from the CMS emphasizes the need for attention to high-quality care that maximizes benefits to patients and eliminates unnecessary costs and utilization.[19] This guidance operationalizes value-based care in terms of both cost and quality by focusing on approaches that are cost-neutral or cost-saving while achieving the same or better outcomes.[13]

Value-based models influence health care delivery by supporting ongoing investments in high-quality care and frequently using incentives intended to reward providers for achieving results through arrangements such as pay-for-performance.[20] Yet, successful adoption of value-based care demands a deeper review of current payment incentives, requiring attention to more fundamental investments in infrastructure, practice transformation, and reimbursement policies.[21] As a result, organizations designed to succeed in fee-for-service models are often ill-equipped to understand and implement value-based services.

Success in value-based programs requires the alignment of stakeholders across the care continuum, including clinicians, patients, policymakers, payers, community and social services partners, information technology, and the biotech industry.[21] For example, in traditional Medicare Accountable Care Organizations, we have witnessed transformative payment and care delivery developments, as organizations establish creative partnerships to improve quality, bend the cost curve, and promote overall outcomes and patient engagement. Examples include health care organization partnerships with food banks and transportation providers. For example, as part of its White House Commitment, Nemours Children's has expanded Cares Closets to more Nemours primary care locations to provide food and other items to families in need, and work with community partners to expand their backpack program, which provides children access to nutritious meals outside of school hours (link to press release: https://nemours.mediaroom.com/2022-09-28-Nemours-Childrens-Health-Commitment-to-Nations-Youth-Highlighted-at-White-House-Conference-on-Hunger-and-Nutrition).

Optimizing pediatric outcomes through value-based care will involve an even broader set of stakeholders than adult health outcomes because of the importance of a multigenerational approach to improving children's health. Thus, stakeholders who play a critical role in the child health care continuum must extend to early childhood, education, and beyond. These cross-sector stakeholders and service providers are critical partners instrumental to the success of pediatric value-based care. These stakeholders must align efforts leveraging data-sharing innovations, insights, and lessons that developed at an accelerated pace during the height of the COVID-19 pandemic.

In this commentary, we describe opportunities to learn from value-based care efforts in Medicare, identify key considerations for optimizing value-based care for pediatric populations, and articulate a clear argument for embedding equity as a foundational imperative for evaluating pediatric value-based care models.

LEARNINGS FROM MEDICARE AND THEIR APPLICATIONS TO PEDIATRIC POPULATIONS

The policy levers potentiating the transition to value-based care at the federal level focus primarily on payment transformation within Medicare. Because this program is federally administered, it is fertile ground for implementing national policy reforms to create financial incentives tied to quality, patient experience, and efficiency standards. Medicare programs such as the hospital value-based purchasing program End-Stage Renal Disease Quality Incentive Program (ESRD_QIP), bundled payments, and many others are part of a nationwide quality strategy aimed at reforming health care delivery systems and payment (Centers for Medicare & Medicaid Services, 2021).[22] CMS value-based programs are essential because they are advancing value-based payment transformation by paying providers based on the quality rather than the quantity of care they provide.

Moving Beyond Fee-for-Service

Early efforts in Medicare value-based care achieved success in addressing inefficiencies or missed opportunities for very high-cost populations. The Medicare Access and Children's Health Insurance Program (CHIP) Reauthorization Act of 2015 (MACRA; P.L. 114-10) was designed to shift Medicare physician payments to be increasingly based on value.[23] Specifically, it established a merit-based incentive payment system (largely based on fee for service [FFS]) and created incentives for the development of, and participation in, Alternative Payment Models (APMs).[24] The law established those eligible clinicians who participate in Advanced APMs will earn a 5% bonus from 2019 through 2024, a provision that advocates are currently seeking to extend.[23] As payment models have evolved, there is an increasing focus on optimizing preventive care among a broader population of Medicare beneficiaries.

A widely accepted framework for characterizing stages along the trajectory from FFS to fully matured value-based care models was updated in 2017 by the Health Care Payment Learning & Action Network.[25] **Fig. 1** is an adaptation of that framework which identifies four categories of increasingly mature payment models ranging from FFS to fully mature population-based payment models, which create accountability and attempt to align financial incentives with improving or optimizing the health of entire populations with the goal of incentivizing further alignment between health care spending and population-level health outcomes.

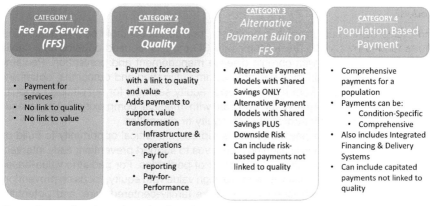

Fig. 1. Categories along the value-based payment continuum. (*Adapted from*: The Alternative Payment Model (APM) Framework. 2017. MITRE Corporation. Accessed October 16, 2022. Accessed: October 29, 2022. https://hcp-lan.org/workproducts/apm-refresh-whitepaper-final.pdf.)

Evolving Medicare payment models from CMS and the Innovation Center increased attention to chronic disease management, preventive care utilization (closing gaps in care), and health-related social needs. CMS also provides opportunities for flexibility to states and payers to utilize existing Medicare funding for a more flexible set of services in models intended to reward patient outcomes instead of the volume of services delivered.

Although these populations can be narrowly defined in some instances, other examples focus on achieving overall population health improvements within geographically defined areas. For example, Maryland's Total Cost of Care All Payer Model seeks to create accountability across payers and providers for optimizing the health of a geographically defined all payer population.[26] This All Payer Model was established through an agreement between CMS and the state of Maryland in 2014, whereby Maryland agreed to achieve specific population health quality targets, while limiting the annual cost growth for all payers over a 5-year term through global hospital budget caps. The Maryland Total Cost of Care model demonstrated success in reducing spending by $88 million in its first year. As of 2021, the model added newly added targets for disparities reduction with other population health and outcomes targets.[27,28] Although this model embodies many key elements and principles of population-focused value-based payments, its narrow focus on Medicare costs and other characteristics of the model may have unintended consequences on pediatric health care delivery infrastructure and child health outcomes.[29]

The CMS Accountable Health Communities (AHC) Initiative produced lessons regarding social needs screening and referral.[30] The model generated a 9% reduction in emergency department visits but did not produce net savings in overall medical expenditures. Additionally, AHC sites were able to connect to social needs of only 15% of all patients. The Medicare ACO REACH Model incorporates health equity through the inclusion of a health equity benchmark adjustment and requirements around identifying and addressing disparities.[31] These additional model components focus on improving participation in new models of care for underserved communities, data capture to inform health equity investments, and fortified screening and referral opportunities to address social determinants of health (SDOH).[32]

Population Health Management: Asthma and Care Coordination as Early Pediatric Models

Early value-based care models in pediatrics include accountable care organizations' efforts funded by CMMI. These Medicaid ACO models focused on avoidable health care costs associated with chronic disease management and prevention. Pediatric models focused on optimizing pediatric asthma utilization and outcomes, optimizing transitions of care (eg, from higher to lower acuity settings) for hospitalized populations, and care coordination for children with medical complexity.[33] These early models did not explicitly address health equity or disparities.

Pediatric value-based payment models represent a critical opportunity to build on lessons from Medicare while aligning incentives to support prevention, early intervention, and family-centered care, all hallmarks of pediatrics. For pediatric value-based care to achieve optimal results, it needs to align value with equity, focus on prevention, address health-related social needs, prioritize family-centered care, and potentiate healthy community transformation and sustained investment. Pediatric payment models will also have to maintain a whole child health approach but measure the life course in shorter segments of time: early childhood, middle childhood, and adolescence (see key elements summary in **Box 2**). Metrics that can tie together various

> **Box 2**
> **Whole child health—defining multi-sector partners**
>
> Whole Child Health is a model that engages multi-sector partners to support the developmental, physical, mental, behavioral, and social needs of children and youth, and to help foster healthy relationships with caregivers, through individual, family-based, and community-level approaches and interventions.[7]
>
> Key Elements
> - Integrated Clinical and Social Delivery Models
> - Health Equity Promotion
> - Centering Families
> - Community Engagement
> - Diverse, Multidisciplinary Workforce
> - Cross-Sector Data Partnerships
> - Financing Reforms that Incentivize Optimal Health
> - Quality Assessment and Improvement

sectors in early childhood education, social services, and behavioral health will be critically important for 0 to 5-year-olds.

Some pediatrics health systems are investing in their own value-based payment efforts. In Nationwide Children's Partners for Kids model, their ACO is serving 400,000 children in value-based care arrangements with their Medicaid Managed Care Organizations. Both financial and quality metrics are tracked alongside a community quality initiative that includes infant mortality, kindergarten readiness, high school graduation, and others.

In Ohio, the Comprehensive Primary Care For Kids model is a voluntary patient-centered medical home model that includes care coordination fees and shared shavings. In addition to pediatric metrics in immunization, preventive care, and screening, the payment model includes a bonus for support of children in foster care, behavioral health linkages, and school support. Cincinnati Children's coordinates pediatric health-focused support with educational institutions to increase the percentage of children reading proficiently or above by 3rd grade in public school and has an accountable care arrangement for 130,000 children covered by Medicaid. These three examples suggest that further accountability for metrics by race, ethnicity, and language strata could allow for robust payment model efforts in other ACO models. They also raise the question of how to account for social complexity or other measures that consider the impact of social conditions on health care utilization and outcomes among populations.

ALIGNING VALUE AND EQUITY

In general, childhood is a time when people are relatively healthy. Yet the experiences, exposures, and environments children encounter as they grow can produce illness, injury, trauma, and even chronic disease that manifests over the life course.[34] Often referred to as the social determinants of health, the political, economic, social, and environmental conditions in which children grow, learn, live, and play can have life-long impacts on health and well-being.[35] Factors such as poverty, education, employment, housing, neighborhood conditions, racism, and discrimination can all impact health directly and indirectly throughout childhood, leaving lasting impacts on health among adults.[36,37]

As one of the other manuscripts in this issue describes, pediatrics has a longstanding tradition of recognizing the need to address social and clinical factors in the interest of children's health and well-being. This includes an imperative to screen for unmet social needs during clinical visits.[38] Despite a concerted focus on identifying and addressing social needs in pediatrics, socioeconomic and racial health disparities persist. At a societal level, interventions that produce healthier community conditions may improve children's mental and physical health and set them on a trajectory of increased economic prosperity and well-being in adulthood.[39–42] Value-based payment may represent an innovative strategy for aligning financial incentives to address health-related social needs for patients and families in ways that also potentiate community-level investments to sustain health and well-being. Over the past several decades, CMS has granted waivers that allow states enhanced flexibility in using federal and state health care dollars to spur payment innovation aimed at improving outcomes for the most vulnerable, including low-income children, covered under Medicaid. For example, in 2018, CMS approved a 1115 Demonstration Waiver for the state of North Carolina Medicaid program to begin in 2019. This waiver provides flexibility to the state for the "Healthy Opportunities Pilot Program" designed to cover non-medical services to address health-related social needs. More recently, the Biden Administration has encouraged states to propose waivers that expand coverage and specifically address health-related social needs. In 2022, CMS approved four state waivers that cover non-medical interventions to support health. In Arizona, Arkansas, Massachusetts, and Oregon, Medicaid will have enhanced flexibility to address housing and nutrition needs. And in Oregon, under the waiver, children will remain continuously enrolled in Medicaid up to the age of 6 years old.

As payers face increasing accountability for performance and delivering results, potentiated by the ACA, many recognize that health disparities are a missed opportunity to produce value through better outcomes. Prioritizing health equity within value-based care is challenging, particularly when accountability is not aligned for payers and providers. Furthermore, the way that populations are defined within pediatric value-based models can vary, depending on payment incentives, which do not always align with achieving impact on the most marginalized or disadvantaged populations who may have limited access to care.[43]

Health equity is defined as "the state in which everyone has the opportunity to attain their full health potential, and no one is disadvantaged from achieving this potential because of social position or other socially determined circumstances".[44] Yet, despite more than a decade of rapid innovation and growing opportunities for flexibility since the ACA, value-based care transformation has failed to produce widespread reductions of health disparities, and thus, has not yet delivered on the promise of advancing health equity.[12]

APMs that attempt to create accountability for the total cost of care for geographically defined populations, such as Maryland's All Payer model, are one example of efforts to align accountability for improving population health and reducing disparities with value-based care. Yet, many challenges create barriers to advancing health equity within these types of models, ranging from lack of access to comprehensive data on the population of interest to questions about social factors that may drive health outcomes or utilization. Data analytics for value-based payment rely heavily on electronic health record and claims data, which present an incomplete picture of overall health, relying inappropriately on utilization patterns as a proxy for disease burden, medical complexity, or risk of poor outcomes.[17,45]

Challenges with cross-sectoral data collection, access, and consent also pose barriers to achieving health equity, including incentives and support for collecting and aligning person-level demographic and outcomes data across health care and social services sectors.[35] Furthermore, the data sources that are available through the health care sector often provide an incomplete picture of the social drivers that impact health including health behaviors, environmental conditions, unmet social needs, access to services and supports, and sociopolitical and interpersonal context.

IN PURSUIT OF WHOLE CHILD'S HEALTH

Given the myriad barriers to advancing health equity from data sources to financial incentives, policy development and implementation to address barriers and create accountability are critical to achieving population health and health equity goals while leveraging value-based care. Policy is an integral lever to support child health equity, aligning incentives across a continuum of sectors, services, and stakeholders working to holistically support children's health and well-being, often referred to as *whole child health*. Although various incentives in the Medicare program have driven a move to value-based care for the adult population, similar incentives are lacking in Medicaid, leaving close to 40% of America's children who are covered under Medicaid behind. The CMMI Integrated Care for Kids (InCK) Model and the Maternal Opioid Misuse (MOM) model coordinate clinical care and social services through payment strategies and integrated care. These new models currently being evaluated have provided some momentum toward child-focused payment reform.[46] However, each predominantly focuses on targeted sub-populations of children with significant chronic disease and social risk. For example, InCK seeks to improve health and reduce avoidable inpatient stays and out-of-home placement for "children with multiple physical, behavioral, or other health-related needs and risk factors.[47]" The MOM model focuses exclusively on pregnant and postpartum women with opioid use disorder and their infants.[48] A pre-implementation phase evaluation report for InCK model was published in August 2022[49] and a similar report for MOM was published in December 2021.[50] These reports describe planning activities and related findings. A full evaluation of model implementation for both InCK and MOM is planned to fully evaluate the model implementation and related impacts.

Numerous barriers stifle efforts to finance and implement more holistic, prevention-focused pediatric APMs that support optimal health and well-being for all children and youth.[46,51] Key barriers include lower potential cost savings for pediatric populations, a longer savings time horizon, wrong-pocket issues[52] where savings from one sector accrue to another, and churn among insurance plans, which limits a payer's opportunities for long-term savings. CMMI's statutory requirements for budget neutrality further exacerbate these challenge.[53]

Despite these barriers, the CMS has encouraged states to innovate by advancing value-based care[13] and addressing health-related social factors through Medicaid Section 1115 waivers and guidance.[54] In January 2021, CMS issued a letter to states outlining opportunities to address social drivers under Medicaid and the CHIP.[55] In August 2022, CMS issued two informational bulletins highlighting existing flexibilities for maximizing Medicaid coverage for services. The bulletins highlight how states can leverage Medicaid (including the early and periodic screening, diagnostic and treatment benefit), CHIP, and other federal programs to provide behavioral health services to children and youth.[56,57] This guidance addresses key areas of cross-sectoral support for *whole child health*, highlighting the role of schools, nutrition, behavioral health, and preventive services. A recent proposed rule from CMS goes beyond flexible guidance on state-level implementation to advocate some national quality standards for Medicaid by establishing mandatory annual reporting requirements around a Core Set of Children's Health Care Quality Measures for Medicaid and CHIP.[58]

This federal guidance must coincide with additional federal investments to incentivize and support states, providers, and payers in achieving readiness to pursue value-based reforms and establish the data infrastructure, and longer time frames needed for the pediatric value-based programs to produce transformational improvements in pediatric population health and child health equity. To this end, Nemours Children's Health has advocated for a pediatric *Whole Child Health* model to be funded through the establishment of a demonstration program at the Center for Medicaid and CHIP Services (CMCS), which does not operate under the same budget neutrality requirements as CMMI. The *whole child health* demonstration could provide implementation support and technical assistance to states for pediatric delivery and payment models that support prevention and health promotion, including developmental, social, and relational health and well-being.

Congress could also offer support through legislation and funding. For example, in draft reports for the Fiscal Year 2023 health appropriations bills, the House and Senate encouraged CMCS to explore a *whole child health* demonstration,[49,59] which is further defined in the KIDS Health Act.[60] This bipartisan, bicameral bill would help states test payment and delivery reforms that integrate prevention and address SDOH for children and youth who are eligible for Medicaid and CHIP. If enacted, it would also provide resources to help states implement innovative multi-sector financing approaches to advance *whole child health*; support workforce training; and enhance health information technology infrastructure, including cross-sector data sharing capabilities. It would also require federal guidance to clarify strategies and best practices for blending and braiding federal funds, including Medicaid, consistent with federal law. Congress has already invested in whole-person health for other populations; for example, the Consolidated Appropriations Act of 2022[61] allocated an additional $10 million, for a total of $83.6 million, to expand a Whole Health Initiative to all Veteran's Administration facilities.[62] Building on this precedent, the *whole child health* Alliance[63] advances models that promote children's optimal health, development, and well-being across the life course and is supporting efforts to advance value-based models for the pediatric population, through Medicaid demonstrations and other incentives, with an emphasis on advancing health equity.

To complement new demonstration models, the Federal government and states could address challenges associated with wrong-pocket issues and churn by better aligning program goals across federal agencies for a specific population such as families with children. Additionally, they could catalyze pooled, multi-sector financing mechanisms such as children's wellness trusts or social impact bonds,[64] both of which incorporate a shared financing approach among multiple stakeholders and could support investments to address SDOH.[65] For example, within the education and early care and education sectors, organizations have blended and braided[66] funds at the state, local, and federal levels to sustain and implement effective programming. Removing budget neutrality to invest in longer-term savings could also help address pervasive and persistent child health disparities through population-based payment models.

When informed by tools such as the Child Opportunity Index,[67] pooled financing mechanisms could meaningfully address resource gaps within communities, promote equity, and directly align with payment models tested under a *whole child health* demonstration. By incorporating place-based indicators of child health and well-being, new funding models could better align resources to communities with the highest unmet social needs among children and families before these conditions produce ill health in adulthood. The Federal Office of Management and Budget could support states by issuing guidance and technical assistance to clarify strategies and best practices for combining funds across sectors. It could also issue guidance on long-term savings associated with improvements in key child physical, mental, emotional, and behavioral health, educational, and other well-being related outcomes. Together, enhanced guidance, demonstration models, Medicaid incentives, and aligned pooled financing mechanisms could provide the support needed to catalyze transformative pediatric models that support whole child health.

Payment models for children and youth can leverage lessons learned through APMs implemented in Medicare populations across multiple settings. Yet to achieve the greatest impact on population health and health equity, these children and youth-focused APMs must prioritize early prevention, cross-sector-collaboration, and health equity. Critical to transformative success are solutions to issues such as the wrong-pocket problem, systemic solutions to ensure adequate funding for social services, and other social support programs. This could include efforts to improve access to additional supports for low-income families such as safe affordable housing and high-quality early childhood education. Because optimizing child health and health equity across the life course can only occur when social and economic conditions in communities can adequately support healthy development, the health care sector cannot fully address unmet needs alone. The health care sector has a critical role to play in ensuring equitable access to health care services of all types from prevention and early intervention to subspecialty and high-acuity hospital-based care. Mobilizing payers, providers, and policymakers can generate a healthier generation, but this promise will only be achieved when accountability and incentives are realigned to support cross-sector efforts with a focus on pediatric populations, prevention, well-being, and equity. Pediatricians have a critical role to play in advocating for the totality of what children and families need to achieve optimal health. Whether it is access to safe and healthy housing, nutritious food, economic opportunity, safe neighborhoods, or nurturing and high-quality learning environments, the voice of pediatricians articulating the meaningful and enduring connections between child health and robust social services and infrastructure to support healthy development is essential if we are to succeed in achieving transformational progress and meaningful results in pediatric value-based care.

CLINICS CARE POINTS

- Fee-for-service models compensate providers for services rendered while value-based payment models can be structured to compensate providers for outcomes achieved

- Value-based care models emphasize quality over utilization and place value on providing effective and efficient care

- The CMS operationalizes value-based care in terms of both quality and cost, emphasizing cost-neutral and cost-saving models that optimize or improve outcomes

- Achieving optimal health and developmental outcomes for pediatric populations requires cooperation and collaboration between pediatricians and multi-sector partners beyond health care, which is embodied in the *Whole Child Health Model* (see **Box 2** for key elements)

DISCLOSURE

The authors have nothing to disclose.

REFERENCES

1. Kindig D, Stoddart G. What Is Population Health? Am J Public Health 2003;93(3): 380–3.
2. Kindig DA. Understanding Population Health Terminology. Milbank Q 2007;85(1): 139–61.
3. Braveman P. What are Health Disparities and Health Equity? We Need to Be Clear. Public Health Rep 2014;129(1_suppl2):5–8.
4. National Academies of Sciences, Engineering, and Medicine. 2017. Communities in Action: Pathways to Health Equity. Washington, DC: The National Academies Press. https://doi.org/10.17226/24624.
5. Porter ME. What Is Value in Health Care? N Engl J Med 2010;363(26):2477–81.
6. Institute of Medicine (National Academies of Science, Engineering, and Medicine). 2001. Crossing the Quality Chasm: A New Health System for the 21st Century. Washington, DC: The National Academies Press. Available at: https://doi.10.17226/10027. Accessed October 11, 2022.
7. Whole Child Health Alliance: Key Elements. White Paper Available at: whole-child-health-alliance-key-elements.pdf (nemours.org). Accessed March 22, 2023.
8. Berwick DM, Nolan TW, Whittington J. The Triple Aim: Care, Health, And Cost. Health Aff (Millwood) 2008;27(3):759–69. https://doi.org/10.1377/hlthaff.27.3.759.
9. Bodenheimer T, Sinsky C. From Triple to Quadruple Aim: Care of the Patient Requires Care of the Provider. Ann Fam Med 2014;12:573–6. https://doi.org/10.1370/afm.1713.
10. Nundy S, Cooper LA, Mate KS. The Quintuple Aim for Health Care Improvement: A New Imperative to Advance Health Equity. JAMA 2022;327(6):521–2.
11. Mate K. On the quintuple aim: why expand beyond the triple aim? Boston, MA: Institute for Healthcare Improvement; 2022. Available at: https://www.ihi.org/communities/blogs/on-the-quintuple-aim-why-expand-beyond-the-triple-aim. Accessed October 11, 2022.
12. Brooks-LaSure C, Fowler E, Seshamani M, Tsai D. Innovation at The Centers for Medicare and Medicaid Services: A Vision for The Next 10 Years. Health Aff Forefr. August 21, 2021. Accessed: October 16, 2022. doi:10.1377/forefront.20210812.211558.
13. Costello A, Smith B. SMD #20-004 RE: value-based care opportunities in Medicaid. Washington, DC: Centers for Medicare & Medicaid Services; 2020. Available at: https://www.medicaid.gov/Federal-Policy-Guidance/Downloads/smd20004.pdf. [Accessed 6 October 2022]. Accessed.
14. Center for Medicare and Medicaid Innovation. ACO Investment Model (AIM) Final Evaluation of Three AIM Performance Years. Available at: https://innovation.cms.gov/data-and-reports/2020/aim-fg-finalannrpt. Accessed December 15, 2022.
15. Institute of Medicine (National Academies of Science, Engineering, and Medicine). 2003. Unequal treatment: Confronting racial and ethnic disparities in health care. Washington, DC: The National Academies Press. Available at: https://doi.org/10.17226/12875. Accessed October 16, 2022.
16. Health Equity | IHI - Institute for Healthcare Improvement. Available at: https://www.ihi.org:443/Topics/Health-Equity/Pages/default.aspx. Accessed October 11, 2022.
17. Obermeyer Z, Powers B, Vogeli C, et al. Dissecting racial bias in an algorithm used to manage the health of populations. Science 2019;366(6464):447–53.

18. Centers for Medicare & Medicaid Services. Innovation center strategy refresh. Washington, DC: Centers for Medicare & Medicaid Services; 2021. Available at: https://innovation.cms.gov/strategic-direction-whitepaper. Accessed October 6, 2022.

19. Allen K. CMS eyes Medicaid alternative payment models (APM) expansion to Control growth in spending. Health Management Associates; 2020. Available at: https://www.healthmanagement.com/blog/cms-eyes-medicaid-alternative-payment-models-apm-expansion-to-control-growth-in-spending/. Accessed October 11, 2022.

20. Cattel DE, Eijkenaar F, Schut FT. Value-based provider payment: Towards a theoretically preferred design. Health Econ Policy Law 2020;15(1):94–112.

21. Boscolo PR, Callea G, Ciana O, et al. Measuring value in health care: A comparative analysis of value-based frameworks. Clin Ther 2020;42(1):34–43.

22. McDonough JE, Adashi EY. The Center for Medicare and Medicaid Innovation-Toward Value-Based Care. JAMA 2022;327(20):1957–8.

23. National Association of ACOs. The ACO Guide to MACRA. 2021. Washington, DC: National Association of ACOs. 2021. ACO-Guide-MACRA21EditionFull Report012721.pdf. Available at: https://www.naacos.com/assets/docs/pdf/macra/2021/ACO-Guide-MACRA21EditionFullReport012721.pdf. Accessed October 13, 2022.

24. Congressional Research Service. The Medicare access and CHIP reauthorization Act of 2015 (MACRA; P.L. 114-10. Washington, DC: Congressional Research Service; 2015. Available at: https://csreports.congress.gov/product/pdf/r/r43962/12.

25. The Alternative Payment Model (APM) Framework. 2017. MITRE Corporation. Available at: https://hcp-lan.org/workproducts/apm-refresh-whitepaper-final.pdf. Accessed October 16, 2022. Accessed: October 29, 2022.

26. Sharfstein JM, Stuart EA, Antos J. Global Budgets in Maryland: Assessing Results to Date. JAMA 2018;319(24):2475–6.

27. Haber S, Beil H, Morrison M, et al. EVALUATION OF THE MARYLAND ALL-PAYER MODEL VOLUME I: FINAL REPORT. :278.

28. Machta R, Peterson G, Rotter J, et al. Evaluation of the Maryland Total Cost of Care Model: Implementation Report. :131.

29. Cheng T. Making Maternal Child Health a Population Health Priority in Maryland. Pediatr Clin North Am 2023;70(1):53–65.

30. Johnson KA, Barolin N, Ogbue C, et al. Lessons from Five Years of The CMS Accountable Health Communities Model. Health Aff Forefr 2022. https://doi.org/10.1377/forefront.20220805.764159.

31. David Pittman BS, Gaus C. ACO REACH Brings Next Era of Medicare Payment Models. Am J Accountable Care. 2022;10(2). Available at: https://www.ajmc.com/view/aco-reach-brings-next-era-of-medicare-payment-models. Accessed October 13, 2022.

32. Innovation Center Strategy Refresh. Centers for Medicare and Medicaid Services. Washington, DC; 2021. Available at: https://innovation.cms.gov/strategic-direction-whitepape. Accessed October 6, 2022.

33. New Payment Model Guidance for Organizations Caring for Children with Complex Medical Conditions: The CARE Award. Children's Hospital Association. Published online April 2017. Available at: https://www.childrenshospitals.org/-/media/files/migration/care_award_payment_model_workbook_061517.pdf. Accessed October 13, 2022.

34. Shonkoff JP, Phillips DA. From Neurons to Neighborhoods: The Science of Early Childhood Development.

35. Social determinants of health. Available at: https://www.who.int/health-topics/social-determinants-of-health. Accessed October 14, 2022.

36. Zambrana RE, Williams DR. The Intellectual Roots of Current Knowledge on Racism and Health: Relevance to Policy and The National Equity Discourse. Health Aff (Millwood) 2022;41(2):163–70.

37. White A, Thornton RLJ, Greene JA. Remembering Past Lessons about Structural Racism — Recentering Black Theorists of Health and Society. N Engl J Med 2021;385:850–5.

38. Garg A, Butz AM, Dworkin PH, et al. Screening for Basic Social Needs at a Medical Home for Low-Income Children. Clin Pediatr (Phila). 2009;48(1):32–6.

39. Chetty R, Hendren N, Katz LF. The Effects of Exposure to Better Neighborhoods on Children: New Evidence from the Moving to Opportunity Experiment. Am Econ Rev 2016;106(4):855–902.

40. Pollack CE, Bozzi DG, Blackford AL, et al. Using the Moving to Opportunity Experiment to Investigate the Long-Term Impact of Neighborhoods on Healthcare Use by Specific Clinical Conditions and Type of Service. Hous Policy Debate 2021;0(0):1–21.

41. Pollack CE, Blackford AL, Du S, et al. Association of Receipt of a Housing Voucher with Subsequent Hospital Utilization and Spending. JAMA 2019;322(21):2115–24.

42. Ludwig J, Sonbanmatsu L, Gennetia L, et al. Obesity, and Diabetes — A Randomized Social Experiment. N Engl J Med 2011;365:1509–19.

43. Fritz CQ, Brittan MS, Keller D. Inpatient Population Health—Defining the Denominator. JAMA Pediatr 2020;174(3):231–2.

44. National Academies of Sciences, Engineering, and Medicine. Communities in action: pathways to health equity. Washington, DC: The National Academies Press; 2017. https://doi.org/10.17226/24624.

45. Lagasse J. The importance of data in value-based care, and how to maximize it. Healthcare Finance News. Available at: https://www.healthcarefinancenews.com/news/importance-data-value-based-care-and-how-maximize-it. Accessed October 14, 2022.

46. Counts NZ, Mistry KB, Wong CA. The Need for New Cost Measures in Pediatric Value-Based Payment. Pediatrics 2021;147(2):e20194037.

47. Integrated Care for Kids (InCK) Model. Available at: https://innovation.cms.gov/innovation-models/integrated-care-for-kids-model. Accessed October 21, 2022.

48. Maternal Opioid Misuse (MOM) Model. Available at: https://innovation.cms.gov/innovation-models/maternal-opioid-misuse-model. Accessed October 21, 2022.

49. Abt Associates, Inc. (2022). Integrated Care for Kids (InCK) Model Evaluation: Report 1. Available at: https://innovation.cms.gov/data-and-reports/2022/inck-model-pre-imp-first-eval-rpt. Accessed December 15, 2022.

50. Esposito, D., Simon, L., Tucker, M., et al (2021). Maternal opioid misuse (MOM) model: Pre-implementation evaluation report. Centers for Medicare & Medicaid Services. Available at: https://innovation.cms.gov/data-and-reports/2022/mom-preimp-report. Accessed December 15, 2022.

51. Gratale D, Viveiros J, Boyer K. Paediatric alternative payment models: emerging elements. Curr Opin Pediatr 2022;34(1):19–26.

52. Butler S. How "Wrong Pockets" Hurt Health. JAMA Forum Archive. 2012-2019. Available at: https://jamanetwork.com/channels/health-forum/fullarticle/2760141. Accessed October 14, 2022.

53. CMMI Model Certifications. CMS. Available at: https://www.cms.gov/Research-Statistics-Data-and-Systems/Research/ActuarialStudies/CMMI-Model-Certifications. Accessed October 14, 2022.

54. Hinton E, Aug 05 LSP, 2021. Medicaid Authorities and Options to Address Social Determinants of Health (SDOH). KFF. Published August 5, 2021. Available at: https://www.kff.org/medicaid/issue-brief/medicaid-authorities-and-options-to-address-social-determinants-of-health-sdoh/. Accessed October 14, 2022.

55. Costello A. SHO# 21-001 RE: Opportunities in Medicaid and CHIP to Address Social Determinants of Health (SDOH). Published online January 7, 2021. Available at: https://www.medicaid.gov/federal-policy-guidance/downloads/sho21001.pdf. Accessed May 22, 2023.

56. Tsai D. Information on School-Based Services in Medicaid: Funding, Documentation and Expanding Services. CMS Informational Bulletin. Published online August 18,2022. Available at: https://www.medicaid.gov/federal-policy-guidance/downloads/sbscib081820222.pdf. Accessed May 22, 2023.

57. Tsai D. Leveraging Medicaid, CHIP, and Other Federal Programs in the Delivery of Behavioral Health Services for Children and Youth. CMCS Informational Bulletin. Published online August 18, 2022. Available at: https://www.medicaid.gov/federal-policy-guidance/downloads/bhccib08182022.pdf. Accessed October 14, 2022.

58. Federal Register: Medicaid Program and CHIP; Mandatory Medicaid and Children's Health Insurance Program (CHIP) Core Set Reporting. Available at: https://www.federalregister.gov/documents/2022/08/22/2022-17810/medicaid-program-and-chip-mandatory-medicaid-and-childrens-health-insurance-program-chip-core-set. Accessed October 14, 2022.

59. Departments of Labor, Health and Human Services, and Education and Related Agencies Appropriations Bill, 2023. REPORT of the Committee on Appropriations House of Representatives. CRPT-117hrpt403.pdf. Accessed October 14, 2022. Available at: https://www.congress.gov/117/crpt/hrpt403/CRPT-117hrpt403.pdf. CRPT-117hrpt403.pdf. Accessed October 14, 2022. https://www.congress.gov/117/crpt/hrpt403/CRPT-117hrpt403.pdf.

60. Carper, Sullivan Lead Colleagues to Introduce Bipartisan, Bicameral Bill to Implement Holistic Approach to Children's Health Care. United States Senator Tom Carper. Published September 29, 2022. Available at: https://www.carper.senate.gov/public/index.cfm/2022/9/carper-sullivan-lead-colleagues-to-introduce-bipartisan-bicameral-bill-to-implement-holistic-approach-to-children-s-health-care. Accessed October 14, 2022.

61. Consolidated Appropriations Act, 2022.; 2022. Available at: https://www.govinfo.gov/content/pkg/CPRT-117HPRT47048/pdf/CPRT-117HPRT47048.pdf. Accessed October 14, 2022.

62. Reddy B, Wisneski LA. Whole Person Health: The Role of Advocacy. Glob Adv Health Med 2022;11. 2164957X221082650.

63. Whole Child Health Alliance. Available at: https://www.nemours.org/about/policy/advocacy/whole-child-health-alliance.html. Accessed October 14, 2022.

64. Social Impact Bond (SIB) Financing: A Pay for Success Strategy. Social Finance. Available at: https://socialfinance.org/social-impact-bonds/. Accessed October 14, 2022.

65. Caring for the Whole Child: A New Way to Finance Initiatives to Improve Children's Health - Manatt, Phelps & Phillips, LLP. Available at: https://www.manatt.com/insights/white-papers/2020/caring-for-the-whole-child-a-new-way-to-finance-in. Accessed October 14, 2022.

66. Braiding and blending funds to promote social determinants of health. Brookings. Published April 17, 2019. Available at: https://www.brookings.edu/events/braiding-and-blending-funds-to-promote-social-determinants-of-health/. Accessed October 14, 2022.
67. Child Opportunity Index (COI). Available at: diversitydatakids.org. https://www.diversitydatakids.org/child-opportunity-index. Accessed October 14, 2022.

Moving Beyond Health Care to Achieve Health Equity

Partnering with Families and Communities to Improve Child Health and Health Equity

Monica J. Mitchell, PhD, MBA[a,b,c,*], Carley Riley, MD[b,d],
Lori E. Crosby, PsyD[a,b]

KEYWORDS

- Community engagement • Partnership • Child • Pediatric • Health equity
- Family voice

KEY POINTS

- Effective partnerships between pediatric health providers, families, and communities can address health-care access and promote child health equity.
- Partnerships between pediatric health providers, families, and communities must foster mutual trust and respect. Communicating transparently is also important.
- Clarifying the goal of partnership between pediatric providers and families and/or communities is important and can range from outreach (disseminating information) to colearning with families to coleading initiatives with community partners.
- Measuring the effectiveness of the partnership and tracking outcomes (eg, meeting shared goals) are important to the success of collaborations between pediatric health providers, families, and communities.

PARTNERING WITH FAMILIES AND COMMUNITIES: CASE STUDY 1

This case study describes how pediatric health providers at Cincinnati Children's foster trust and respect while developing a sustainable community partnership that addresses pediatric health and health equity. This partnership highlights best practices and guiding principles important to engaging families and communities, discussed later in this article, including developing shared goals (**Table 1**).

The First Ladies Partnership with Cincinnati Children's Hospital is an example of a sustainable community partnership that is addressing pediatric health and promoting health equity.

[a] Division of Behavioral Medicine, Cincinnati Children's Hospital Medical Center, 3333 Burnet Avenue, MLC 7039, Cincinnati, OH 45229, USA; [b] Department of Pediatrics, University of Cincinnati College of Medicine, Cincinnati, OH, USA; [c] Community Relations, Children's Hospital Medical Center, Cincinnati, OH, USA; [d] Division of Critical Care, Cincinnati Children's Hospital Medical Center, 3333 Burnet Avenue, MLC 2005, Cincinnati, OH 45229, USA
* Corresponding author. Division of Behavioral Medicine, Cincinnati Children's Hospital Medical Center, 3333 Burnet Avenue, MLC 7039, Cincinnati, OH 45229.
E-mail address: Monica.Mitchell@cchmc.org

Pediatr Clin N Am 70 (2023) 683–693
https://doi.org/10.1016/j.pcl.2023.04.001
0031-3955/23/© 2023 Published by Elsevier Inc.
pediatric.theclinics.com

Table 1
Guiding principles and best practices for community engagement[4]

Best Practices and Guiding Principles	Strategies for Ensuring Successful Community Engagement	Example of Successful Community Engagement
Establish trust and respect	• Spend time in the community • Engage in active listening and understanding of family and community perspective • Share decision-making power and incorporate ideas	• Community and family members share ideas about child health needs and ways to address them together • Health partners visit a local food bank to learn more about addressing food insecurity
Develop equitable relationships and shared goals	• Incorporate ideas (or buy in) from partners • Ensure mutual benefit for partners • Leverage complementary strengths or assets from each partner • Work together to establish clear and measurable goals that will guide the partnership and define its success	• Family and community partners agree that they will partner to address food insecurity and develop 3 goals that will be measured and tracked • A decision-making committee is established that includes family and community partners
Build on the strengths and resources of the community	• Coordinate and collaborate across health and community programs with similar missions to increase impact • Use strength-based language rather than focusing on deficits and problems	• Health and community partners use their strengths to create a food clinic in a primary care clinic • The focus is on the opportunity to increase food access and link families to resources to address basic needs, rather than exclusively framing the problem as one of poverty, hunger, and one that residents need to solve
Communicate effectively and transparently	• Ensure partners have a "voice" despite real or perceived power differences • Incorporate family and community voice in planning and discussion • Communicate openly about the potential benefits and limitations of the collaboration	• Partners are valued and feel open to providing ideas • Ideas are prioritized to inform partnership goals and outcomes • Benefits and limitations are discussed at the onset and throughout the partnership
Measure the outcomes of the partnership, understanding that learning is an iterative process	• Regularly assess the partnership to determine how well the collaboration is working • Ensure quality improvement mindset and practices are part of the design to make changes as needed and progress	• Health partners and the food bank assessed trust, communication, and other aspects of the partnership • Other outcomes were assessed, including how children and families benefitted from the food clinic

(continued on next page)

Table 1 (*continued*)		
Best Practices and Guiding Principles	**Strategies for Ensuring Successful Community Engagement**	**Example of Successful Community Engagement**
		• Quality improvement supported learning and continuous progress
Include partners in the sharing and dissemination	• Include all partners in all phases of the collaboration, including the dissemination and celebration of milestones and results	• Outcomes and progress were regularly shared with partners • Partnership results and successes were disseminated through community media and peer-reviewed publications

See Refs.[10–14]

First Ladies for Health is an organization comprising leading women in the church and the first lady of the city (the mayor's wife). The organization's mission is to "empower people to make informed choices about health." Early in the partnership, a shared goal was established between The First Ladies and community partners to engage families in the event, especially those from Black/African American and Latino communities, and to increase pediatric uptake of the flu vaccine. Partners agreed that to accomplish this goal, it would be important to increase awareness and address vaccine hesitancy and related myths with churches and surrounding communities. Pediatric health providers from Cincinnati Children's would also work with partners (eg, churches, health department) to provide children and families with vaccines and health screenings during an annual Family Health Day—an event hosted at several community locations on a single day. Health and community partners work together on the planning, communication, and implementation of the event. Health Day's successes include increases in attendance, pediatric health screenings, and flu

Table 2 Levels of community involvement, communication, and impact[14–17]		
Level	**Engagement**	**Relational Outcomes**
Inform	Provide information; coordinate outreach	Develop communication channels and outreach networks
Consult	Get ideas, feedback, and information from the community	Community members and expertise may inform how decisions are made
Involve	Community members actively participate, and their ideas are considered	Bidirectional communication and cooperation are established
Collaborate	Partner with communities, ideally from the initiation of the idea until the completion of the project	Partners foster trust and develop collaborative solutions
Shared leadership	Community partners have power in the collaboration and influence final decisions	Bidirectional leadership is established to ensure the community has shared representation and leadership

vaccinations during the 8 years of the partnership.[1] Consistent with the goal, more than 90% of those attending the event, identified as Black/African American or Latino. During the course of the collaboration, partners have expanded to include coronavirus disease 2019 research and vaccinations and pediatric mental health. Other win–wins for health and community partners include obtaining collaborative grants and coauthoring presentations and publications. Community partnerships such as the First Ladies for Health collaboration help to overcome barriers related to the social determinants of health (SDoH; eg, transportation, income, access, and trust), which are so critical to improving pediatric health. The First Ladies partnership also helps to build trust between the Black community and health-care providers and supports pediatric health providers in taking steps to understand and address historical racism. Another case example is discussed in this article.

BACKGROUND

Pediatric health providers are increasingly working with families and community partners to effectively address pediatric health disparities and advance health equity.[2] When pediatric health providers and institutions partner with community organizations, their collaborative efforts can be an effective way to disseminate health education and promote positive health behaviors.[3] These partnerships are especially effective when they are well structured and responsive and when there is mutual trust and respect.[4] Community partnerships and collaborations support pediatric health providers in extending traditional care models to facilitate access and community-based care delivery. When building community partnerships, pediatric health providers are working actively in *communities*, commonly defined as "a group of people with diverse characteristics who are linked by social ties, share common perspectives, and engage in joint action in geographic locations or settings."[5] Partnerships with communities may include health departments, schools, and others community organizations that allow pediatricians and other pediatric health providers to assist children and families who may have difficulties accessing health care.[6] In meeting children and families "where they are," more children can receive pediatric care services, including preventative primary and mental health care.[7] These partnerships also allow health-care systems to engage in collaborative efforts to address the SDoH and well-being beyond the traditional boundaries of the health-care system. Working with families and communities to codesign partnerships from the onset increases the likelihood that these pediatric programs will be relevant and effective.[8]

This article will discuss the importance of pediatric health providers and institutions collaborating with families and communities to improve child health and health equity. Key components of effective partnerships will also be discussed. Finally, models for family and community partnerships will be summarized, as well as how practitioners might establish sustainable partnerships.

ENSURING EFFECTIVE ENGAGEMENT WHEN PARTNERING IN COMMUNITIES

Best practices for establishing effective community partnerships are well documented and include working with partners to (1) establish trust and respect, (2) develop equitable relationships and shared goals, (3) build on the strengths and resources of the community, (4) communicate effectively and transparently, (5) measure the outcomes of the partnership, understanding that learning is an iterative process, and (6) include partners in the sharing, dissemination, and celebration of results.[9] These principles will be discussed and how they can be successfully applied in family and community-pediatric partnerships.

MODELS FOR PARTNERING WITH COMMUNITIES TO IMPROVE HEALTH

Community engagement has been effectively used to improve pediatric outcomes. One model that has been applied is the Public Participation Spectrum that was developed by the International Association for Public Participation (IAP).[15] This model has been adapted for Community engagement.[16,17] The IAP and others referencing their model, generally describe 5 stages for increasing involvement in communities to improve health promotion and outcomes (**Table 2**).

McNeill and colleagues[17] completed an analysis of 37 studies that used the IAP model with children and families for patient-oriented clinical research. The article concluded that the majority of these studies (23% or 78%) engaged children and families at the "Involve" level. A total of 7 (10.8%) engaged children and families at the "Consult" level, with 3 (8.1%) at the "Inform" level. None of the studies reviewed met the criteria for "Shared Leadership." This analysis provides an understanding of where pediatric healthcare-community partnerships are currently with regards to the stepwise model to achieve community engagement at the highest levels, including working with community partners to make decisions together. Although there has not been a similar analysis of IAP's model to examine the level of engagement of community partners in pediatric research or practice, we can see from a range of studies[18–23] that connections are most often made at the "Inform," "Consult," and "Involve" levels, similar to the findings in the McNeill and colleagues article.

As it relates to the IAP model, pediatric institutions and providers are broadening efforts to provide information to communities about the health services offered.[24–26] They are also increasing awareness of topics related to health equity (eg, asthma, obesity, diabetes) and how communities might access services through community-based models (eg, primary care, school-based health).[21] Community members are asked to provide their perspectives and consultation on important topics that are priorities for pediatric health providers and institutions, and in many cases for communities and residents.

The application of the IAP model for community engagement[15] provides the opportunity for partners to consider what level of engagement is intended and appropriate for a respective partnership and to clarify the goals and intent of the collaboration at the onset. This way, there is transparency in communication and trust can be established. The guiding principles are applied, and the partnership structure is clear to all partners. As an example, the goal of community members serving on the Institutional Review Board (IRB) may be for them to "consult" or to be "involved" (the goal may not be for "shared leadership" in this circumstance). Communicating to the community member about why their participation is valued is important. Community members might be told that "some IRB protocols involve community engagement and their voice as a community member is important as decisions are made." In this example, the collaborative relationship between pediatric health providers and the community is set up to be strong because of the respect, transparency, and open communication that is established at the beginning of the relationship.

The Assessing Community Engagement (ACE) Conceptual model is another framework for understanding how community engagement can serve as a driver of health and health equity.[25] This model, developed by the Organizing Committee for the ACE brought together by The National Academy of Medicine and Robert Wood Johnson Foundation, outlines 4 drivers of health and health equity advanced through meaningful community engagement: (1) strengthened partnership and alliances, (2) expanded knowledge, (3) improved health + health care programs and policies, and (4) thriving communities. The framework, summarized in **Table 3**, also describes

Table 3
Health equity through transformed systems for health: Model for achieving health equity through meaningful community engagement (summary of the model)[27]

Strengthened Partnerships and Alliances	Expanded Knowledge	Improved Health, Health Care Programs, Policies	Thriving Communities
• Diversity and inclusivity • Partnerships and opportunities • Acknowledgment, visibility and recognition • Sustained relationships • Mutual value • Trust • Shared power • Structural support for community engagement	• New curricula, strategies, and tools • Bidirectional learning • Community ready Information	• Community-aligned solutions • Actionable, implemented, recognizable solutions • Sustainable solutions	• Physical + mental health • Community capacity + connectivity • Community power • Community resiliency • Life quality + well-being

Community Engagement Core Principles (Crosscutting Across the 4 Key Drivers)
Co-equal, Co-created, Ongoing, Shared Governance, Multi-knowledge, Equitably Financed, Culturally-Centered, Inclusive, Bi-directional, Trust

core principles of community engagement that cut across these 4 drivers: trust, bidirectional and culturally centered relationships, inclusion, shared governance, equitability in financing, sustainability, and colearning.

Diversity, equity, and inclusion as well as social, economic, and political factors are central to the ACE model, which calls for community-aligned solutions. In this, community-engaged efforts to improve health equity should ensure that shared goals are culturally responsive. One way to do this is by including pediatric health providers who represent the cultural values of the community when possible (providers who live in and/or are trusted by the community, those who speak the same language when the community does not speak English, and so forth). Moreover, as this framework makes apparent, diversity and inclusion must be core to partnership discussions as community engagement strategies are being developed, implemented, and evaluated. When working in communities, socioecological and cultural factors are closely tied to the health of the community.[28] For this reason, topics such as racism, poverty, income, housing, and other social influences of health will inevitably come up in partnership discussions. When they do, partners will need to feel comfortable discussing these topics, managing them sensitively, and incorporating them into the design as appropriate (eg, barriers to care, SDoH, race and mistrust related to vaccine hesitancy, and so forth).[29] Through these discussions, when health providers share values with the community and when trust is built, new knowledge can be created and disseminated (materials, curricula), as proposed in the model.[27] The final outcome described in the model is the cocreation of thriving communities, including improved mental and physical health and well-being for children and families. Importantly, this goal is shared by pediatric health providers and the community (**Table 3** for a Summary of the Model). The box below summarizes organizations that health providers can consider when partnering to advance child health and health equity.

Community-Based Partners and Resources to Consider:
  Civic organizations (Junior League, and so forth)
  Diversity organizations (Urban League, Hispanic Chamber)
  Faith-based organizations
  Foodbanks
  Funders, foundations (United Way, and so forth)
  Health organizations (eg, Health Departments)
  Housing authority, homeless coalitions
  Hospitals, clinics, primary care offices
  Linguistic, rural, income, access considerations
  Maternal and child health organizations
  Preschools/childcare centers
  Schools and universities
  Social service organizations (YMCA, Recreation Centers)
  Organizations and programs specific to your community

TOOLS FOR ASSESSING COMMUNITY ENGAGEMENT AND PARTNERSHIP IN PEDIATRIC HEALTH

ACE and partnership is essential to improving their effectiveness but identifying evaluation tools can challenging. There are several published tools that allow partners to evaluate whether the partnership is meeting its intended health impact goals, as well as achieving guiding principles related to trust, respect, communication, and inclusion. Publicly available tools/toolkits are summarized in **Table 4**.

Pediatric health and quality improvement data (eg, trends in flu vaccinations) may also provide information on whether community partnership goals are being met and progress is being made.

PARTNERING WITH FAMILIES AND COMMUNITIES: CASE STUDY 2

This case study will describe how pediatric health providers have partnered with families and community partners to host an annual Sickle Cell Research and Education Day that promotes education, clinical care and advocacy among pediatric patients, their family members, and the broader community.[34,35] This partnership highlights best practices and guiding principles important to family and community engagement (summarized previously in this article), including ensuring trust, demonstrating respect, and developing shared goals.

Sickle Cell Research and Education Day is an annual event that was started in 2002, and one that is hosted in the community by Cincinnati Children's Hospital in collaboration with other community partners such as the Sickle Cell Alliance Foundation, Hoxworth Blood Center, and the Urban League of Greater Cincinnati.[34] The event was started in response to the need for greater family and youth engagement in research and clinical care and opportunities. The event also provides the opportunity to build trust with patients and families and reduce stigma related to sickle cell disease in the community. For this reason, family and youth engagement are key to the design, implementation, and sustainability of the event. The event has 3 goals: (1) increase trust and participation in Sickle Cell Disease (SCD) clinical research, (2) improve knowledge of sickle cell care management among youth and caregivers, and (3) ensure that youth and caregiver voice and ideas shape the event. The Research Day event has taken place for more than 15 years and includes a caregiver/community symposium, youth symposium, and children's program, growing its attendance from

Table 4
Community partnership and engagement assessment tools[3]

Description of Assessment/Tool	References
Institutional Community Engagement (ICE) Self-Assessment: Seven institutions receiving Clinical and Translational Science Awards, led by the University of Rochester, collaborated to develop the ICE Self-Assessment. This measure helps institutions map community engagement activities by structure, process, and outcome measures and to track activities over time. ICE assesses health impact as well as institutional commitment to community-engaged scholarship[30]	Vitale K, N GL, Abraido-Lanza AF, Aguirre AN, Ahmed S, Esmond SL, Evans J, Gelmon SB, Hart C, Hendricks D, McClinton-Brown R, Young SN, Stewart MK, Tumiel-Berhalter LM. Community Engagement in Academic Health Centers: A Model for Capturing and Advancing Our Successes. J Community Engagem Scholarsh. 2018;10(1):81–90. Epub 2018 Feb 14. PMID: 30581538; PMCID: PMC6301056.
Community Engagement and Participation Checklist: Policy Link developed a 34-item checklist to assess community engagement and equity because it relates to 5 areas: (1) building trust and accountable relationships, (2) develop shared vision for community change, (3) build partnerships with public agencies, (4) develop and sustain capacity, and (5) translate community vision into policy change. The measure is meant to be a guide and not prescriptive[31]	Policy Link: Community Engagement & Participation Checklist Addressing Disparities for Healthier Places www.policylink.org/resources-tools
Community engagement in an academic medical center: The authors provide a model for evaluating the effectiveness of community engagement, which includes ways that the partnership (1) improves the health of the community, (2) increases the academic partner's capacity for community engagement, and (3) increase practices in community engagement and public health[32]	Szilagyi PG, Shone LP, Dozier AM, N GL, Green T, Bennett NM. Evaluating community engagement in an academic medical center. Acad Med. 2014 Apr;89(4):585–95. https://doi.org/10.1097/ACM.0000000000000190.
Readiness for community-based participatory research: Evaluating the readiness to partner might be a first step. The authors provide a framework for evaluating whether the academic and community partner are "ready" and have the capacity to partner. The article also discusses what it would take to develop an effective partnership (eg, relational and technical skills, and so forth)[33]	Andrews JO, Newman SD, Meadows O, Cox MJ, Bunting S. Partnership readiness for community-based participatory research. Health Educ Res. 2012 Aug;27(4):555–71. https://doi.org/10.1093/her/cyq050.

30 to more than 500 participants. Successful outcomes include less than 75% of participants rate high satisfaction and trust for research. More than 75% of youth and caregivers complete research studies that enroll participants during the research day event.[34] Another positive outcome is attendees learn about completed research studies and clinical care advances each year. Families also have the opportunity to update contact information and make appointments, removing well-documented barriers to care and communication in this pediatric population. The Research and

Education Day model has been replicated in other SCD Centers and in other pediatric chronic diseases. The SCD Research and Education Day model can be applied to primary and specialty care and how we can include youth and family voices in clinical care and research recruitment and retention.[34–36]

SUMMARY AND IMPLICATIONS FOR PEDIATRIC HEALTH PROVIDERS

There are benefits when pediatric health providers, institutions, and community partners work together and establish trust, respect, communication, and shared goals. Communicating clearly and transparently about the goals and potential of the partnership is important (eg, outreach as the goal versus shared leadership as the expectation). Examples of community partners include health departments, schools, faith-based organizations, pediatric physician networks, social service organizations, and/or other community organizations that allow for pediatric health providers and pediatric institutions to increase access, address SDoH, and potentially meet children and families "where they are." These partnerships may also allow for children who are underserved or who live in underresourced communities to be reached.[37] When community-based partnerships are based on shared goals and outcomes and mutual respect, collaborations are especially sustainable and effective. These partnerships are also critical to addressing child health disparities and closing child health equity gaps. Best practice models serve as examples for health providers and institutions who want to establish successful partnerships.

CLINICS CARE POINTS TO SUPPORT FAMILIES, COMMUNITIES, AND CHILD HEALTH EQUITY

> Pediatric health professionals can better integrate families and communities in care by the following:
>
> - Providing health education and pediatric health prevention and wellness care beyond the walls of the hospital and in places where children and families live.
> - Develop strategies to increase trust between providers and parents, especially when discussing topics such as immunizations and vaccinations. Increase providers' cultural understanding of how to build stronger relationships with families and communities.
> - Health providers, practices, and institutions may also coordinate with community partners and organizations to deliver comprehensive care. Schools, health departments, and others play important roles in addressing SDoH.

DISCLOSURE

This work was funded in part by the CCTST at the University of Cincinnati is funded by the National Institutes of Health (NIH) Clinical and Translational Science Award (CTSA) program, grant UL1TR001425. The content is solely the responsibility of the CCTST and does not necessarily represent the official views of the NIH.

REFERENCES

1. Corley AMS, Gomes SM, Crosby LE, et al. Partnering With Faith-Based Organizations to Offer Flu Vaccination and Other Preventive Services. Pediatrics 2022; 150(3). e2022056193.

2. Council on Community Pediatrics. Community Pediatrics: Navigating the Intersection of Medicine, Public Health, and Social Determinants of Children's Health. Pediatrics 2013;131(3):623–8.

3. Beck AF, Marcil LE, Klein MD, et al. Pediatricians Contributing to Poverty Reduction Through Clinical-Community Partnership and Collective Action: A Narrative Review. Acad Pediatr 2021;21(8S):S200–6. PMID: 34740429.

4. Tsopelas L, Fleegler EW, Lorenzi M, et al. Community Asthma Initiative to Improve Health Outcomes and Reduce Disparities Among Children with Asthma. MMWR Suppl 2016;65(1):11–20.

5. MacQueen KM, McLellan E, Metzger DS, et al. What is community? An evidence-based definition for participatory public health. Am J Public Health 2001;91(12): 1929–38. PMID: 11726368; PMCID: PMC1446907.

6. Nishiguchi EP, Kadunc K, Lee A, et al. Assessing 5-Year Outcomes of an Academic Pediatrics-Community Partnership Focused on Rural Child Health. Prog Community Health Partnersh 2021;15(2):243–53.

7. Beck AF, Marcil LE, Klein MD, et al. Pediatricians contributing to poverty reduction through clinical-community partnership and collective action: a narrative review. Academic Pediatrics 2021;21(8):S200–6.

8. Butler AM, Hilliard ME, Comer-HaGans D. Review of Community-Engaged Research in Pediatric Diabetes. Curr Diab Rep 2018;18(8):56.

9. Williamson HJ, Chief C, Jiménez D, et al. Voices of Community Partners: Perspectives Gained from Conversations of Community-Based Participatory Research Experiences. Int J Environ Res Public Health 2020;17(14):5245.

10. Israel BA, Coombe CM, Cheezum RR, et al. Community-based participatory research: a capacity-building approach for policy advocacy aimed at eliminating health disparities. Am J Public Health 2010;100(11):2094–102.

11. Israel BA, Schulz AJ, Parker EA, et al. Review of community-based research: assessing partnership approaches to improve public health. Annu Rev Public Health 1998;19:173–202.

12. Centers for Disease Control and Prevention (CDC). Principles of Community Engagement, Second Edition. Washington, DC: NIH Publication; 2011.

13. Wilkins CH, Alberti PM. Shifting Academic Health Centers From a Culture of Community Service to Community Engagement and Integration. Acad Med 2019; 94(6):763–7. PMID: 30893063; PMCID: PMC6538435.

14. Fawcett S, Schultz J, Watson-Thompson J, et al. Building multisectoral partnerships for population health and health equity. Prev Chronic Dis 2010;7(6):A118. Epub 2010 Oct 15. PMID: 20950525; PMCID: PMC2995607.

15. The Extent of Public Participation. Report by the International Association for Public Participation (IAP2). 2014.cma.org/pm.

16. Raderstrong J, Robinson TB. The why and how of working with communities through collective impact. Community Dev 2015;42(2):181–93.

17. De Leiuen Cherrie, Arthure Susan. Collaboration on Whose Terms? Using the IAP2 Community Engagement Model for Archaeology in Kapunda, South Australia. J Community Archaeol Herit 2016;3(2):81–98. https://doi.org/10.1080/20518196.2016.1154735.

18. McNeill M, Noyek S, Engeda E, et al. Assessing the engagement of children and families in selecting patient-reported outcomes (PROs) and developing their measures: a systematic review. Qual Life Res 2021;30:983–95.

19. Cummings K, Kang RJ, Tseng CH, et al. Academic-community partnerships improve outcomes in pediatric trauma care. J Pediatr Surg 2015;50(6):1032–6. Epub 2015 Mar 14. PMID: 25812442.

20. Skelton JA, Palakshappa D, Moore JB, et al. Community engagement and pediatric obesity: Incorporating social determinants of health into treatment. J Clin Transl Sci 2019;4(4):279–85.
21. Davis KG. Integrating Pediatric Palliative Care into the School and Community. Pediatr Clin North Am 2016;63(5):899–911. PMID: 27565367.
22. Walls TA, Hughes NT, Mullan PC, et al. Improving Pediatric Asthma Outcomes in a Community Emergency Department. Pediatrics 2017;139(1):e20160088. Epub 2016 Dec 8. PMID: 27940506.
23. Goldman MP, Auerbach MA, Garcia AM, et al. Pediatric Emergency Medicine ECHO (Extension for Community Health Care Outcomes): Cultivating Connections to Improve Pediatric Emergency Care. AEM Educ Train 2020;5(3):e10548. https://doi.org/10.1002/aet2.10548.
24. Carter CG, Thompson LA, Silverstein JH, et al. Pediatrics after-hours: a twenty-year academic-community partnership for acute care delivery. J Pediatr 2015; 166(4):788–9.
25. Smith SM, Quadri M, Lowry KW. Community Outreach Among Employees of an Academic Children's Hospital. J Community Health 2021;46:413–9.
26. Tweed J. Caring for Kids: Bridging Gaps in Pediatric Emergency Care Through Community Education and Outreach. Crit Care Nurs Clin North Am 2017;29(2): 143–55.
27. Aguilar-Gaxiola S, Ahmed SM, Anise A, et al. Assessing Meaningful Community Engagement: A Conceptual Model to Advance Health Equity through Transformed Systems for Health: Organizing Committee for Assessing Meaningful Community Engagement in Health & Health Care Programs & Policies. NAM Perspect 2022;2022. https://doi.org/10.31478/202202c.
28. Fanta M, Ladzekpo D, Unaka N. Racism and pediatric health outcomes. Curr Probl Pediatr Adolesc Health Care 2021;51(10):101087.
29. Trent M, Dooley DG. Dougé J; Section on Adolescent Health. Council on Community Pediatrics; Committee on Adolescence. The Impact of Racism on Child and Adolescent Health. Pediatrics 2019;144(2):e20191765.
30. Vitale K, Newton GL, Abraido-Lanza AF, et al. Community Engagement in Academic Health Centers: A Model for Capturing and Advancing Our Successes. J Community Engagem Scholarsh 2018;10(1):81–90.
31. Policy Link. Community Engagement & Participation Checklist Addressing Disparities for Healthier Places. www.policylink.org/resources-tools.
32. Szilagyi PG, Shone LP, Dozier AM, et al. Evaluating community engagement in an academic medical center. Acad Med 2014;89(4):585–95.
33. Andrews JO, Newman SD, Meadows O, et al. Partnership readiness for community-based participatory research. Health Educ Res 2012;27(4):555–71.
34. Hines J, Mitchell MJ, Crosby LE, et al. Engaging Patients With Sickle Cell Disease and Their Families in Disease Education, Research, and Community Awareness. J Prev Interv Community 2011;39(3):256–72.
35. Crosby LE, Strong H, Johnson A, et al. The Teen Symposium: Engaging adolescents and young adults with sickle cell disease in clinical care and research. Clin Prac in Pediatr Psychol 2020;8(2):139–49.
36. Valenzuela JM, Vaughn LM, Crosby LE, et al. Understanding the experiences of youth living with sickle cell disease: a photovoice pilot. Fam Community Health 2013;36(2):97–108.
37. Tobin Tyler E. Medical-Legal Partnership in Primary Care: Moving Upstream in the Clinic. Am J Lifestyle Med 2017;13(3):282–91.

Addressing Social Determinants of Health in Practice

Melissa R. Lutz, MD, MHS[a], Arvin Garg, MD, MPH[b],
Barry S. Solomon, MD, MPH[c],*

KEYWORDS

- Social determinants of health • Social risks • Social needs • Pediatrics

KEY POINTS

- Major pediatric organizations recommend screening for and providing interventions to address social determinants of health in the clinical setting.
- There are several social risk-screening tools designed for use in pediatrics but there are limited published data on their validity and efficacy.
- Screening for social risks can have unintended negative consequences and families may decline assistance based on their perception of need, fear of repercussions, or earlier experiences.
- Partnerships with community-based organizations and the use of linking services (ie, volunteers, community health workers, social workers, care coordinators, and case managers) are critical for connection to resources.

BACKGROUND: A BRIEF HISTORY

Pediatrics has a long-standing history of treating the "whole person" and acknowledging factors beyond physical health that contribute to an individual's well-being. The patient-centered medical home model was pioneered in pediatrics and pediatric guidelines, such as Bright Futures, include various anticipatory guidance topics that center on the social, emotional, and mental health of not only the patient but also their family. In 2016, in response to the continued high rate of childhood poverty, 2 major pediatric organizations advocated to formalize the way in which we address social determinants of health (SDoH) in the clinical setting. The American Academy of

[a] Department of Pediatrics, Johns Hopkins University School of Medicine, 200 North Wolfe Street, Room 2088, Baltimore, MD 21287, USA; [b] Department of Pediatrics, Child Health Equity Center, UMass Chan Medical School, UMass Memorial Children's Medical Center, 55 Lake Avenue North, Suite S5-856, Worcester, MA 01655, USA; [c] Department of Pediatrics, Johns Hopkins University School of Medicine, 200 North Wolfe Street, Room 2055, Baltimore, MD 21287, USA
* Corresponding author.
E-mail address: bsolomon@jhmi.edu

Pediatr Clin N Am 70 (2023) 695–708
https://doi.org/10.1016/j.pcl.2023.03.006
0031-3955/23/© 2023 Elsevier Inc. All rights reserved.
pediatric.theclinics.com

Pediatrics (AAP) released a policy statement recommending that pediatricians "screen for risk factors within SDoH during patient encounters"[1] and the Academic Pediatric Association published a review article that identifies specific SDoH domains and lists several screening tools.[2]

A few years later, an ad-hoc committee from the National Academy of Sciences, Engineering, and Medicine released a report calling for the integration of services addressing social needs and SDoH into the delivery of health care. This report refers to the "5 A's": awareness, adjustment, assistance, alignment, and advocacy. At the individual level, health-care providers should assist patients and adjust care to account for their social needs while aligning with communities and advocating for policy change at the community level. Awareness of the importance of SDoH should occur at both levels.[3] In a 2018 review of published SDoH interventions, Beck and colleagues presented a conceptual framework to explain how both positive and negative social, environmental, structural, economic, and political factors affect behaviors and physiologic functions, which affect health outcomes for individuals, households, and populations across the life span (**Fig. 1**).[4]

Since then, many pediatric primary care clinics have adopted processes for SDoH screening, and there is now a large and growing body of literature examining the influence of social factors on physical and mental health. However, despite the high level of current interest in the topic, there is no consensus for how to best address SDoH in the clinical setting. This review seeks to summarize the current pediatric literature, including both the strengths and weaknesses of current practices, opportunities for further research, and evidence-informed practical strategies for clinicians.

CLINICAL CASE: SOCIAL DETERMINANTS OF HEALTH IN CONTEXT

The following clinical case illustrates the influence of social drivers on health and highlights the importance of addressing these issues in clinical practice.

Ali is a 5-year-old girl who is presenting to your primary care clinic with her mother for a follow-up visit. She was born at 25 weeks' gestation and has chronic lung disease, retinopathy of prematurity, severe dysphagia, and global developmental delay.

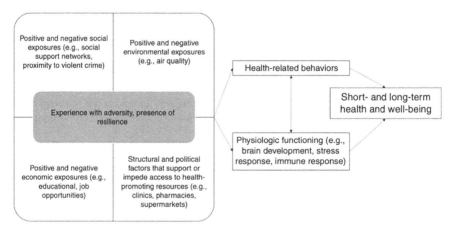

Fig. 1. Conceptual framework summarizing the relationship between structural and social exposures and health outcomes across the life span. (Beck, A.F., Cohen, A.J., Colvin, J.D. et al. Perspectives from the Society for Pediatric Research: interventions targeting social needs in pediatric clinical care. Pediatr Res 84, 10–21 (2018). https://doi.org/10.1038/s41390-018-0012-1.)

She was last seen for a well-child visit 4 months ago and at that time was instructed to follow-up with various subspecialists including her pulmonologist, ophthalmologist, gastroenterologist, speech language pathologist, and occupational therapist. Today you discover that she saw her speech pathologist and occupational therapist a few times but she has not seen them recently and she has not yet seen any of the subspecialists. She also lost 5 lbs in the interim. At the end of the visit, her mother asks if the clinic still has any bags of food available. After some discussion, you learn that her parents often run out of food before the end of the month, do not have a reliable form of transportation, and given recent loss of employment, they are at risk of being evicted from their apartment and of having their utilities shut-off. For these reasons, they have had trouble making it to her various follow-up appointments and have been unable to purchase the supplemental nutritional formula she had received in the past.

How can we, as pediatric professionals, do a better job identifying and addressing social drivers of health to optimize the health and well-being of our patients and their families?

IMPLEMENTING SOCIAL RISK AND SOCIAL NEEDS SCREENING

There are several social risk-screening tools designed for use in pediatric settings. These tools use validated questions to identify risks in specific social domains (eg, The Hunger Vital Sign to detect food insecurity). "Social risks" refer to individual-level or household-level adverse factors that could negatively influence health, which differ from "social needs" that reflect a family's own priorities and are revealed by self-report.[5] Screening tools can facilitate efficient identification of risks but should be followed up with a discussion about the family's needs and desire for assistance. Busy clinicians and practices must also weigh adding SDoH screening to other psychosocial screenings already being performed including, adverse childhood experiences, postpartum depression, preconception care needs, and others. Although social needs can be elucidated without use of a screening tool, implementing screening tools into a clinical workflow promotes wider and more uniform distribution and increases referrals to community agencies for basic needs, including food, employment, transportation, education, and housing.[5,6]

In pediatrics, screening tools are generally intended to be completed by the patient's parent, with parent defined to include both parents and other legal guardians for the purpose of this article. Commonly screened domains include financial stability, education, food security, transportation, employment, and the physical environment (ie, housing, utilities, neighborhood). The screeners are brief, typically containing fewer than 15 questions, and accessible to a broad audience, including individuals with low literacy levels and non-English speakers. Screeners should include questions most relevant for the patient population, as this can vary across different communities. For example, in a study examining social needs of families in 18 pediatric practices across the United States, the highest reported needs of Spanish speaking parents related to food access, whereas more speakers that are English requested help with childcare enrollment.[7] In some cases, social risk screening questions are also embedded into other broader screening tools, such as the Survey of Well-Being in Young Children (SWYC), which also contains developmental and behavioral screening questions.[8]

Screening tools are administered using various modalities (verbal, paper, and electronic) but several studies have shown that parents tend to prefer paper or electronic screening tools compared to verbal screening. Using a device, such as a computer or tablet, is not only easier and faster than completing screening verbally, but is also more private. Many parents express reluctance to discuss sensitive information, such as social needs, in front of their children or with clinical staff due to feelings of shame and fear of judgment.[9] Newer innovations allow for screening questions to be incorporated into the electronic health record (EHR) or sent to patients before the visit to simplify the process even further, but to our knowledge, the effectiveness of such methods have not yet been published in the literature. **Table 1** summarizes the key properties of various published pediatric screening tools and **Table 2** displays examples of specific social needs included within commonly screened SDoH domains.

Regardless of modality, screening should be performed in a private setting (eg, examination room) where the patient and parent feel comfortable and supported. Screening should be approached with compassion, empathy, and respect. Often, the pediatric primary care office provides this type of environment, where a trusting longitudinal relationship has already been established.[10] In earlier studies, parents preferred to be screened in the primary care office rather than in the emergency department.[11] However, in a more recent study, Tedford and colleagues show that screening in the emergency department can capture individuals who do not present to primary care regularly or those who are seen in primary care but still have unmet social needs. Specifically, they found Spanish-speaking caregivers of pediatric patients presenting to the emergency department had twice the odds of having at least one unmet need compared with English speaking caregivers.[12]

Furthermore, interest in receiving resources is higher when the purpose of screening is clearly explained before asking screening questions. A brief prompt using normative language at the beginning of the screener is helpful and is even more effective when accompanied by a verbal explanation by clinic personnel.[13] Similarly, parents who were asked about their desire for assistance before screening are more likely to accept assistance from the clinic.[14,15] As a household's needs can change over time, it is currently recommended by some that parents complete screening at all health maintenance visits.[16] However, as screening becomes more popular in subspecialty clinics, emergency departments, and inpatient settings, further research will be necessary to determine the optimal frequency of screening. Although parents should always be given the option to decline screening, repeated screening could cause additional stress and practices may unnecessarily duplicate efforts to assist families.

Despite the widespread use of social risk screening tools in pediatric clinical care settings, there is very little published data to support the validity of the commonly used tools. In a systematic review, Sokol and colleagues identified 17 studies using 11 screeners and only 3 (WE CARE, IHELP, and SEEK) included an assessment of validity and/or reliability.[17] Oldfield and colleagues explored the internal consistency and construct validity of the WE CARE tool. They found that interrater reliability between adolescents and their parents was high (82%). However, there were discrepancies between positive and negative screens comparing 3 domains in the WE CARE and Accountable Health Communities tools (housing, food, and utilities), suggesting that responses vary depending on how the question is asked.[17–19] As there is no "gold standard" screening method, sensitivity, specificity, and superiority cannot be determined. Furthermore, to our knowledge, current published literature focuses primarily on their pragmatic properties and there are no published studies examining the validity of the other pediatric screening tools, which will be an important future direction for research.

RESPONDING TO POSITIVE SCREENS

Whether a practice decides to use an existing screening tool or create their own, it is vital that they are prepared to respond appropriately to all risks identified. There are

Table 1
Social risk and social needs screening tools used in pediatrics

	Screening Tool					
	Health Leads	iHELP	MLP	SEEK	SWYC	WE CARE
Year created	2016	2007	2015	2007	2010	2007
Number of social risk questions	10	14	10	9	9	10
Asks about desire for assistance	X	X		X		X
Reading level (grade)	6th	7th	NR	4th–5th	10th	9th
Completion time	NR	NR	NR	3 min	10 min	<5 min
Administration method	Paper	Verbal	Paper	Paper Electronic Verbal	Electronic Paper	Paper Verbal
Additional languages				Spanish, Chinese, Swedish, Vietnamese	Spanish, Burmese, Nepali, Portuguese, Arabic	
SDoH Domains						
Economic stability	X	X	X			X
Education	X	X	X		X	X
Social and community context	X	X	X	X	X	
Health and clinical care			X	X		
Neighborhood and physical environment	X	X	X	X	X	X
Food	X	X	X	X	X	X

Abbreviations: iHELLP, Income, Housing, Education, Legal status, Literacy, Personal Safety Questionnaire; MLP, Medical-Legal Partnership; SEEK, Safe Environment for Every Kid; SWYC, Survey of Well-being of Young Children; WE CARE, Well Child Care, Evaluation, Community Resources, Advocacy, Referral, Education.

Data from Henrikson NB, et al. Psychometric and pragmatic properties of social risk screening tools: A systematic review. *American Journal of Preventive Medicine.* 2019;57(6):S13 and De Marchis EH, Brown E, Aceves BA, Loomba V, Molina M, Cartier Y, Wing H, Gottlieb LM. *State of the Science on Social Screening in Healthcare Settings.* 2022. San Francisco, CA: Social Interventions Research and Evaluation Network.

Table 2
Social needs included within commonly screened SDoH domains

SDoH Domain	Social Needs
Economic stability	• Poor housing conditions (eg, mold, mice, cockroaches, lead paint, water leaks) • Homelessness, inability to pay rent, risk for eviction • Financial strain • Employment or job training • Transportation • Utilities assistance
Education	• Special education needs • Childcare (eg, head start enrollment) • Parent literacy • Interest in obtaining a high school equivalency degree or attending vocational school or college
Social and community context	• Interpersonal violence • Parent tobacco use, substance use • Social support
Health and clinical care	• Child and parent health insurance • Parent access to primary care provider • Maternal preconception care needs • Parental depression
Neighborhood and physical environment	• Community violence • Access to safe recreational space
Food	• Food insecurity (eg, Hunger Vital Sign) • Urgent food need (onsite food pantry) • Women, Infants, and Children (WIC) and Supplemental Nutrition Assistance Program (SNAP) enrollment
Other	• Citizenship status • Power of attorney and guardianship • Safety supplies (eg, smoke alarm, car seat, stair gates) • Parental stress and parenting support • Clothing

various types of interventions that require different levels of staff and community involvement, as summarized in **Fig. 2**.

At the most basic level, it is useful to develop or have access to a database or directory of community resources that can easily be provided to families. Because it is difficult to keep up with the frequently changing availability of resources, clinics should take advantage of publicly available regional directories and national resources.

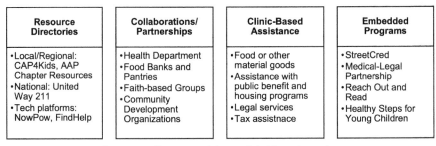

Resource Directories	Collaborations/ Partnerships	Clinic-Based Assistance	Embedded Programs
•Local/Regional: CAP4Kids, AAP Chapter Resources •National: United Way 211 •Tech platforms: NowPow, FindHelp	•Health Department •Food Banks and Pantries •Faith-based Groups •Community Development Organizations	•Food or other material goods •Assistance with public benefit and housing programs •Legal services •Tax assistnace	•StreetCred •Medical-Legal Partnership •Reach Out and Read •Healthy Steps for Young Children

Fig. 2. Interventions for responding to positive social risk and needs screens.

CAP4Kids is a website designed and maintained by the Children's Advocacy Project that has a variety of social and developmental resources and parent printouts for 16 cities throughout the United States (https://cap4kids.org/). Local AAP chapters also typically provide lists for regional resources. National resources include the United Way's 211, which can be accessed via their website, phone, or text (https://www.211.org/). Individuals can work with United Way representatives who connect them to local resources, including urgent needs such as food and housing. Larger practices may elect to purchase subscriptions for software platforms such as NowPow (https://nowpow.com/nowpow-platform) and Findhelp, previously known as Aunt Bertha (https://www.findhelp.org) that can link families to resources.

Next, practices should form cross-sector partnerships with community groups and other organizations because this not only helps to keep directories up to date, but also facilitates open communication for warm referrals. Ideally, community sites can message the practice to inform them of a successful resource connection to close the referral loop. In addition to resource referral, clinics may also offer material goods, such as nonperishable food or fresh produce, newborn items, home safety items, and so forth. Local nonprofit organizations are often eager to collaborate with clinicians to distribute these materials. Clinics can also provide services such as assistance with enrollment for public benefit programs, including the Supplemental Nutrition Assistance Program (SNAP); Special Supplemental Nutrition Program for Women, Infants, and Children (WIC); Temporary Assistance for Needy Families (TANF); Child Tax Credit, and housing programs. There are several nationally recognized programs that are embedded within the clinic setting to provide specific services, including medical-financial partnerships, such as StreetCred, which provides tax preparation services (https://www.mystreetcred.org/), the Medical-Legal Partnership (https://medical-legalpartnership.org/), Reach Out and Read (https://reachoutandread.org/), and the Healthy Steps program (https://www.healthysteps.org/).

Responding to positive screens does not need to be the job of the clinician alone but protocols involving support staff should be established within the clinic to streamline screening and referral processes. "Linking services," which involve volunteers, community health workers, social workers, care coordinators, and case managers are invaluable in facilitating connection to resources.[20,21] Formal patient navigation programs, such as those modeled after Health Leads,[22] have also been shown to decrease health-care utilization by decreasing risk of hospitalizations[23] and increasing adherence to recommended well-child visits.[24,25] Patient navigation is traditionally performed in clinic but if the space or resources are not available to do so, services can be carried out using telephone calls or video visits. Although an in-person patient navigator can remind providers to make referrals during the clinic visit, both in-person and remote patient navigation are effective.[26] In some cases, parents even preferred to receive resources via text message or email to in-person consultation with a care coordinator.[18]

Another promising strategy is to provide support for parents to navigate resources on their own. Previously, web-based screening has led to higher positivity rates on social risks screening[27] and including a built-in database of services facilitated resource connection.[28] In a recent mixed-methods intervention study, comparing self-navigation to in-person assistance, 77% of participants in the self-navigation group engaged with assistance and 85% of those participants followed up with resources, compared with 14% and 33%, respectively, in the in-person assistance group.[29]

Above all, the ability to follow through with provided resources is a priority. The process of social risk and/or social need identification and resource referral is complex and even those interested in receiving resources can be lost to follow-up due to missed phone calls or appointments, lack of transportation or childcare, and time constraints.[30] In a pilot study assessing use of an SDoH program serving an ethnically diverse pediatric population, families with non-US citizens or caregivers with limited English proficiency were at high risk of being lost to follow-up. However, those families who engaged in the program used community services more than their peers.[31] When making resource referrals, we should consider the unique language and cultural needs of families from diverse backgrounds. In general, families find it easier to connect with resources when immediate solutions exist and are available, resources are integrated into the health-care system, and when there is a direct pathway for connection.[32]

CONCERNS AND POTENTIAL UNINTENDED CONSEQUENCES

Several studies have demonstrated there is often a disparity between the number of individuals who screen positive and those who request or seek assistance.[11,15,33] Some parents who screen negative, either because they are truly not at risk or due to concerns about disclosing sensitive information, may want help connecting to resources. Others who screen positive for social risks may not be ready to receive help in the moment.[34] Recent qualitative work has also elucidated several common themes that could explain why parents choose not to accept assistance in the clinical setting (Fig. 3).

The first major theme relates to the individual's perception of their own needs. They may have more pressing needs or priorities (social, medical, or other) that take precedence over the risk factors identified on their clinic's screening tool.[29,35] Alternatively, they may think that their own need is not as severe as the needs of other families and do not want to take resources that could be allocated elsewhere.[9] Furthermore, the parent's level of activation, or ability to navigate resources independently, and the perceived urgency of the need affect desire to receive assistance. In an assessment of a resource connection program at Rainbow Babies and Children's Hospital, parents

Perception of Need
- More pressing needs or other priorities
- Belief that other families need resources more
- Ability to navigate resources independently

Negative Repercussions
- Questions about confidentiality
- Concerns about referral to law enforcement, immigration officials and/or child protective services
- Fear of judgment, stigmatization, or discrimination
- Feelings of shame

Prior Experiences
- Already receiving assistance
- Prior negative experiences with resources
- Difficulties connecting with resources in the past
- Not eligible for assistance
- Limited availability of resources
- Lack of tailored services (i.e., language concordant or medically tailored services)

Fig. 3. Barriers to receiving resources in the clinical setting.

with more urgent needs, which were most commonly shelter or utilities, were more likely to stay involved in the program, whereas those individuals with high levels of activation, or confidence in their ability to obtain resources on their own, were less likely to remain involved with the program.[35]

Second, many cite fear of negative consequences of screening results as a barrier to receiving assistance. Although the majority of parents surveyed are not concerned about the confidentiality of their screening results, some still express concerns about how their information could be used or shared[36] and are not comfortable with documentation of results in the EHR.[34] Many express fears of being reported to law enforcement, immigration officials, or child protective services based on the results of their screens.,[37] Even those who are not concerned about external referrals may still be concerned about judgment, stigmatization, and/or discrimination by their health-care provider.[9] In 2 studies of verbal screening, participants preferred to be screened by nurses, community health workers, or patient navigators over clinicians because these individuals bridged cultural gaps and have the time and expertise to respond to their needs.[21] Despite efforts to implement uniform processes and normalize the practice of screening, this is still a sensitive topic and some parents report feeling shame in having to respond positively to a social risk screen and thus do not answer questions honestly.[38] Because of these factors, screening is often not a linear process; only a small number of parents who are screened are able to engage with resources, which further accentuates inequities, as demonstrated **Fig. 4**.[39]

Finally, families' current or earlier experiences with resources are often overlooked in the screening-referral process. Often, parents know about available resources and may already be receiving assistance.[36] Conversely, they may have had negative experience with the resources that are offered or had difficulty connecting with the resource in the past. Social support programs often have strict eligibility criteria and burdensome application processes that can deter parents from applying on their own. Moreover, due to limited availability and capacity of services in the health-care setting, parents report low confidence that the offered resources will benefit them, especially

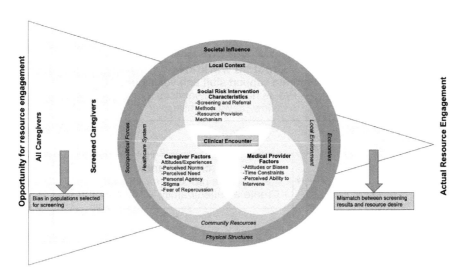

Fig. 4. Pathway from screening to resource engagement. (Figure reproduced with permission from Cullen et al, "Pediatric Social Risk Screening: Leveraging Research to Ensure Equity" *Academic Pediatrics.* 2022;22: 190-192.)

if they are seeking tailored assistance such as language concordant resources or medically tailored services.[37,39]

In recent years, with increased attention to addressing systemic racism and reducing health disparities, funders, private insurers, and federal agencies have begun providing financial support for interventions to address SDoH. Many hospitals and health systems have become "anchor institutions" by collaborating and investing in their local communities.[40] The shift toward value-based care in state Medicaid managed care organizations and accountable care organizations has led to the creation of clinician incentives for SDoH screening and linkage to services.[41] Although many are in favor of widespread adoption of this change, we must ensure our community partners have the capacity and resources to handle additional referrals. In addition, providing payment for SDoH screening and intervention could result in a more paternalistic approach, a loss of family autonomy, and less shared decision-making.[42] We will need to work with our local professional societies and advocacy groups to be sure that clinician, family, and community partner perspectives are considered in payment reform discussions.

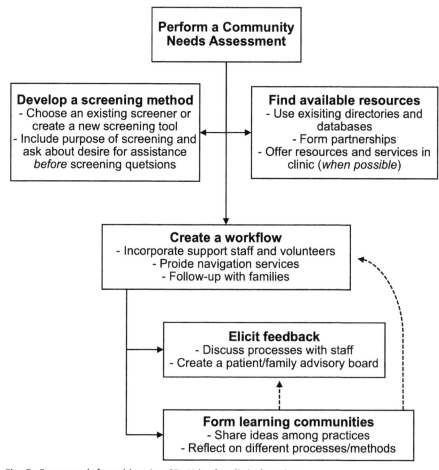

Fig. 5. Framework for addressing SDoH in the clinical setting.

Due to these concerns, some have questioned whether we should universally offer resources instead of screening parents in clinic,[5] and there are ongoing studies to examine alternative methods. Cullen and colleagues propose that the types of resources offered can be selected based on needs identified in Community Health Needs Assessments or population-level data, rather than individual screening results.[38] This approach has been used to address intimate partner violence in the past, where education is provided using standard scripts and then resources provided to all patients for themselves or to be passed on to a friend.[33] However, this strategy does not allow a provider to tailor resources to an individual's need, so a hybrid or tiered approach may be most successful. Nevertheless, offering resources upfront can help to start the conversation about social needs and facilitate effective social risk screening.

SUMMARY

Addressing SDoH in the clinical setting is consistent with our collective values as pediatric professionals and is a crucial component of our holistic approach to pediatric care. Current methods for screening and resource provision hold a lot of potential, but there are specific strategies we can implement to make these processes more effective and avoid critical pitfalls related to trust, respecting families' lived experiences, and family autonomy. There is not a one-size-fits-all approach; protocols can and should be adapted depending on practice size (single provider practices vs those with anchor institutions), setting, community needs, and availability of resources within the clinic and in the community. Before implementing screening, practices must establish connections with community programs and agencies so resources can be provided for all risks identified. Additional research in diverse patient populations is needed to assess the influence of screening tools on improving pediatric health and health-care utilization outcomes, determine the appropriate frequency of screening, evaluate innovative methods for screening and resource provision, and understand the impact of financial incentives for screening. As we work to advance the ways in which we approach SDoH, it is vital that we continue to engage with and learn from our patients, support staff, community stakeholders, and colleagues (**Fig. 5**).

CLINICS CARE POINTS

- Addressing SDoH in clinical practice is well aligned with our priorities as pediatric professionals.

- Screening tools are helpful to identify social risks but should be followed with more in-depth conversations to discuss a household's needs.

- Clinics should be prepared to intervene (ie, provide resources or referrals) on any social risks identified through screening, which can be facilitated by forming cross-sector partnerships and incorporating linking services into their workflow.

- After creating a workflow, it is important to continue to engage with and learn from patients, support staff, community stakeholders, and colleagues and adapt processes accordingly.

DISCLOSURE

The authors have nothing to disclose.

REFERENCES

1. Poverty and child health in the united states.Pediatrics (Evanston). 2016;137(4); e20160339. Available at: https://www.ncbi.nlm.nih.gov/pubmed/26962238.
2. Chung, EK., Siegel BS, Garg, A, et al. Screening for social determinants of health among children and families living in poverty: A guide for clinicians. Current problems in pediatric and adolescent health care. 2016;46(5):135-153. Available at: https://www.clinicalkey.es/playcontent/1-s2.0-S1538544216000341.
3. National Academies of Sciences, Engineering, and Medicine, Division HaM, Services, Board on Health Care, Health, Committee on Integrating Social Needs Care into the Delivery of Health Care to Improve the Nation's. Integrating social care into the delivery of health care. Washington, DC: National Academies Press; 2019.
4. Beck AF, Cohen AJ, Colvin JD, et al. Perspectives from the society for pediatric research: Interventions targeting social needs in pediatric clinical care. Pediatr Res 2018;84(1):10–21. Available at: https://www.ncbi.nlm.nih.gov/pubmed/2979 5202.
5. Garg A, Brochier A, Messmer E, et al. Clinical approaches to reducing material hardship due to poverty: Social risks/needs identification and interventions. Acad Pediatr 2021;21(8S):S154–60. Available at: https://www.ncbi.nlm.nih.gov/pubmed/34740423.
6. Garg A, Butz AM, Dworkin PH, et al. Improving the management of family psychosocial problems at low-income children's well-child care visits: The WE CARE project. Pediatrics (Evanston) 2007;120(3):547–58.
7. Polk S, Leifheit KM, Thornton R, et al. Addressing the social needs of Spanish- and English-speaking families in pediatric primary care. Acad Pediatr 2020; 20(8):1170–6.
8. The survey of well-being of young children. Available at: https://pediatrics.tufts medicalcenter.org/the-survey-of-wellbeing-of-young-children/overview.Updated 2022. Accessed August 30, 2022.
9. Cullen D, Attridge M, Fein JA. Food for thought: A qualitative evaluation of caregiver preferences for food insecurity screening and resource referral. Acad Pediatr 2020;20(8):1157–62.
10. Byhoff E, De Marchis EH, Hessler D, et al. Part II: A qualitative study of social risk screening acceptability in patients and caregivers. Am J Prev Med 2019;57(6): S38–46.
11. De Marchis EH, Hessler D, Fichtenberg C, et al. Part I: A quantitative study of social risk screening acceptability in patients and caregivers. Am J Prev Med 2019; 57(6):S25–37.
12. Tedford NJ, Keating EM, Ou Z, et al. Social needs screening during pediatric emergency department visits: Disparities in unmet social needs. Acad Pediatr 2022. https://doi.org/10.1016/j.acap.2022.05.002.
13. Nederveld AL, Duarte KF, Rice JD, et al. IMAGINE: A trial of messaging strategies for social needs screening and referral. Am J Prev Med 2022;63(3):S164.
14. De Marchis EH, Hessler D, Fichtenberg C, et al. Assessment of social risk factors and interest in receiving health Care–Based social assistance among adult patients and adult caregivers of pediatric patients. JAMA Netw Open 2020;3(10): e2021201.
15. Bottino J, Rhodes ET, Kreatsoulas C, et al. Food insecurity screening in pediatric primary care: Can offering referrals help identify families in need? Acad Pediatr

2016;17(5):497–503. Available at: https://www.clinicalkey.es/playcontent/1-s2.0-S1876285916304685.

16. Garg A, Dworkin PH. Applying surveillance and screening to family psychosocial issues: Implications for the medical home. J Dev Behav Pediatr 2011;32(5):418.

17. Sokol R, Austin A, Chandler C, et al. Screening children for social determinants of health: a systematic review. Pediatrics 2019;144(4):e20191622.

18. Oldfield BJ, Casey M, Decew A, et al. Screening for social determinants of health among children: Patients' preferences for receiving information to meet social needs and a comparison of screening instruments. Population Health Management 2021;24(1):141.

19. Gottlieb L, Fichtenberg C, Alderwick H, et al. Social determinants of health: What's a healthcare system to do? J Healthc Manag 2019;64(4):243–57. Available at: https://www.ncbi.nlm.nih.gov/pubmed/31274816.

20. Emengo VN, Williams MS, Odusanya R, et al. Qualitative program evaluation of social determinants of health screening and referral program. PLoS One 2020; 15(12).

21. Garg A, Marino M, Vikani AR, et al. Addressing families' unmet social needs within pediatric primary care. Clin Pediatr 2012;51(12):1191–3. Available at: https://journals.sagepub.com/doi/full/10.1177/0009922812437930.

22. Pantell MS, Hessler D, Long D, et al. Effects of in-person navigation to address family social needs on child health care utilization: A randomized clinical trial. JAMA Netw Open 2020;3(6):e20644.

23. Arbour MC, Floyd B, Morton S, et al. Cross-sector approach expands screening and addresses health-related social needs in pri- mary care. Pediatrics 2021;148. e2021050152.

24. Hill S, Topel K, Li X, et al. Engagement in a social needs navigation program and health care utilization in pediatric primary care. Acad Pediatr 2022;22(7):1221–7.

25. Messmer E, Brochier A, Joseph M, et al. Impact of an on-site versus remote patient navigator on pediatricians' referrals and families' receipt of resources for unmet social needs. J Prim Care Commun Health 2020;11. 2150132720924252. Available at: https://journals.sagepub.com/doi/full/10.1177/2150132720924252.

26. Gottlieb LM, Tirozzi KJ, Manchanda R, et al. Moving electronic medical records upstream. Am J Prev Med 2015;48(2):215–8. Available at: https://www.clinicalkey. es/playcontent/1-s2.0-S0749379714003754.

27. Hassan Areej, Scherer EA, et al. Improving social determinants of health. Am J Prev Med 2015;49(6):822–31. Available at: https://www.clinicalkey.es/playcontent/1-s2. 0-S074937971500207X.

28. Cohen AJ, Isaacson N, Torby M, et al. Motivators, barriers, and preferences to engagement with offered social care assistance among people with diabetes: A mixed methods study. Am J Prev Med 2022;63(3):S152.

29. Tablazon IL, Palakshappa D, OBrian FC, et al. Perspectives of caregivers experiencing persistent food insecurity at an academic primary care clinic. Acad Pediatr 2021. https://doi.org/10.1016/j.acap.2021.07.025.

30. Uwemedimo OT, May H. Disparities in utilization of social determinants of health referrals among children in immigrant families. Front Pediatr 2018;6:207.

31. Lian T, Kutzer K, Gautam D, et al. Factors associated with patients' connection to referred social needs resources at a federally qualified health center. J Prim Care Commun Health 2021;12:1–10. Available at: https://journals.sagepub.com/doi/full/10.1177/21501327211024390.

32. Bittner JC, Thomas N, Correa ET, et al. A broad-based approach to social needs screening in a pediatric primary care network. Acad Pediatr 2021;21(4):694–701.

33. Ray KN, Gitz KM, Hu A, et al. Nonresponse to health-related social needs screening questions. Pediatrics (Evanston) 2020;146(3):e20200174. Available at: https://search.proquest.com/docview/2449275922.

34. Ronis SD, Masotya M, Birkby GM, et al. Screening families in primary care for social and economic needs: Patients' urgency and activation for social care navigation. Am J Prev Med 2022;63(3):S122.

35. Hamity C, Jackson A, Peralta L, et al. Perceptions and experience of patients, staff, and clinicians with social needs assessment. TPJ 2018;22(4S):18.

36. Fichtenberg CM, De Marchis EH, Gottlieb LM. Understanding patients' interest in healthcare-based social assistance programs. Am J Prev Med 2022;63(3):S109.

37. Pfeiffer EJ, De Paula CL, Flores WO, et al. Barriers to patients' acceptance of social care interventions in clinic settings. Am J Prev Med 2022;63(3):S116.

38. Cullen D, Wilson-Hall L, McPeak K, et al. Pediatric social risk screening: Leveraging research to ensure equity. Acad Pediatr 2022;22(2):190–2.

39. Schoenthaler AM, Gallager RP, Kaplan SA, et al. From screening to the receipt of services: A qualitative examination. Am J Prev Med 2022;63(3):S144.

40. Koh HK, Bantham A, Geller AC, et al. Anchor institutions: best practices to address social needs and social determinants of health. Am J Public Health 2020;110(3):309–16.

41. Melzer Sanford M. Addressing social determinants of health in pediatric health systems: balancing mission and financial sustainability. Curr Opin Pediatr 2022; 34(1):8–13.

42. Garg A, Homer CJ, Dworkin PH. Addressing social determinants of health: challenges and opportunities in a value-based model. Pediatrics 2019r;143(4): e20182355.

Pursuing a Cross-Sector Approach to Advance Child Health Equity

Alexandra M.S. Corley, MD, MPH[a,b,]*, Adrienne W. Henize, JD[b],
Melissa D. Klein, MD, MEd[c,d,e], Andrew F. Beck, MD, MPH[a,b,f]

KEYWORDS

- Cross-sector partnerships • System of care • Social determinants of health
- Health equity

KEY POINTS

- Child health experts include educators, legal advocates, childcare providers, government leaders, benefits agencies, community organizations, clinicians, and many others.
- A team of child health professionals, linked by codesigned partnerships, is necessary to establish an equitable, effective, outcomes-focused system of care.
- Systems of care address the needs of a defined population with a shared vision for outcome measurement, evaluation, and improvement.

ILLUSTRATIVE CASE

Imagine you are seeing two siblings, aged 9 months and 3 years, for well-child visits in primary care. They arrive in clinic 30 minutes after their scheduled appointment time. Their mother is apologetic, noting that she was delayed at the hospital because her third child, a 6-year-old, is admitted with an asthma exacerbation. She was late picking up her other children from their grandparents' house, where they were being watched. As a result, the family missed the bus transfer on the way to clinic.

[a] Department of Pediatrics, University of Cincinnati College of Medicine, 3333 Burnet Avenue MLC 7035, Cincinnati, OH 45229, USA; [b] Division of General & Community Pediatrics, Cincinnati Children's Hospital Medical Center, 3333 Burnet Avenue MLC 7035, Cincinnati, OH 45229, USA; [c] Department of Pediatrics, University of Cincinnati College of Medicine, 3333 Burnet Avenue MLC 2011, Cincinnati, OH 45229, USA; [d] Division of General & Community Pediatrics, Cincinnati Children's Hospital Medical Center, 3333 Burnet Avenue MLC 2011, Cincinnati, OH 45229, USA; [e] Division of Hospital Medicine, Cincinnati Children's Hospital Medical Center, 3333 Burnet Avenue MLC 2011, Cincinnati, OH 45229, USA; [f] Division of Hospital Medicine, Cincinnati Children's Hospital Medical Center, 3333 Burnet Avenue MLC 7035, Cincinnati, OH 45229, USA
* Corresponding author. Department of Pediatrics, University of Cincinnati College of Medicine, 3333 Burnet Avenue MLC 7035, Cincinnati, OH 45229.
E-mail address: alexandra.corley@cchmc.org

Pediatr Clin N Am 70 (2023) 709–723
https://doi.org/10.1016/j.pcl.2023.03.008
0031-3955/23/© 2023 Elsevier Inc. All rights reserved.
pediatric.theclinics.com

You begin the visit, empathetically acknowledging this parent's challenges. You describe routine screenings and immunizations planned for each child. Their mother is glad that you will check the infant's lead level, as both older children have a history of lead poisoning. The family has not moved from the affected apartment, a unit (and building) plagued by poor upkeep, pests, and mold. The mother describes continued issues getting the landlord to help. She also asks for advice on getting the children into daycare or preschool. She is having difficulty navigating enrollment processes. There is an urgency to this request as her workplace does not tolerate missed hours, and extended family members may not be able to watch the younger children much longer. She is also concerned because her 6-year-old still cannot read and has missed many days due to his asthma symptoms. The school advised that he repeat first grade without any testing or delineation of individualized approaches to educational intervention.

As you contemplate responses to this complexity, you find yourself feeling comfortable with immunizations, blood draws, and asthma controller medications. You are less comfortable navigating public transportation schedules, housing ordinances, early childhood education programs, educational law, and more. The "system" of care—the confluence of people, organizations, and support structures that work together to meet the needs of children and families—comes into a sharper view.[1]

> Pediatric clinicians may find themselves less comfortable navigating social complexity than medical complexity.

INTRODUCTION

Clinical practice is increasingly complex. To provide safe, effective, and equitable care, clinicians must be able to efficiently identify pertinent information and coproduce treatment plans that work for patients and families and can be adapted where needed.[2] Clinicians must also know when to seek the advice and services of others.

Expertise of a range of professionals, when brought into the clinical setting, can meaningfully improve outcomes.[3] Routinely, a primary care clinician may seek the counsel of a consulting subspecialist, for example, referring a child to a cardiologist for a heart murmur. We suggest that these connections should extend beyond the walls of the health care system to a system of care inclusive of community consultants, experts, and partners.[4]

The Healthy People 2030 defines the social determinants of health (SDH) as "the conditions in the environments where people are born, live, learn, work, play, worship, and age that affect a wide range of health, functioning, and quality-of-life outcomes and risk."[5] Profound inequities in child health outcomes are driven by differential exposures and experiences related to these determinants, most of which occur outside the health care system.[6-12] Yet, there has been a long-standing gap in how health care systems identify and then seek to address the SDH.[13-15] We suggest that there is an urgent need to move toward a more balanced approach to medical and social determinants through multidisciplinary connection.[16-18]

System of Care

It is estimated that only 10% to 20% of our health is influenced by clinical care.[19] Still, care for children is generally problem-focused and siloed into single institutions or sectors. For example, all three children from the above case may interact with multiple health care providers while simultaneously trying to navigate various social service agencies. Working through the complexities of separate medical and social systems requires time and resources that are often inequitably distributed. However, what if we start thinking about these systems not as separate entities but as an intercon- nected system of care and support?

The system of care that influences child health and well-being is dynamic, and an intentional network of support persons, groups, and structures with the purpose of meeting the unique needs of children and their families.[20] To achieve child health eq- uity, systems of care must be tailored to the needs of children and their caregivers, thoughtfully integrated into communities, and guided by practices steeped in cultural humility.[21] Leaning on these shared values, systems of care allow agencies that may otherwise be isolated to collaborate. If we consider the various settings in which chil- dren live, learn, and grow, it becomes clear that child health experts include more than just pediatric clinicians or health care stakeholders. Educators, legal experts, child- care providers, government leaders, benefits agencies, community organizations, and many others affect the well-being and trajectories of children.

Child health experts include more than just pediatric clinicians; educators, legal advocates, childcare providers, government leaders, benefits agencies, community organizations, and many others affect the well-being and trajectories of children.

If we only consider clinical stakeholders, we will always fall short.

The system of care responsible for child health must be multidisciplinary, community-focused, and truly cross-sector. If we only consider clinical stakeholders in thinking about child health, we will always fall short. Cross-sector relationships be- tween pediatric clinicians and other professionals, and bridges between health care and community settings, must be intentionally created, thoughtfully maintained, and continuously refined. Herein, we will define a "system of care." We will then provide strategies to build and sustain cross-sector partnerships with stakeholders squarely within this system. We will cite examples of partnerships that have positively affected child health and well-being, a non-exhaustive list representative of what may be avail- able across communities. Finally, we will raise questions and opportunities for further research and innovation.

SYSTEM OF CARE AND SYSTEM OF HEALTH

If population health[22] outcomes are largely driven by factors outside the health care system, it behooves us to consider a health system that is wider than clinics and hos- pitals.[23] We encourage the following steps to capture an inclusive system of care and the system of health.[24]

First, the population must be defined. This may vary depending on care setting or aim, but stakeholders must be able to define the population in question and visualize themselves and their roles in this definition. This could include all patients within a certain clinic registry or all children within a defined geography.[25] By agreeing on the population, stakeholders will be able to enumerate a denominator to which activ- ities will be directed. Second, stakeholders must define shared measures, shared out- comes, including numerators attached to improvement activities, or interventions. When clinical and community partners come together, they can continually return to their quantified shared population and shared outcomes. What percentage of children within a clinic registry are engaged with a community partner? How many newborns are enrolled in public benefits like Special Supplemental Nutrition Program for Women, Infants, and Children (WIC) in a timely fashion? A critical third step in getting started, once numerators and denominators are in place, is for stakeholders to build a tracking system to follow measures over time. They may consider a shared dashboard to depict progress, needs and wants, and successes and challenges enabled by partnership.

An Inclusive *System of Care*: How to Get Started
1. Define the population
2. Identify shared improvement measures
3. Build a tracking system

The three children in our case may be three of 10,000 children cared for by a clinic or 1000 in a neighborhood. Numerators that capture their lived experience, risks, and assets could include the presence (or absence) of safe and stable public housing, enrollment (or non-enrollment) in high-quality childcare and school settings, and access to health-promoting resources such as food pantries or green space. Each of these assets and risks contributes to larger denominators that represent the population shared by partners who may be well served by a shared measurement infrastructure that enables partners to quickly see themselves as part of the larger system of health: within a given city or neighborhood, the percentage of children living in safe, stable housing, enrolled in high-quality childcare, having their educational needs met, and who are food secure. Such an approach will support deepened situational awareness[26–28] and cross-community connections critical to improved care delivery and ultimately, better, more equitable outcomes.[29–32]

Such a system is illustrated in **Fig. 1**. The largest frame depicts the city of Cincinnati. Neighborhoods are colored various shades of gray, illustrative of the percentage of individuals living below the federal poverty level. Such a "geomarker" depicts an SDH relevant to health outcomes and inequities.[25] One can zoom in to take a closer look at a specific neighborhood, considering risks and assets that are present on the ground. One can zoom in still further to consider the household or child, enveloped by a system of providers who, together, work to change hard-to-move shared

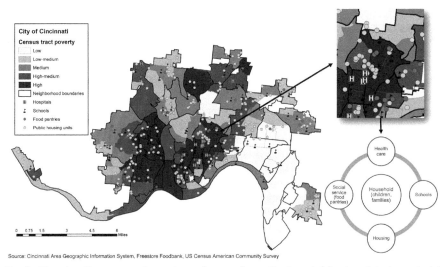

Source: Cincinnati Area Geographic Information System, Freestore Foodbank, US Census American Community Survey

Fig. 1. Mapping the cross-sector system of care—from city, to neighborhood, to household.

outcomes. Next, we will delineate the steps needed to develop and sustain impactful health-relevant, cross-sector partnerships.

DEVELOPING AND SUSTAINING CROSS-SECTOR PARTNERSHIPS

The Healthy People 2030 groups the SDH into five domains: economic stability; education access and quality; health care access and quality; neighborhood and built environment; and social and community context.[5] Many outside of the health care system have expertise in SDH-relevant processes and policies. They are well-positioned to mitigate negative impacts and augment positive impacts that the SDH promulgate. Clinical-community partnerships have the potential capability to interrupt the cycle of poverty that often perpetuates acute care needs for symptoms or conditions that should be preventable (eg, lead poisoning, asthma exacerbations, behavioral health needs).

The Healthy People 2030 SDH domains touch the family introduced in the case above. The mother is employed, but she does not have reliable transportation to bring her children to the clinic. Family members help care for her children, which may not be sustainable. This mother is struggling to navigate complex processes to enroll her younger children in high-quality childcare/preschool. She is worried about her oldest child's potential to succeed in school, but she does not know how to advocate for appropriate educational supports. Her two older children have a history of lead poisoning and asthma, but she has been unable to move or successfully engage with her landlord to remedy in-home triggers. You can begin to see how an effective system of care that includes high-quality education and employment, secure housing, and nonprofit resources to meet basic needs is essential if these children and this family are to thrive. A system with direct links from the clinic to the broader caring community can be built by assessing patients' risks and assets, prioritizing risks collaboratively with the patient and family, determining and developing appropriate interventions with cross-sector partners, and operationalizing interventions through strategic integration into the clinical setting and partner workflow.[30]

Assessing patients' risks and needs is essential to identify those that are most important to the family and amenable to intervention through cross-sector collaboration. Tools such as the Results Oriented Management and Accountability scale[33] and the Arizona Self-Sufficiency Matrix[34] identify, measure, and record improvement in families' assets, capacity, and needs. These and other tools give families the agency to identify where they see their current state and what they want to prioritize for their family moving forward.[35] Clinicians can use social screeners[36] and well-recognized frameworks such as Maslow's Hierarchy of Needs to work with families to identify, prioritize, and address risks and then map them to effective community interventions (**Fig. 2**).

Successful interventions that use cross-sector collaboration depend on, first, understanding which community partners share the health care partner's vision for healthy, thriving children and families. This can be done by objectively surveying the community landscape, ideally with input from community members and families that may be better positioned than clinicians to understand available assets and resources. Next, partners can align on goals for the work they hope to do together. This will often require codesign of measures and a joint management structure. Partners may need to delineate when and how to share data, ensuring that governance and confidentiality rules are followed. Partners may also wish to collaboratively seek funding to help the venture move forward faster. Ideally, collaboration enhances capacity and provides mutual benefit to each partner. For example, a primary care

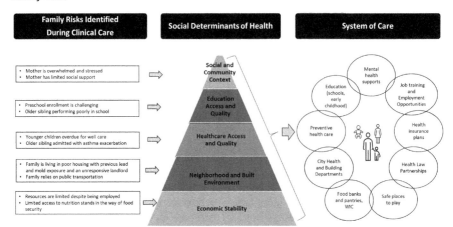

Fig. 2. Integration of family risks and social determinants of health into a system of care.

clinic's partnership with a regional food bank to establish an in-clinic food pantry supports the clinic's desire to mitigate patients' food insecurity and the food bank's mission to alleviate child hunger.[37] Collective action can be accelerated by consistently using human-centered design, community organizing, and quality improvement methods and by ensuring that the right voices are at the table from the beginning. Indeed, partnerships are likely to be strongest when families can meaningfully participate in their design, implementation, and evaluation.[38,39]

Successful cross-sector collaborations depend on:
1. Understanding the shared vision between health care and community partners
2. Collaboratively aligning goals, codesigning measures, and managing oversight together

---

Meaningful and effective integration of cross-sector interventions into clinical workflow is essential. Curricula for medical students or residents increasingly include training on the SDH and poverty. This may be in the form of experiential learning[40–42] with supplemental didactic instruction. However, such training may be insufficient. Clinicians will often still need additional training and experience working with and learning from community partners to effectively complete meaningful social histories and recognize and use appropriate community resources.[43] Depending on the clinical setting, education can be directed toward trainees (eg, nursing or medical students, residents, and fellows), care management team members, or other frontline staff that can connect families to help. Encouraging innovation in the electronic health record offers further opportunity to integrate cross-sector work into clinical settings. For example, the SDH Wheel in Epic Healthy Planet, Epic Systems' accountable care and population management system module[44] includes social screening prompts, visibility of risks across care settings, and the potential for closed-loop communication between health care and community partners through referral platforms such as Findhelp[45] and WellSky.[46] Action at clinical sites can be complemented by networked approaches or coalitions that incorporate shared principles, aims, and drivers in pursuit of system transformation.

EXAMPLES OF CROSS-SECTOR PARTNERSHIPS

Examples of cross-sector partnerships are highlighted in **Table 1**. Partnerships can take many forms, a diverse array whose full recitation is beyond the scope of this

Table 1
Examples of cross-sector partnerships

Name	Goals	Partners	Measures and Impact
Clinically integrated partnerships			
Child-focused legal aid partnership—eg, Child HeLP[49]	Resolve legal issues that undermine health and well-being in children and families	Legal aid advocates, clinical providers (eg, primary care centers)	• Number of referrals by referring provider and clinical site • Number and type of cases opened • Number and type of positive legal outcomes • Number of children and families impacted in referred households • Dollars recovered in back and adjusted future public benefits for families
Maternal-focused legal aid partnership—eg, M-HeLP	Improve maternal and newborn health outcomes through legal advocacy	Legal aid advocates, clinical providers (eg, obstetric practice, primary care centers)	• Number of patients screened for potential legal needs • Percentage of patients identified with health-harming legal need • Number of referrals • Number and type of cases opened • Engagement in prenatal care • Percentage of infants born preterm • Newborn legal assessment • Newborn adherence to preventative care
Embedded food pantry with formula program[37]	Minimize food insecurity and formula stretching among families with infants and children	Local food bank and associated food pantries, primary care centers	• Number of referrals by clinical site • Number of children and families impacted in referred households • Age of children in referred households

(continued on next page)

Table 1
(continued)

Name	Goals	Partners	Measures and Impact
Reading programs[63]	Promote early literacy skills by providing books to children to enhance school success	Primary Care Centers, Dolly Parton Imagination Library, Reach Out and Read	• Number of children enrolled in Reach Out and Read • Number of children enrolled in Imagination Library • Number of books provided • Age of children in referred households • How often parents read to their children at home
Kindergarten captain/early childhood specialists	Enhance connections between children and high-quality preschools	Primary Care Centers, Preschools, Local School Districts	• Number of children referred • Number of children enrolled in high-quality preschool • Kindergarten readiness
Coordinated awareness and assistance partnerships			
Special Supplemental Nutrition Program for Women, Infants, and Children (WIC)	Ensure healthy food availability for women, infants, and children ≤5 years	WIC state agencies, health departments, primary care centers, community centers, and so forth	• Number of referrals • Number of participants • Vouchers provided (number; value)
Housing risk identification program—eg, CLEAR[54]	Mitigate housing risks among patients admitted with asthma	Cincinnati Health and Building Departments, inpatient asthma unit	• Number of referrals • Percent of referrals that result in healthy homes visit • Percent of visits that result in orders for housing code violation abatement • Percent of orders that result in improved housing conditions

Community-connected learning

Community learning network—eg, All Children Thrive[31]	To bring stakeholders together to collaborate, learn, formulate and answer questions, encourage discovery, and implement findings to cocreate an environment where children thrive	Community leaders, families, local agencies, and health care providers	• Population health outcomes (eg, hospitalizations) • School achievement outcomes (eg, 3rd grade reading) • Process and outcome measures stratified by race, ethnicity, socioeconomic status • Capabilities built • Percent of activities that are coproduced with parents, families, partners
Value-based payment plans—eg, Cincinnati Children's HealthVine or Nationwide Children's Partners for Kids	To promote equitable, high-value outcomes among Medicaid enrollees	Clinical practices, Medicaid Managed Care, patients, and families	• Population health outcomes (eg, hospitalizations, achievement of preventive milestones • Medicaid claims, costs

article. Some partnerships connect to patients and families within the clinical setting; others connect within community setting (eg, homes, schools, child welfare, juvenile justice, and community agencies). Certain partnerships are clinically integrated, whereas others use learning network structures to share in the pursuit of solutions.[4] Such collaborative networks, or coalitions, can also prompt policy innovations that extend the reach of partnerships from single encounters to entire populations.

Clinically Integrated Partnership Programs

Medical-Legal, or Health-Law, Partnerships link a clinical partner with legal advocates, experts in addressing the legal needs of low-income people. The Cincinnati Child Health-Law Partnership (Child HeLP) was launched in 2008 as a clinically integrated partnership, connecting pediatric primary care centers (PPCCs) at Cincinnati Children's Hospital Medical Center (CCHMC) with the Legal Aid Society of Greater Cincinnati (LASGC)[47] to address social and environmental risks that may be amenable to legal remedies. The Maternal Health-Law Partnership (M-HeLP) is an analogous partnership launched in 2017 between one of Cincinnati's largest obstetrical practices, the CCHMC PPCCs, and LASGC. M-HeLP aims to improve maternal and newborn health outcomes based on an integrated system of screening, assessment, and referral for legal advocacy for pregnant individuals. Both Child HeLP and M-HeLP address civil legal needs, catalyze system-level change through joint advocacy, and educate health professionals about the SDH.[48–50] According to the National Center for Medical-Legal Partnership, there are 450 such partnerships across 49 states and the District of Columbia.[51]

To address infant food insecurity, the PPCCs established two clinically integrated nutrition programs. Keeping Infants Nourished and Developing, a collaboration with the Freestore Foodbank[52] (the region's largest food bank), provides formula to infants living in food insecure households. To further address food insecurity, the PPCCs also collaborated with this same food bank to open primary care-embedded food pantries. Any family who indicates food insecurity during a visit can obtain 3 days of shelf-stable food for their entire family. In addition, families are often linked with other in-clinic interventions or community-based resources to address the underlying challenges they face.[53]

Coordinated Awareness and Assistance Partnerships

Several programs also exist that could coordinate awareness and assistance directed toward a range of social determinants. An example is the Collaboration to Lessen Environmental Asthma Risks (CLEAR). CLEAR connects children hospitalized with asthma who also have an adverse, asthma-related housing exposure (eg, pests, mold) to health department sanitarians expert in both healthy housing education and housing code enforcement. Referrals are generated from the electronic health record to such community-based experts who then respond.[54] By making this link, we coordinate awareness of healthy housing capabilities within the region with assistance. Such coordination also facilitates pattern recognition—awareness of patterns of adverse housing and assistance that extends from individual patients to tenants of the same building complex.

Community-Connected Learning

Cincinnati's All Children Thrive (ACT) Learning Network[55] was established in 2015, connecting hundreds of pediatric clinicians with individuals, families, and agencies from across the city, aligned around established goals. ACTs shared measures focus on three thematic areas—excellent and equitable health outcomes; safe and supported families; and pathway to full potential. Early on, a focus was placed on bringing families, all of whom live in neighborhoods with suboptimal child health outcomes into ACT. Parent perspectives have been critical in the drive to integrate sectors and promote development of the network's central principles: children are at the center of our work; equity is foundational; relationships, trust, and working together are essential; we all teach, we all learn; and daily work is action-oriented and result-focused. These principles encourage active engagement, promoted through capability building, and shared understanding of issues and problems. ACT uses quality improvement methods and codesign to rapidly spur learning and action. Key enablers include quality improvement experts, data analysts, and community engagement specialists.[31]

Further, coalitions such as Children's HealthWatch[56] that successfully advocated for statewide expansion of tax credits to support at-risk families and Vot-ER[57] that works to integrate voter education and registration into health care settings offer health care and community partners opportunities to advocate for policy changes that can positively affect thousands of families. Such coalitions have only grown in importance, as value-based payment schema have expanded. Partnerships with Medicaid Managed Care Organizations incentivize collaboration with primary care practices to enable prevention. The active use of claims and electronic health record data inform and drive better, more equitable outcomes.[58–60] This economic shift toward value is likely to promote innovation in the realm of clinical–community partnership, providing new opportunities to invest in interventions outside of the health care system. Reimbursing for community-connected activities, investing in healthy housing, or paying for transportation all are now possible.[61,62]

RESEARCH QUESTIONS, CHALLENGES, AND OPPORTUNITIES FOR INNOVATION

Cross-sector partnerships are increasingly seen as a beneficial adjuvant to clinical care. As more partnerships emerge, strategies to evaluate their clinical and nonclinical impact are critical. What are the "right" outcomes to assess as we seek to evaluate such partnerships? Who determines which outcomes are most important? What happens if a partnership moves one outcome but not another? Many of the problems that such partnerships are trying to solve evolved over decades if not centuries. How can we balance the urgency to act with patience, with the reality that we may not see the changes we seek overnight?

Many of these questions are influenced by the fundamental imbalance in spending between health care and social care sectors.[13,14] As value-based payment mechanisms become more common, there are additional opportunities to consider how and where meaningful health-relevant investments might be made. Novel payment mechanisms represent one potential way to overcome the significant challenge of financial sustainability. Co-identifying and then comanaging such challenges will be important to ensure joint solutions. Indeed, we ought to consider where to direct cost savings and reinvestment.[62] We encourage strategic investments that strengthen codesigned inclusive partnerships and enable population health innovation spaces that are truly collaborative.[39]

SUMMARY

In revisiting the case with the mother of three young children, we can recall how that family was affected by the SDH. Consider their care experience and what determines whether their path bends toward illness or wellness. Excellent, evidence-based clinical care is necessary, but not sufficient to promote wellness. Meaningful connection to cross-sector community partners can extend the reach of the clinician and care provided, improving equitable outcomes for children, households, and communities.

CLINICS CARE POINTS

- Child health experts include parents and a wide array of community-based experts who together compose a child health system.
- To establish a right-sized system of care for children, define the population and desired outcomes, establish measures of interest, and identify stakeholders to track these data over time.
- Finding cross-sector collaborators can start with identifying a shared vision for healthy children and families.

DISCLOSURE

The authors have no relevant disclosures to report.

ACKNOWLEDGMENTS

The authors would like to thank all the clinical–community partners who have been vital to the development and lasting impact of our partnership programs. This work was supported, in part, by the Agency for Healthcare Research and Quality (AHRQ, 1R01HS027996-01A1).

REFERENCES

1. Roth LR. Redefining "Medical Care. Cornell J Law Public Policy 2017;27(1):65–106.
2. Roy B, Riley C, Sears L, et al. Collective Well-Being to Improve Population Health Outcomes: An Actionable Conceptual Model and Review of the Literature. Am J Health Promot 2018;32(8):1800–13.
3. Cheng TL, Emmanuel MA, Levy DJ, et al. Child Health Disparities: What Can a Clinician Do? Pediatrics 2015;136(5):961–8.
4. Liu PY, Beck AF, Lindau ST, et al. A Framework for Cross-Sector Partnerships to Address Childhood Adversity and Improve Life Course Health. Pediatrics 2022; 149(Suppl 5).
5. Social Determinants of Health. Office of Disease Prevention and Health Promotion, Office of the Assistant Secretary for Health, Office of the Secretary, U.S. Department of Health and Human Services. Healthy People 2030 Web site. Available at: https://health.gov/healthypeople/priority-areas/social-determinants-health. Published 2022. Accessed September 15, 2022.
6. Akinbami LJ, Moorman JE, Garbe PL, et al. Status of childhood asthma in the United States, 1980-2007. Pediatrics 2009;123(Suppl 3):S131–45.
7. Akinbami LJ, Moorman JE, Liu X. Asthma prevalence, health care use, and mortality: United States, 2005-2009. Nat Health Stat Rep 2011;(32):1–14.
8. Beck AF, Moncrief T, Huang B, et al. Inequalities in Neighborhood Child Asthma Admission Rates and Underlying Community Characteristics in One US County. J Pediatr 2013;163(2):574–80.
9. Beck AF, Florin TA, Campanella S, et al. Geographic Variation in Hospitalization for Lower Respiratory Tract Infections Across One County. JAMA Pediatr 2015; 169(9):846–54.

10. Gupta RS, Zhang X, Sharp LK, et al. Geographic variability in childhood asthma prevalence in Chicago. J Allergy Clin Immunol 2008;121(3):639–45.e1.
11. Wright RJ, Subramanian SV. Advancing a multilevel framework for epidemiologic research on asthma disparities. Chest 2007;132(5 Suppl):757S–69S.
12. Krieger N. Health Equity and the Fallacy of Treating Causes of Population Health as if They Sum to 100. Am J Public Health 2017;107(4):541–9.
13. Bradley EH, Elkins BR, Herrin J, et al. Health and social services expenditures: associations with health outcomes. BMJ Qual Saf 2011;20(10):826–31.
14. Bradley EH, Canavan M, Rogan E, et al. Variation In Health Outcomes: The Role Of Spending On Social Services, Public Health, And Health Care, 2000-09. Health Aff (Millwood) 2016;35(5):760–8.
15. Brewster AL, Brault MA, Tan AX, et al. Patterns of Collaboration among Health Care and Social Services Providers in Communities with Lower Health Care Utilization and Costs. Health Serv Res 2017. https://doi.org/10.1111/1475-6773.12775.
16. Berkowitz SA, Baggett TP, Edwards ST. Addressing Health-Related Social Needs: Value-Based Care or Values-Based Care? J Gen Intern Med 2019;34(9):1916–8.
17. Boozary AS, Shojania KG. Pathology of poverty: the need for quality improvement efforts to address social determinants of health. BMJ Qual Saf 2018;27(6):421–4.
18. Yaeger JP, Kaczorowski J, Brophy PD. Leveraging Cross-sector Partnerships to Preserve Child Health: A Call to Action in a Time of Crisis. JAMA Pediatr 2020;174(12):1137–8.
19. Hood CM, Gennuso KP, Swain GR, et al. County Health Rankings: Relationships Between Determinant Factors and Health Outcomes. Am J Prev Med 2016;50(2):129–35.
20. BA S, RM F. Caring for severely emotionally disturbed children and youth. Principles for a system of care. Child Today 1988;17(4):11–5.
21. Stroul B, Blau G, Friedman R. Updating the system of care Concept and Philosophy. Washington, DC: Georgetown University Center for Child and Human Development, National Technical Assistance Center for Children's Mental Health; 2010.
22. Kindig D, Stoddart G. What is population health? Am J Public Health 2003;93(3):380–3.
23. Sampath BRJ, Baldoza K, Mate K, et al. Whole system quality: a Unified approach to building responsive, Resilient health care systems. Boston: Institute for Healthcare Improvement; 2021.
24. Anderson AC, O'Rourke E, Chin MH, et al. Promoting Health Equity And Eliminating Disparities Through Performance Measurement And Payment. Health Aff (Millwood) 2018;37(3):371–7.
25. Beck AF, Sandel MT, Ryan PH, et al. Mapping Neighborhood Health Geomarkers To Clinical Care Decisions To Promote Equity In Child Health. Health Aff (Millwood) 2017;36(6):999–1005.
26. Endsley MR. Measurement of Situation Awareness in Dynamic-Systems. Hum Factors 1995;37(1):65–84.
27. Endsley MR. Toward a Theory of Situation Awareness in Dynamic-Systems. Hum Factors 1995;37(1):32–64.
28. Beck AFHD, Kahn RS, Taylor SC, et al. Rapid, Bottom-Up Design of a Regional Learning Health System in Response to COVID-19. Mayo Clin Proc 2021.
29. Siegel B, Erickson J, Milstein B, et al. Multisector Partnerships Need Further Development To Fulfill Aspirations For Transforming Regional Health And Well-Being. Health Aff (Millwood) 2018;37(1):30–7.

30. Henize AW, Beck AF, Klein MD, et al. A Road Map to Address the Social Determinants of Health Through Community Collaboration. Pediatrics 2015;136(4):e993–1001.
31. Kahn RS, Iyer SB, Kotagal UR. Development of a Child Health Learning Network to Improve Population Health Outcomes; Presented in Honor of Dr Robert Haggerty. Acad Pediatr 2017;17(6):607–13.
32. Wesson DE, Kitzman HE. How Academic Health Systems Can Achieve Population Health in Vulnerable Populations Through Value-Based Care: The Critical Importance of Establishing Trusted Agency. Acad Med 2018;93(6):839–42.
33. Results Oriented Management and Accountability. Available at: https://nascsp.org/csbg/csbg-resources/roma/. Published 2022. Accessed November 22, 2022.
34. US Department of Housing and Urban Development. Self Sufficiency Matrix: Using HMIS to Benchmark Progress. Available at: https://www.hudexchange.info/resource/1562/self-sufficiency-matrix-using-hmis-to-benchmark-progress-sample. Published 2022. Accessed November 22, 2022.
35. Garg A, Toy S, Tripodis Y, et al. Addressing social determinants of health at well child care visits: a cluster RCT. Pediatrics 2015;135(2):296–304.
36. Chung EK, Siegel BS, Garg A, et al. Screening for Social Determinants of Health Among Children and Families Living in Poverty: A Guide for Clinicians. Curr Probl Pediatr Adolesc Health Care 2016;46(5):135–53.
37. Beck AF, Henize AW, Kahn RS, et al. Forging a pediatric primary care-community partnership to support food-insecure families. Pediatrics 2014;134(2):e564–71.
38. Beck AF, Marcil LE, Klein MD, et al. Pediatricians Contributing to Poverty Reduction Through Clinical-Community Partnership and Collective Action: A Narrative Review. Acad Pediatr 2021;21(8S):S200–6.
39. Parsons A, Unaka NI, Stewart C, et al. Seven practices for pursuing equity through learning health systems: Notes from the field. Learn Health Syst 2021;5(3):e10279.
40. Lichtenstein C, de la Torre D, Falusi O, et al. Using a Community Bus Tour for Pediatric Residents to Increase Their Knowledge of Health Disparities. Acad Pediatr 2018;18(6):717–9.
41. Klein M, Alcamo A, Beck A, et al. Can a video curriculum on the social determinants of health affect residents' practice and families' perceptions of care? Academic pediatrics 2014;14(2):159–66.
42. Lazow M, Real F, Ollberding N, et al. Modernizing Training on Social Determinants of Health: A Virtual Neighborhood Tour is Noninferior to an in-Person Experience. Academic pediatrics 2018;18(6):720–2.
43. Klein M, Kahn R, Baker R, et al. Training in social determinants of health in primary care: does it change resident behavior? Academic pediatrics 2011;11(5):387–93.
44. Corporation ES. Coordinated Care Management. Available at: https://www.sfdph.org/dph/files/wpcfiles/Epic_Coordinated_Care_Management.pdf. Published 2019. Accessed September 15, 2022.
45. Findhelp CSCfHC. Findhelp: a Public Benefit Corporation;. Available at: https://go.findhelp.com/ohio. Published 2022. Accessed September 15, 2022.
46. Wellsky. Social Care Coordination - WellSky. Available at: https://wellsky.com/social-care-coordination/. Published 2022. Accessed September 15, 2022.
47. Legal Aid Society of Greater Cincinnati. Available at: https://lascinti.org/. Published 2022. Accessed September 23, 2022.
48. Beck AF, Klein MD, Schaffzin JK, et al. Identifying and treating a substandard housing cluster using a medical-legal partnership. Pediatrics 2012;130(5):831–8.

49. Klein MD, Beck AF, Henize AW, et al. Doctors and lawyers collaborating to HeLP children–outcomes from a successful partnership between professions. J Health Care Poor Underserved 2013;24(3):1063–73.

50. Beck AF, Henize AW, Qiu T, et al. Reductions In Hospitalizations Among Children Referred To A Primary Care-Based Medical-Legal Partnership. Health Aff (Millwood) 2022;41(3):341–9.

51. The Partnerships. National Center for Medical-Legal Partnerships. Available at: https://medical-legalpartnership.org/partnerships/. Published 2022. Accessed September 15, 2022.

52. Freestore Foodbank. @FreestoreFB. Available at: https://freestorefoodbank.org/. Published 2022. Accessed September 25, 2022.

53. Burkhardt MC, Beck AF, Conway PH, et al. Enhancing accurate identification of food insecurity using quality-improvement techniques. Pediatrics 2012;129(2): e504–10.

54. Beck A, Simmons J, Sauers H, et al. Connecting at-risk inpatient asthmatics to a community-based program to reduce home environmental risks: care system redesign using quality improvement methods. Hosp Pediatr 2013;3(4):326–34.

55. All Children Thrive. Available at: https://actcincy.org. Published 2022. Accessed September 23, 2022.

56. Watch CsH. Home - Children's HealthWatch. Available at: https://childrenshealthwatch.org/home-2/. Published 2022. Accessed September 16, 2022.

57. Vot-ER. Home - Vot-ER. @vot_er_org. Available at: https://vot-er.org/. Published 2022. Updated 2020-05-09. Accessed September 16, 2022.

58. Boye KB, Chang DI. Case Study: Nationwide Children's Hospital: An Accountable Care Organization Going Upstream to Address Population Health,. NAM Perspectives, Discussion Paper. Washington, DC: National Academy of Medicine; 2017. Discussion Paper. https://doi.org/10.31478/201704g. Discussion Paper.

59. Weier RC, Gardner W, Conkol K, et al. Partners for Kids Care Coordination: Lessons From the Field. Pediatrics 2017;139(Suppl 2):S109–16.

60. Kelleher K, Reece J, Sandel M. The Healthy Neighborhood, Healthy Families Initiative. Pediatrics 2018;142(3).

61. Galloway I. Using pay-for-success to increase investment in the nonmedical determinants of health. Health Aff (Millwood) 2014;33(11):1897–904.

62. Sandhu S, Alderwick H, Gottlieb LM. Financing Approaches to Social Prescribing Programs in England and the United States. Milbank Q 2022;100(2):393–423.

63. Szumlas GA, Petronio P, Mitchell MJ, et al. A Combined Reach Out and Read and Imagination Library Program on Kindergarten Readiness. Pediatrics 2021;147(6).

Addressing Structural Racism in Pediatric Clinical Practice

Marciana Laster, MD, MSCR[a,b], Daniel Kozman, MD, MPH[a,c],
Keith C. Norris, MD, PhD[a,d],*

KEYWORDS

• Pediatrics • Racism • Child health • Disparities • Race • Ethnicity

KEY POINTS

- Racial and ethnic disparities in children are strongly driven by discriminatory laws, policies, and practices that create and perpetuate inequities in the allocation of health-affirming resources and opportunities, also known as structural racism.
- Both structural and interpersonal racism can adversely impact a child's biological and psychological functioning.
- By integrating strategies that address the impact of structural racism along the life course into clinical care, we can optimize our potential to mitigate both existing disparities and the intergenerational transmission of many health and social disadvantages, thereby improving the health of minoritized children, families, and communities.

INTRODUCTION

The health of children and families is strongly influenced by the array of economic, political, and social factors in which they are born, grow, live, work, worship, and age. This includes the neighborhood and physical environment, access to quality education, health literacy, nutrition, green space exposure, socioeconomic status, level of trust in the medical community, health insurance status, and access to care. These factors and more are called the social determinants of health (SDoH),[1–3] which are detailed in Melissa R. Lutz and colleagues' article, "Addressing Social Determinants of Health in Practice," in this issue. By better understanding the SDoH and the

[a] David Geffen School of Medicine, University of California, Los Angeles, CA, USA; [b] Division of Pediatric Nephrology, UCLA Department of Pediatrics, 10833 Le Conte Avenue, MDCC A2-383, Los Angeles, CA 90095-1752, USA; [c] UCLA Department of Medicine, Section of Medicine-Pediatrics & Preventive Medicine; [d] Division of General Internal Medicine and Health Services Research, UCLA Department of Medicine, 1100 Glendon Avenue, Suite 710, Los Angeles, CA 90024, USA
* Corresponding author. Division of General Internal Medicine and Health Services Research, UCLA Department of Medicine, 1100 Glendon Avenue, Suite 710, Los Angeles, CA.
E-mail address: kcnorris@mednet.ucla.edu

Pediatr Clin N Am 70 (2023) 725–743
https://doi.org/10.1016/j.pcl.2023.03.010
0031-3955/23/© 2023 Elsevier Inc. All rights reserved.
pediatric.theclinics.com

downstream implications of exposure to suboptimal health-affirming structures and systems on specific disease conditions, we can both improve population health and advance health equity.[4] Studies of racial and ethnic differences in health outcomes have largely focused on access to care and experiences of individual-level racial discrimination, with solutions targeting health care financing, equitable allocation of and access to quality care, availability of language interpreters, community-based care, strategies to address bias and other approaches to reduce disparities.[5] However, over the last few decades, there has been a shift from a focus on personally mediated racism to elucidating system-level factors. When race-based discriminatory laws drive the inequitable allocation of many of the SDoH to different communities and families, policies and practices, it is termed structural racism.[6–8]

In fact, it is structural racism that leads to racial and ethnic inequities in health-affirming resources, and structural racism is the major factor in the development and perpetuation of racial and ethnic health disparities, adversely affecting the health and well-being of generations of American Indians, African Americans, and other minoritized (socio-politically marginalized and/or excluded) groups.[7,8] Children's mental, physical, and spiritual growth and development are especially susceptible to the impact of inequities in the SDoH.[9] Structural racism impacts child health through a variety of mechanisms, from physical and emotional violence to the violence of deprivation and constrained dreams.[10] Thus, health disparities are the result of the intersection of a complex set of systems (health and health care) and a very complex problem (racism).[11]

Optimizing the health of all children requires an understanding of the many ways structural racism directly and indirectly impacts children's health and the practice of pediatric medicine.[9,12] It is critical for pediatric clinicians to not only understand the importance of how racism can impact the health of their patients but to be aware of the intersectionality of race and other identities that are commonly discriminated against. Pediatric clinicians must often navigate the discrimination their patients suffer by sex, religious affiliation, immigrant status, family composition, sexuality, ability/disability, and other identities. The intersection of these stressors can have a powerful direct influence on children and their families leading to psychosocial problems, maladaptive beliefs and behaviors, and ultimately adverse health outcomes. In this commentary, we will explore the genesis of structural racism and the steps that pediatric clinicians and other child health professionals can take to increase their awareness of the role of racism, especially structural racism, on the children they care for and their families, and how to help leverage health system and community-based resources when needed.

RACE, ETHNICITY, AND HEALTH DISPARITIES

Despite its official status in government, research, and health professions, the term race is a misnomer and there is only the human race or *Homo sapiens*.[13] In the United States (and many other countries), race is used instead as the socio-political interpretation of how one looks in a "race"-conscious society.[14,15] Racial discrimination has evolved into a system to control power based on how groups of people look (racism) and then expanded to marginalize and/or exclude other people as well (eg, ethnicity as defined by culture/language/religion).[14,15] Of note, the definition of race is inconsistent, changing across space and time.[13] Although there are well-known biologic associations with race or ethnicity, these associations are wrongly interpreted as causal. This is due to false narratives of race as biologic with innate group differences in physiology, biology, intellect, and other attributes as originally defined by Carl Linnaeus in the 1700s.[16,17]

Unfortunately, persistent race-based views in medicine have their origin in the false and widespread belief that race and ethnicity have innate distinguishing biologic properties and personal attributes, termed race essentialism.[18] This has led to race and ethnicity often being used inappropriately in medicine and clinical decision-making. As group-level social variables that are inconsistently characterized, and unordered with no direct relation to any medical or physiologic process, neither race nor ethnicity can directly inform us of anything specific about individuals (**Box 1**).

Each person from a given racial and/or ethnic group is not the same, nor are they equally different from other racial and/or ethnic groups. Ancestry informative markers can be consistently measured, but are also unordered with no direct relation to any medical or physiologic process and therefore cannot directly inform us of anything specific about individuals. By contrast, gene polymorphisms (eg, cystic fibrosis, sickle cell anemia) may be directly related to a disease state and, in clinically relevant cases, can be used to help directly inform clinical treatment.[20]

Racial and ethnic health disparities are group-level health differences, that with rare exceptions adversely affect minoritized populations (eg, disease prevalence, health outcomes), and would not exist in an equitable and just society.[21] Racial and ethnic health disparities are primarily driven by inequities in the allocation of health-affirming resources and opportunities due to structural racism and related systemic biases.[22] Importantly, they are not related to innate group differences, as there are no relevant innate health differences across racial and ethnic groups.

DEFINING RACISM AND BIAS

There are multiple forms of racism (including structural racism) and biases, which manifest in unique ways across the life course with important health implications for pediatric patients and families. Racism in the United States has origins in colonialism and imperialism, in which race (and sex)-based inequality were institutionalized into law, policies, and practices, leaving a legacy of racism and segregation that continues to impact health today.[23] Dr. Camara Jones reminds us that racism is not isolated incidents or acts based on racial discrimination (**Box 2**).[24]

Box 1
The use of race and ethnicity in medicine[18,19]

- Simply put, race is how society sees you and racism is what society does to you based on how it sees you.

- Race and ethnicity are not risk factors for poor health. They are risk factors for racism, and racism is a risk factor for poor health.

- Race and ethnicity should not be used to direct a specific treatment, but, as social constructs, should be considered with the social history to help inform potential risks, early screening, etc.

- Race and ethnicity and even ancestry informative markers may have group-level biologic associations but do not have innate biologic properties outside of phenotype.

- Group differences in race, ethnicity, or ancestry informative markers cannot be validly assigned to each group member as a race or ethnic or even an ancestry informative marker-based modifier in a formula or algorithm.

- Known differences in the prevalence of racial or ethnic group associations with disease-related gene polymorphisms can be used in ordering a differential diagnosis, but should not be used to exclude a diagnosis.

> **Box 2**
> **What is racism?**[14,15,24,25]
>
> - Racism is not isolated incidents or acts based on racial discrimination, but "a system of structuring opportunity and assigning value based on the social interpretation of how one looks (which is what we call race)."
> - Racism operates at three levels: (i) structural/institutional, (ii) personally mediated, and (iii) internalized.
> - Importantly, defining racism as a system—and not a series of isolated incidents or acts based on an innate character flaw or personal moral failing—helps start important conversations, as we are no longer trying to divide the room into who is racist and who is not.
> - In this way, we can focus our efforts on systems and actions that perpetuate inequities and their downstream effects on health.

At an individual-level, narratives of perceived inherent group differences based on identity (racial, sex, religion, gender identity, socioeconomic status/class, etc.) are best described as biases, prejudices, and stereotypes (beliefs) or microaggressions and discrimination (behaviors). Further, these beliefs can turn into individual-level discriminatory actions such as microaggressions, which are the subtle verbal and non-verbal insults often done unconsciously. Such beliefs often perpetuate a dominant stereotype so they go uninterrupted, subsequently leading to overt discrimination and unequal treatment of members of groups based on an ostracized identity, and support for race-based discriminatory policies and practices that are the foundation of structural racism.[26] For many minoritized children, the impact of racism and discrimination on health across one's life course begins with maternal exposures and their impact on the prenatal environment, followed by early childhood and then adolescence experiences.[9]

STRUCTURAL RACISM AND HEALTH INEQUITIES

Structural racism is defined as "the totality of ways in which societies foster racial discrimination, through mutually reinforcing inequitable systems (in housing, education, employment, earnings, benefits, credit, media, health care, criminal justice, and so on).[8] This in turn reinforces discriminatory beliefs, values, and distribution of resources, which together affect the risk of adverse health outcomes."[8] One of the greatest and long-lasting impacts of structural racism in pediatrics is through its maintenance of child poverty.[27] Child poverty distributes along racial-ethnic lines with 31% of Black children and 23% of Hispanic children experiencing poverty as compared to 11% of White children in 2021.[28] Child poverty is manifest as housing instability, food insecurity, and economic stagnation, all of which impact the ability to access and maintain quality medical services. Decades-long policies and practices have prevented wealth building and social mobility among minoritized populations and relegated them to environments with limited health care access and direct toxic exposures affecting health. Unfair practices such as redlining, systematic destruction of minority-owned neighborhoods, and the seizure of minority-owned property using Eminent Domain have limited land ownership and the wealth inherent to it. These practices have affected the trajectory of its victims for generations and contribute to the maintenance of child poverty within minoritized groups.[10,29]

The downstream effects of structural racism underlie numerous disparate pediatric health outcomes. For instance, Black infants have higher rates of premature birth with higher rates of prematurity-related comorbidities including sepsis, intraventricular hemorrhage (IVH), and retinopathy of prematurity.[29–31] IVH, in particular, has been associated with racial segregation, a consequence of structural racism that limits access to high-quality neonatal intensive care unit (NICU) care.[29,32] Even within high-quality NICUs, Black and Hispanic mothers reported language discrimination and ineffective communication. Although biases mediated toward Asian and White mothers were not reported in this study, Asian and White mothers reported witnessing differences in the amount of respect and attention given by clinicians to mothers of lower educational or socioeconomic backgrounds.[33] Another example of disparate health outcomes resulting from structural racism is racial differences in the prevalence and management of pediatric asthma. Not only is asthma more prevalent in Black children, but also rates of emergency department visits and hospitalization are higher in previously redlined communities and communities of low opportunity.[34,35]

Structural racism can adversely impact childhood development through not only biological embedding, but also the intergenerational transmission of risk and protective factors that create and perpetuate disparities. Given the intergenerational nature of trauma, it is extremely important that pediatricians and their team consider the role of structural racism and associated traumas on caregiving, child development, family dynamics, and developmental changes over time in response to multiple exposures. Disparities may also be perpetuated through intergenerational transmission of biologic and socio-political factors on the health of children and their families.[36,37] Prenatal and early postnatal social support, enhanced prenatal medical care, and other related strategies are consistent resilience factors in attenuating the intergenerational transmission of multiple health disparity conditions, from obesity to cardiac disease to mental health and more.[38–42] Interventions to directly address the clinical impact of racial discrimination on intergenerational health and/or clinical disease states are needed, while efforts to achieve social and racial justice continue. In the end, the ongoing and lingering effects of prior racial legislative laws/policies/practices continue to manifest as a system of violence ranging from physical and emotional violence to the violence of deprivation and constrained dreams for a disproportionate number of minoritized children and families (**Box 3**).

Minoritized children and adolescents not only experience racial discrimination directly, but indirectly as bystanders through prejudice or discrimination that is experienced by friends, families, and strangers. Unfortunately, children and adolescents may have both physiologic and psychological responses as bystanders to racism and the impact can continue long after the initial encounter.[9] Further, the downstream impact of structural racism on the SDoH, including the disparate manner in which health systems and providers may fail to equitably offer guideline-driven and evidenced-based quality care, may lead to disparities in child development, health, and wellness.

As noted earlier, structural racism is a level of racism that is embedded in the laws, policies, and practices in our society and institutions, and it does not require a racially biased individual to perpetuate it.[47] No one alive today owned an enslaved person through the transatlantic slave trade or created White supremacy ideology (belief of innate racial superiority of the White race) or structural racism. Unfortunately, many conversations immediately identify all White people as the perpetrators of structural racism and label all people who are not anti-racist as racist, missing the many nuances of race and racism, and leading to many people who are not actively racist being offended and stopping necessary dialogue. The reality is that, at an individual level, it is not a person's identity that is important, but their actions. As an example, many White people work to dismantle structural racism while many non-White people actively support/promote White supremacy narratives and policies. It has been common to place people in two groups relative to racism: anti-racist and racist. Another

---

Box 3
Key mechanisms through which structural racism impacts child health[27,31,36,41,43–46]

- Psychological and biologic trauma from negative social messaging, increased perceived/actual personally mediated discrimination, persistent implicit and explicit racial biases, and microaggressions.

- Residential segregation and disproportionately placing minority children in disinvested communities that are wrought with poor educational opportunities, limited access to quality health care, increased exposure to natural disasters, environmental toxins, poor quality nutrition, and limited safe play space.

- Limited opportunities for parents by limiting access to quality education and employment which manifests daily as limited transportation, limited time off work, and other barriers to accessing quality care for their children.

- In utero and childhood traumatic events such as exposure to poverty, race-based bias and discrimination, parental incarceration, substance use, domestic violence, separations, abuse and neglect, and familial displacement can adversely impact fetal development during pregnancy as well as subsequent transition to adulthood, becoming an important modulator of physical and mental disease.

- Intergenerational trauma such as the impact of a traumatic experience(s) that inflict negative social, psychological, and biological consequences (eg, epigenetics) not only on one generation, but also on subsequent generations for children and their families, and entire communities.

---

perspective is that everyone can and does make three choices, especially related to structural racism (**Box 4**).

Disaggregating people who are passive regarding structural racism from those who actively promote it can help maintain a dialogue with a large group of unaware or uneducated people who could become powerful anti-racists. Also, by focusing on racism as a system and structural racism as a level of racism that is historically embedded and now essentially autonomous, we can better use our efforts to target systems and when relevant, individuals by their actions and not their identity. With that understanding, it becomes easier to examine and address structural racism as a foundational influence on child development and its role in health across the life course. This understanding is necessary to develop progress toward health equity and most effectively intervene in health disparities, though the actions needed at a societal level are not trivial (**Table 1**).

THE INFLUENCE OF RACISM AND BIAS ON BIOLOGICAL AND PSYCHOLOGICAL FUNCTIONING

Racism and bias, including structural racism, may impact biological and psychological functioning in children and parents. The influence of structural racism on parents may

---

Box 4
Choices one can make related to structural racism

- Actively support and/or promote structural racism policies and practices, and White supremacy ideology and narratives (in which case one would appropriately be labeled a racist)

- Passively support structural racism policies and practices by doing nothing (apathetic toward racial oppression—not helpful, but not actively racist)

- Actively work to dismantle structural racism related policies and practices (anti-racist)

Table 1
Potential societal-level interventions for addressing structural racism in pediatrics

Key Pediatric-Related Adverse Societal Factors	Potential Societal-Level Interventions
1 Low Socioeconomic Status (SES)	• Programs to address income inequality (eg, living wage vs minimal wage) • Unrestricted income supplements for low-income earners • Housing vouchers for low-income earners • Expand childcare resources such as preschool • Jobs that are friendly to and supportive of workers with young children who need frequent medical care
2 Limited or Absent Health Insurance and/or Access to Care	• Re-establish full funding for the Affordable Care Act (ACA) Navigator Program, which provides free, one-on-one assistance to help people understand their ACA health insurance options and enrollment • Expansion and/or revision of the ACA benefits to create a more universal health care system • Establish more federally qualified health centers (FQHCs) and expansion of early specialty care among FQHCs
3 Low Level of Educational Attainment	• Restructure public education to provide equal funding to all public schools rather than basing funding on community-level wealth which is inherently inequitable
4 Limited Health Literacy	• Implement age-specific health and wellness educational programs in K-12 to promote a national culture of health
5 Poor Nutrition	• Governmental incentives (eg, tax credit) to food suppliers/retailers for providing affordable access to healthy foods • Address food apartheid (system of systemic injustice that divides those with access to an abundance of nutritious food and those who have been denied that access) by de-incentivizing availability to non-nutritious foods (eg, fast foods) and incentivize food industry leaders to implement culturally and literacy tailored affordable and healthy fresh foods to low-income, high-risk families
6 Limited Green Space Exposure	• Create more parks with walking space such as ready access to sidewalks, parks, and more in the communities at highest risk • Create spaces on school premises to support outdoor activities and reinstate physical education curriculum • Health-informed traffic patterns and urban planning (eg, to accommodate cyclists, sidewalks to promote walking) in high-risk communities

(continued on next page)

Table 1
(continued)

	Key Pediatric-Related Adverse Societal Factors	Potential Societal-Level Interventions
7	Environment	• Reduce placement of alcohol and tobacco outlets, factories, refineries, and toxic landfills in minoritized communities • Enhance environmental toxin-related abatement activities
8	Distrust of the Medical Institution	• Acknowledge historical injustices such as unethical research practices that have disproportionately targeted patients from racial and ethnic minority communities • Making amends for these past injustices through direct compensation to affected individuals and their families and/or via indirect investments into communities lacking health resources • Ensure equitable and ethical participation of populations presently underrepresented in clinical research within pediatric clinical trials that inform clinical guidelines pertinent to all communities • Revise media portrayal and narratives of racial and ethnic minority communities to avoid depicting them in sub-human narratives, and erase the subtle subconscious cues from a myriad of levels of being less than, unwelcomed, patronized, or worse that permeate all society including systems of health resources and health care

have downstream effects, including maladaptive psychological and cognitive/executive functioning that influence adolescent and parental choices and actions.[48] Exposures to racism and bias are major forms of psychosocial stress for minoritized groups, representing an additional burden on top of the other daily psychosocial stressors that most people face. Structural racism-related stressors include, but are not limited to, deeply entrenched socioeconomic and political injustices that contribute to a greater daily individual and family burden of stressors that are not inherent for low-income White counterpart children and families.[11,47,49,50] The subsequent state of distress (or stress as used in common parlance) is characterized by exaggerated and/or prolonged psychological and biologic responses to maintain homeostasis.[51,52] Structural racism-related stress or distress may be summarized as the cumulative impact of repeated experience with social and/or economic adversity, racism, and political marginalization, culminating in "wear and tear" which has been termed weathering.[53,54] These stressors activate a number of neuro-hormonal and physiologic systems,[52,54] including, but not limited to, the sympathetic nervous system,[52,54] activation of endocrine pathways and inflammatory cytokines,[52,54–56] altered immune regulation and oxidative stress-responsive signaling,[55,57,58] and epigenetic changes.[45,59–62] This cumulative physiologic burden or allostatic load may contribute to disparities in many chronic diseases such as early elevation of blood pressure and cardiac disease, early diabetes, refractory asthma, greater risk for somatic mutations and cancer, and more.[54,63–67] The higher prevalence, earlier onset, and/or greater severity of many of these common chronic conditions among racial and ethnic minorities reinforces the linkage between the additional burden of stress and health disparities that occur along the life course.[49,68–71]

In regards to cognitive and executive functioning, Keating and colleagues[48] reported recent discrimination in a group of 319 young adults (mean age 29 years) and was negatively associated with cognitive flexibility and working memory, reinforcing the adverse impact of racism on young adults to achieve their potential in educational outcomes as well as to follow provider recommendations for health.

ADDRESSING STRUCTURAL RACISM OF HEALTH SYSTEMS AND CLINICAL INSTITUTIONS

It is also paramount to understand how structural racism, locally in clinical contracts, health system policies, health care locations, and messaging, impacts our families' ability to meaningfully and longitudinally engage with their health care team and develop strategies to mitigate its impact (**Table 2**). In seeking to achieve a payer mix with the highest reimbursement rates, many health systems, including many nonprofit organizations, very heavily prioritize maintaining as high a proportion of privately insured patients as possible. In the United States, over 45 million children (34.9%) are publicly insured through Medicaid or the Children's Health Insurance Program (CHIP), with 38.4% and 20.6% of those being Hispanic and non-Hispanic Black-identified children despite their comprising only 25.6% and 12.7% of the pediatric population, respectively.[72] Moreover, minoritized children with special health needs are two to three times as likely to be only insured with Medicaid or CHIP, and their families are five times more likely to report being sometimes or often unable to afford enough to eat.[73] Unfortunately, the access to quality care for many of these patients is limited. Institutional strategy regarding payer contracting, community marketing, and chosen locations often positions the health system, hospitals, and/or clinics to preferentially or solely engage wealthier populations, with minimal presence in under-resourced and minoritized communities. This structurally manifests in a de facto second-class system, with the most marginalized racial and ethnic groups being much more commonly cared for in heavily under-resourced and understaffed clinical settings, further contributing to lower quality care and worse health outcomes.[74]

Clinicians must actively engage with their institutional leaders to advocate for an institutional strategy that is not satisfied with the status quo of this two-tiered system, but instead proactively seeks ways to provide access to clinical resources and quality care that meet the health needs of these marginalized communities (see **Table 2**). Clinicians must also engage state and federal legislators to close the gap between public and private insurance reimbursement rates, as well as to expand eligibility for public insurance coverage to all children regardless of legal documentation status. Meanwhile, it is also incumbent upon the health care team to proactively connect families to local navigators for counseling regarding their eligibility for securing health insurance and other health-related benefits which mitigate the structural racism inherent to disparate insurance, location, and transportation accessibility.

Beyond physical accessibility, linguistic and cultural accessibility must also be ensured in our clinical institutions. Many pediatric clinicians still rely on using family members to communicate with patients and families with limited English proficiency, with nearly half reporting doing so and only modest improvement in recent decades with increased phone interpreter use.[75] Meanwhile, the family may need to interact with many other members of the health team who also may not consistently utilize appropriate interpreter services to schedule appointments and access resources. Language concordance must in turn be preserved not only in any posted

Table 2
Potential health system and clinical institution-level interventions for addressing structural racism in pediatrics

	Key Pediatric-Related Adverse Societal Factors	Potential Health System/Clinical Institution-Level Interventions
1	Low Socioeconomic Status (SES)	• Health systems can convene, catalyze, mobilize, and partner to create solutions such as Medical-Financial Partnerships, Medical-Legal Partnerships, behavioral health services, and more to help mitigate the impact of low SES on child outcomes • Increase provider awareness of the impact of low SES on pediatric outcomes and potential patient resources such as social workers and community-based organizations
2	Limited or Absent Health Insurance and/or Access to Care	• Quality improvement programs with incentives to providers/multidisciplinary teams with high rates of implementing evidence-based pediatric care • Promote treatment decisions that rely on evidence-based guidelines, are timely, and are made using a shared decision approach to integrate patients' individual preferences, prognoses, and comorbidities (eg, quality improvement incentives) • Utilize lay health educators, patient navigators, and/or engagement of community-based and allied health professionals, especially for developmental screening, mental health, and well-child-care services • Align pediatric management with the Chronic Care Model to emphasize patient-/family-centered care, integrated long-term treatment approaches to childhood comorbidities, and ongoing collaborative communication and team goal setting (eg, multidisciplinary care team) • Create new convenient provider locations in low-income communities and/or use of mobile clinics • Improve ease to navigate the health system (eg, signage in multiple languages, parking) • Electronic health record and portal messaging in multiple languages
3	Low Level of Educational Attainment	• Educational materials to enhance pediatric care messaging including the use of novel strategies such as novellas or other short stories, brief videos, and the use of social or digital media
4	Limited Health Literacy	• Enhance therapeutic alliance-based interventions to improve medication adherence by incorporating cultural adaptation, face-to-face delivery mode, shared decision-making, patient/family activation, patient-/family-centered goal setting, etc. • Multidimensional support programs with nurses and pharmacists to discuss medical concerns, medications, and care coordination

(continued on next page)

Table 2
(continued)

Key Pediatric-Related Adverse Societal Factors	Potential Health System/Clinical Institution-Level Interventions
	• Multidisciplinary care teams with goal-setting discussions (including patient, family, and caregivers)
5 Poor Nutrition	• Electronic health record alerts based on patient address to identify patients/families living in a food swamp or desert • Referral to a dietician trained in structural competency and equity who can connect qualified families to Supplemental Nutrition Assistance Program (SNAP), or Special Supplemental Nutrition Program for Women, Infants and Children (WIC) • Health system clinic-based food pantries
6 Limited Green Space Exposure	• Connecting patients/families to local community-based organizations (CBOs), churches, etc. with walking groups or other structured exercise activities such as the Diabetes Prevention Program
7 Environment	• Reduce placement of alcohol and tobacco outlets, factories, refineries, and toxic landfills in minoritized communities • Enhance environmental toxin-related abatement activities
8 Distrust of the Medical Institution	• Collaboration with community members and existing community sites to develop a broader narrative of trust • Engage social support networks such as family or close friend-/confidant-based interventions to assist in implementing and increasing adherence to pediatric care recommendations for lifestyle, nutritional, and pharmacologic interventions • Ensure reasonable racial/ethnic and linguistic concordance of providers and staff and in materials provided to the local patient population • Culturally and linguistically tailored referrals to CBOs to address social risks • Enhance research recruitment with an emphasis on better racial and ethnic concordance between research team members and local community • Use multidisciplinary teams to increase time and depth of encounters with patients from "health providers"

clinic signs and health education materials, but also within electronic health records and portal messaging.[76]

Patients and their families may also implicitly receive other signals that the clinical space has not been designed for access by or inclusion of those sharing their own particular race or ethnicity. Ensuring that posted images and patient-facing materials clearly reflect serving and valuing a diverse patient population is critical, and may result in stronger intentions to increase engagement in healthier behaviors.[77] Another consequential but historically devalued and neglected aspect of health care delivery is the lack of representation of marginalized populations within the clinician workforce. This underrepresentation can impact both the quality of care delivery as well as health outcomes. Studies have demonstrated that race-concordant visits are more likely to be longer in time spent and are associated with more patient-positive affect, with higher reported patient ratings of care,[78] while expectant mother–physician racial concordance is associated with a significant improvement in Black infant mortality.[79] Organizations must rigorously work to foster the training, recruitment, and retention of clinicians of underrepresented backgrounds to ensure their clinician group better reflects the racial and ethnic makeup of their locally marginalized communities.

Addressing Structural Racism in Pediatric Clinical Practice

A series of intensifying calls have been made from across the United States to take meaningful action to address racism.[80] It is past the time for pediatric clinicians and the broader medical community to collectively stand up to racism and compel the nation's health care system to make antiracism as integral to health care success as addressing childhood obesity and asthma.[81] Since structural racism operates through multiple pathways, attempts to address its downstream effects on health can be overwhelming for an individual practitioner. Dr Benjamin Danielson recently highlighted the fact that children and families of minoritized groups consistently face both structural and interpersonal racism in health care, as well as the downstream inequities in the SDoH that drive racial and ethnic health disparities.[81] Both implicit and explicit racial biases, mistrust, lack of dignity and respect, as well as punitive policies and systems such as child welfare involvement further worsen health outcomes for minoritized pediatric patients and their families. As racism in the United States has formally been named a public health crisis, there are actions, especially within the health system, pediatric clinicians who care for many of the most vulnerable patients can take to improve their health (**Box 5**, see **Table** 2).[9,12,24,81]

An area ripe for the application of an anti-racist lens is in the gold standard of pediatric care, the pediatric medical home. First introduced by the American Academy of Pediatrics in 1967, this has evolved into a model of providing pediatric care that is accessible, family-centered, continuous, comprehensive, coordinated, compassionate, and culturally effective.[82] Although this model is intended to improve medical care in pediatrics, its impact is felt differentially across racial-ethnic groups. For instance, evidence shows that Black, Hispanic and/or impoverished children are

---

Box 5
Steps pediatric clinicians can take to help address the impact of racism on their patients[81]

- Call out racism in health care systems and beyond.

- Advocate for health systems to implement policies and practices to mitigate the many downstream impacts of structural racism such as lack of access to quality medical care, poverty, poor nutrition, exposure to environmental toxins, mental health disorders, and more.

- Discuss and counsel families on the effects of exposure to interpersonal racism as victims and bystanders (as well as the role of discrimination and intersectionality in many cases).

- Create an environment of inclusion from the level of the health system to colleagues and staff in the office where all people are treated with dignity and mutual respect.

- Use tenets of family- and patient-centered approaches while ensuring high-quality care is delivered through a race-conscious and not a race-blind or race-based lens.

less likely to experience family-centered and continuous medical care—two major tenants of the medical home model.[83,84] This reality likely reflects the formation of this model without proper consideration of structural racism and the limitations it imposes on the accessibility and continuity of health care. For instance, the model, as first introduced, fails to highlight difficulties experienced by impoverished and minoritized families such as limited transportation, food insecurity, and housing instability all of which interact to directly impact the accessibility of care. Therefore, the proper implementation of the medical home among all pediatric patients must be considered and addressed, as well as other, barriers. One way to overcome this limitation, as proposed by Lilijenquist and Coker, is the incorporation of non-clinical members and community resources into the health care team (see **Table 2**).[84] This practice can help to relieve the burden of saturated pediatric clinics and take advantage of resources from community-based organizations (eg, Head Start programs) that are accessible and reflective in background and identification to pediatric patients and families. One example of this is the *Healthy Steps for Young Children* intervention, which leveraged non-clinician developmental specialists to provide developmental screening, assessment, and guidance and resulted in increased adherence to developmental screening and vaccination.[85] Not only is such resource-shifting effective, it also allows for the freeing of clinician time to build rapport, provide medical knowledge, and anticipatory guidance. Time invested in these areas can go far in building the clinician–family relationship, particularly in pediatric clinics serving families among whom medical mistrust is a barrier to medical care.[86]

Although a team-based approach is essential to the comprehensive care of patients who experience racism and poverty, it remains critical that pediatric clinicians gain personal knowledge about the impact of structural racism on the patient.[87] This includes taking a self-inventory of explicitly and implicitly held beliefs about racial groups which are rooted in stereotypes and lead to bias. It also involves learning and understanding how the SDoH impact health and health care. Further, the physician should provide an avenue to discuss the SDoH, racism and other issues that drive health and the patient's ability to engage fully in health care recommendations (**Box 6**).[87]

After this assessment, it is important to validate the experience of patients and families to avoid re-traumatization. The clinician must also leave the door open for continued relationship building. Additionally, when possible, patients/families should be referred to appropriate resources such as Medical-Financial Partnerships (Marcil L.E., Hole M.K., Jackson J., et al., Anti-Poverty Medicine Through Medical-Financial Partnerships: A New Approach to Child Poverty. Acad Pediatr. 2021 Nov-Dec;21(8S):S169-S176), legal aid to battle housing or employment discrimination,

---

Box 6
Strategies pediatric clinicians might use for initiating conversations around race[87,88]

- An introductory statement such as *"As your physician, I would like to create a safe space for you to discuss key life experiences that contribute to your mental and physical health. Would you be comfortable talking with me about some of your experiences?"*

- If the patient answers "Yes" clinicians can ask: *"What life experiences do I need to understand to help you reach your health goals?"*

- If the patient is open to discussing these and related issues, follow-up open-ended questions might be: *"How are you doing during this challenging time?"* or *"How are you feeling about what's going on in the world/our country right now as it relates to health care, health resources and/or racism?"* or how often do you think about your race?

sources for fresh foods, etc. This requires that the clinic and medical staff become familiar with and establish connections to resources within the community in which they serve. By integrating strategies that address structural racism and life course perspectives, we optimize our potential to mitigate existing disparities and the intergenerational transmission of many health and social disadvantages, thereby, improving the health of minoritized children, families, and communities.[89]

CLINICS CARE POINTS

- Avoid prescribing treatments based solely on a patient's race or ethnicity.
- Closely interrogate all clinical algorithms for the use of race or ethnicity and eliminate from your practice any resulting disparate treatment of patients based on these algorithms.
- Membership in a racial or ethnic group that has a disproportionately high prevalence of disease or disease-related complications should prompt further exploration of social history (including disease-related SDoH) and family history to help inform more specific potential risks, need for screening, and more.
- In general, higher group-level risk should prompt more frequent follow-up and monitoring for your patient.
- Do not assign group stereotypes to an individual patient.
- Known differences in the prevalence of racial or ethnic group associations with disease-related gene polymorphisms can be used in ordering a differential diagnosis, but should not be used to exclude a diagnosis.

DISCLOSURES

K.C. Norris is a consultant for Atlantis Health Care Inc. for dialysis quality improvement.

ACKNOWLEDGMENTS

K.C. Norris is supported in part by National Institutes of Health, United States (NIH) grants P30AG021684, UL1TR000124, and P50MD017366; M. Laster is supported in part by NIH grant K23DK123378. The contents of this work are solely the responsibility of the authors and do not necessarily represent the official views of the NIH.

REFERENCES

1. Commission on Social Determinants of Health. Closing the gap in a generation: health equity through action on the social determinants of health: final report of the commission on social determinants of health. Geneva, Switzerland: World Health Organization; 2008.
2. Singh GK, Daus GP, Allender M, et al. Social determinants of health in the United States: addressing major health inequality trends for the nation, 1935-2016. International Journal of MCH and AIDS 2017;6:139.
3. Magnan S. Social Determinants of Health 201 for Health Care: Plan, Do, Study, Act. NAM Perspect; 2021.
4. Braveman P, Arkin E, Orleans T, et al. What is health equity? Behavioral science & policy 2018;4(1):1–4.
5. Smedley BD, Stith AY, Nelson AR. Racial and ethnic disparities in diagnosis and treatment: a review of the evidence and a consideration of causes. Unequal

treatment: Confronting racial and ethnic disparities. In: in health care. Washington, DC: National Academies Press; 2003.

6. Wilkerson I. Caste: the origins of our discontents. New York, NY: Random House; 2020.

7. Bailey ZD, Feldman JM, Bassett MT. How structural racism works — racist policies as a root cause of U.S. Racial health inequities. N Engl J Med 2020. https://doi.org/10.1056/NEJMms2025396.

8. Bailey ZD, Krieger N, Agénor M, et al. Structural racism and health inequities in the USA: evidence and interventions. Lancet 2017;389:1453–63.

9. Jindal M, Trent M, Mistry KB. The intersection of race, racism, and child and adolescent health. Pediatr Rev 2022;43:415–25.

10. Jones CP. Addressing violence against children through anti-racism action. Pediatric Clinics 2021;68:449–53.

11. Griffith DM, Mason M, Yonas M, et al. Dismantling institutional racism: theory and action. Am J Community Psychol 2007;39:381–92.

12. Trent M, Dooley DG, Dougé J. The impact of racism on child and adolescent health. Pediatrics 2019;144. https://doi.org/10.1542/peds.2019-1765.

13. Marshall E. DNA studies challenge the meaning of race. Science (New York, N.Y.) 1998;282:654–5.

14. Jones CP. Confronting institutionalized racism. Phylon 2002;50:7–22.

15. Jones CP. Invited commentary:"race," racism, and the practice of epidemiology. Am J Epidemiol 2001;154:299–304.

16. Linnaeus C. Systema naturae, 1735: facsimile of the first edition with an introduction and a first English translation of the" Observationes". De Graaf; 1964.

17. Ford CL, Harawa NT. A new conceptualization of ethnicity for social epidemiologic and health equity research. Soc Sci Med (1982) 2010;71:251–8.

18. Mohottige D, Boulware LE, Ford CL, et al. Use of race in kidney research and medicine: concepts, principles, and practice. Clin J Am Soc Nephrol 2022;17:314–22.

19. Robinson WS. Ecological correlations and the behavior of individuals. Am Sociol Rev 1950;15:351–7.

20. Witzig R. The medicalization of race: scientific legitimization of a flawed social construct. Ann Intern Med 1996;125(8):675–9.

21. Alvidrez J, Castille D, Laude-Sharp M, et al. The national institute on minority health and health disparities research framework. Am J Public Health 2019; 109:S16–20.

22. Norris K, Nissenson AR. Race, gender, and socioeconomic disparities in CKD in the United States. J Am Soc Nephrol 2008;19:1261–70.

23. Beech BM, Ford C, Thorpe RJ, et al. Poverty, racism, and the public health crisis in America. Front Public Health 2021;9. https://doi.org/10.3389/fpubh.2021.699049.

24. Jones CP. Toward the science and practice of anti-racism: launching a national campaign against racism. Ethn Dis 2018;28:231–4.

25. Jones CP. Levels of racism: a theoretic framework and a gardener's tale. Am J Public Health 2000;90:1212–5.

26. Capers Qt, Clinchot D, McDougle L, et al. Implicit racial bias in medical school admissions. Acad Med 2017;92:365–9.

27. Heard-Garris N, Boyd R, Kan K, et al. Structuring poverty: how racism shapes child poverty and child and adolescent health. Academic Pediatrics 2021;21:S108–16.

28. Kids Count Data Center. The Annie E. Casey Foundation. Available at: @https://datacenter.kidscount.org/data/tables/44-children-in-poverty-by-race-andethnic-ity?loc=1&loct=1 - detailed/1/any/false/2048,1729,37,871,870,573,869,36,868,867/10,11,9,12,1,185,13/324,323. Accessed 21 September, 22.

29. Fanta M, Ladzekpo D, Unaka N. Racism and pediatric health outcomes. Curr Probl Pediatr Adolesc Health Care 2021;51:101087.

30. Wallace ME, Mendola P, Kim SS, et al. Racial/ethnic differences in preterm perinatal outcomes. Am J Obstet Gynecol 2017;216:306.e1–12.

31. March of Dimes Foundation. 2020 March of Dimes report card. Available at: https://www.marchofdimes.org/peristats/tools/reportcard.aspx. Accessed 10 November, 2022.

32. Murosko D, Passerella M, Lorch S. Racial segregation and intraventricular hemorrhage in preterm infants. Pediatrics 2020;145. https://doi.org/10.1542/peds.2019-1508.

33. Glazer KB, Sofaer S, Balbierz A, et al. Perinatal care experiences among racially and ethnically diverse mothers whose infants required a NICU stay. J Perinatol 2021;41:413–21.

34. Nardone A, Casey JA, Morello-Frosch R, et al. Associations between historical residential redlining and current age-adjusted rates of emergency department visits due to asthma across eight cities in California: an ecological study. Lancet Planet Health 2020;4:e24–31.

35. Beck AF, Huang B, Wheeler K, et al. The child opportunity index and disparities in pediatric asthma hospitalizations across one ohio metropolitan area, 2011-2013. J Pediatr 2017;190:200–6.e1.

36. Fortuna LR, Tobón AL, Anglero YL, et al. Focusing on racial, historical and intergenerational trauma, and resilience: a paradigm to better serving children and families. Child Adolesc Psychiatr Clin N Am 2022;31:237–50.

37. Slopen N, Heard-Garris N. Structural racism and pediatric health—a call for research to confront the origins of racial disparities in health. JAMA Pediatr 2022;176:13–5.

38. Sauder KA, Ritchie ND. Reducing intergenerational obesity and diabetes risk. Diabetologia 2021;64:481–90.

39. Katzow MW, Messito MJ, Mendelsohn AL, et al. Protective Effect of Prenatal Social Support on the Intergenerational Transmission of Obesity in Low-Income Hispanic Families. Child Obes 2022. https://doi.org/10.1089/chi.2021.0306.

40. Buchheim A, Ziegenhain U, Kindler H, et al. Identifying risk and resilience factors in the intergenerational cycle of maltreatment: results from the TRANS-GEN study investigating the effects of maternal attachment and social support on child attachment and cardiovascular stress physiology. Front Hum Neurosci 2022;16:890262.

41. Ahmad SI, Shih EW, LeWinn KZ. Intergenerational transmission of effects of women's stressors during pregnancy: child psychopathology and the protective role of parenting. Front Psychiatry 2022;13:838535.

42. Swetlitz C, Lynch SF, Propper CB, et al. Examining maternal elaborative reminiscing as a protective factor in the intergenerational transmission of psychopathology. Res Child Adolesc Psychopathol 2021;49:989–99.

43. Fall CH. Fetal malnutrition and long-term outcomes. Nestle Nutr Inst Workshop Ser 2013;74:11–25.

44. Sebastiani G, Navarro-Tapia E, Almeida-Toledano L, et al. Effects of antioxidant intake on fetal development and maternal/neonatal health during pregnancy. Antioxidants 2022;11. https://doi.org/10.3390/antiox11040648.

45. van Steenwyk G, Roszkowski M, Manuella F, et al. Transgenerational inheritance of behavioral and metabolic effects of paternal exposure to traumatic stress in early postnatal life: evidence in the 4th generation. Environ Epigenet 2018;4: dvy023.

46. Hanson JL, Chandra A, Wolfe BL, et al. Association between income and the hippocampus. PLoS One 2011;6:e18712.

47. Williams DR, Mohammed SA. Racism and health I: pathways and scientific evidence. Am Behav Sci 2013;57. https://doi.org/10.1177/0002764213487340.

48. Keating L, Kaur A, Mendieta M, et al. Racial discrimination and core executive functions. Stress Health 2022;38:615–21.

49. Thorpe RJ, Jr, Norris KC, Beech BM and Bruce MA. Chapter 10. Racism Across the Life Course,Racism: Science & Tools for the Public Health Professional. APHA Press; Washington, DC. https://ajph.aphapublications.org/doi/abs/10.2105/9780 875533049ch10

50. Williams DR. Race, socioeconomic status, and health. The added effects of racism and discrimination. Ann N Y Acad Sci 1999;896:173–88.

51. Cohen S, Janicki-Deverts D, Miller GE. Psychological stress and disease. JAMA 2007;298:1685–7.

52. McEwen BS. Protective and damaging effects of stress mediators. N Engl J Med 1998;338:171–9.

53. Geronimus AT. The weathering hypothesis and the health of African-American women and infants: evidence and speculations. Ethn Dis 1992;2:207–21.

54. Geronimus AT, Hicken M, Keene D, et al. Weathering" and age patterns of allostatic load scores among blacks and whites in the United States. Am J Public Health 2006;96:826–33.

55. Thames AD, Irwin MR, Breen EC, et al. Experienced discrimination and racial differences in leukocyte gene expression. Psychoneuroendocrinology 2019;106: 277–83.

56. Brody GH, Yu T, Miller GE, et al. Discrimination, racial identity, and cytokine levels among African-American adolescents. The Journal of Adolescent Health 2015; 56:496–501.

57. O'Connell MA, Hayes JD. The Keap1/Nrf2 pathway in health and disease: from the bench to the clinic. Biochem Soc Trans 2015;43:687–9.

58. Tu W, Wang H, Li S, et al. The anti-inflammatory and anti-oxidant mechanisms of the Keap1/Nrf2/ARE signaling pathway in chronic diseases. Aging and disease 2019;10:637–51.

59. Nicholas SB, Kalantar-Zadeh K, Norris KC. Socioeconomic disparities in chronic kidney disease. Adv Chron Kidney Dis 2015;22:6–15.

60. Dirven BCJ, Homberg JR, Kozicz T, et al. Epigenetic programming of the neuroendocrine stress response by adult life stress. J Mol Endocrinol 2017;59:R11–31.

61. Barcelona de Mendoza V, Huang Y, Crusto CA, et al. Perceived racial discrimination and DNA methylation among African American women in the InterGEN study. Biol Res Nurs 2018;20:145–52.

62. Dehaene S, Kerszberg M, Changeux J-P. A neuronal model of a global workspace in effortful cognitive tasks. Proc Natl Acad Sci U S A 1998;95:14529–34.

63. LaVeist TA. Minority populations and health: an introduction to health disparities in the United States, 4. San Francisco, CA: John Wiley & Sons; 2005.

64. Duru OK, Harawa NT, Kermah D, et al. Allostatic load burden and racial disparities in mortality. J Natl Med Assoc 2012;104:89–95.
65. Seeman TE, Singer BH, Rowe JW, et al. Price of adaptation–allostatic load and its health consequences. MacArthur studies of successful aging. Arch Intern Med 1997;157:2259–68.
66. Forde AT, Crookes DM, Suglia SF, et al. The weathering hypothesis as an explanation for racial disparities in health: a systematic review. Ann Epidemiol 2019;33:1–18.e13.
67. McEwen BS, Stellar E. Stress and the individual. Mechanisms leading to disease. Arch Intern Med 1993;153:2093–101.
68. Umberson D, Thomeer MB, Williams K, et al. Childhood adversity and men's relationships in adulthood: life course processes and racial disadvantage. J Gerontol B Psychol Sci Soc Sci 2016;71:902–13.
69. Paradies Y, Ben J, Denson N, et al. Racism as a determinant of health: a systematic review and meta-analysis. PLoS One 2015;10:e0138511.
70. Priest N, Doery K, Truong M, et al. A systematic review of studies examining the relationship between reported racism and health and wellbeing for children and young people. Soc Sci Med 2013;95:115–27.
71. Paradies Y, Truong M, Priest N. A systematic review of the extent and measurement of healthcare provider racism. J Gen Intern Med 2014;29:364–87.
72. Access in Brief: Children's Experiences in Accessing Medical Care. November 2021. Available at: https://www.macpac.gov/wp-content/uploads/2016/06/Access-in-Brief-Childrens-Experiences-in-Accessing-Medical-Care.pdf.
73. Williams E, Musumeci M. Children with Special Health Care Needs: Coverage, Affordability, and HCBS Access. Oct 4, 2021. Kaiser Family Foundation. Available at: https://www.kff.org/medicaid/issue-brief/children-with-special-health-care-needs-coverage-affordability-and-hcbs-access/.
74. 2019 national healthcare quality and disparities report. Rockville, MD: Agency for Healthcare Research and Quality; 2020. AHRQ Pub. No. 20(21)-0045-EF.
75. DeCamp LR, Kuo DZ, Flores G, et al. Changes in language services use by US pediatricians. Pediatrics 2013;132:e396–406.
76. Casillas A, Perez-Aguilar G, Abhat A, et al. Su salud a la mano (your health at hand): patient perceptions about a bilingual patient portal in the Los Angeles safety net. J Am Med Inf Assoc 2019;26:1525–35.
77. Buller MK, Bettinghaus EP, Fluharty L, et al. Improving health communication with photographic images that increase identification in three minority populations. Health Educ Res 2019;34:145–58.
78. Cooper LA, Roter DL, Johnson RL, et al. Patient-centered communication, ratings of care, and concordance of patient and physician race. Ann Intern Med 2003;139:907–15.
79. Greenwood BN, Hardeman RR, Huang L, et al. Physician–patient racial concordance and disparities in birthing mortality for newborns. Proc Natl Acad Sci U S A 2020;201913405. https://doi.org/10.1073/pnas.1913405117.
80. Dreyer BP, Trent M, Anderson AT, et al. The death of george floyd: bending the arc of history toward justice for generations of children. Pediatrics 2020;146.
81. Danielson B. Confronting racism in pediatric care. Health Aff 2022;41:1681–5.
82. Available at: https://www.aap.org/en/practice-management/medical-home/medical-home-overview/what-is-medical-home/., W. i. a. M. H. A. A. o. P.
83. Diao K, Tripodis Y, Long WE, et al. Socioeconomic and racial disparities in parental perception and experience of having a medical home, 2007 to 2011-2012. Academic Pediatrics 2017;17:95–103.

84. Liljenquist K, Coker TR. Transforming well-child care to meet the needs of families at the intersection of racism and poverty. Academic Pediatrics 2021;21:S102–7.
85. Minkovitz CS, Strobino D, Mistry KB, et al. Healthy steps for young children: sustained results at 5.5 years. Pediatrics 2007;120:e658–68.
86. Coker TR, Keller D, Davis S, et al. APS/SPR virtual chat: race, racism, and child health equity in academic pediatrics. Pediatr Res 2022;91:1669–76.
87. Diop MS, Taylor CN, Murillo SN, et al. This is our lane: talking with patients about racism. Women's Midlife Health 2021;7:7.
88. Jones CP, Truman BI, Elam-Evans LD, et al. Using "socially assigned race" to probe white advantages in health status. Ethn Dis 2008;18:496–504.
89. Andersen SH, Richmond-Rakerd LS, Moffitt TE, et al. Nationwide evidence that education disrupts the intergenerational transmission of disadvantage. Proc Natl Acad Sci U S A 2021;118. https://doi.org/10.1073/pnas.2103896118.

Addressing Health Literacy in Pediatric Practice
A Health Equity Lens

Tiffany A. Stewart, MD[a], Eliana M. Perrin, MD, MPH[b],
Hsiang Shonna Yin, MD, MS[a,c,*]

KEYWORDS

- Health literacy • Health equity • Health communication • Universal precautions

KEY POINTS

- The majority of parents in the US face health literacy challenges, and low health literacy is considered an important mediator of income- and race/ethnicity-associated health disparities.
- Low health literacy has been linked to poor health knowledge, less optimal health behaviors, and worse child health-related outcomes across domains of health.
- Pediatricians and other health care providers can take many steps to integrate a health literacy approach into their clinical practice to support the ability of families to take action on health recommendations, setting the stage for improved child health outcomes and advancing health equity.

Two cases illustrate the importance of health literacy in clinical pediatrics.

Case 1: A 2-year-old female presents to the clinic for a routine well-child check. Upon the evaluation of the growth chart, the pediatrician notices that her weight has been steadily increasing in percentile since about 4 months of age, and has now crossed several percentile lines, and her current BMI is 95%ile. In discussion with the father regarding her BMI, he smiles and says, "95% is an 'A', right? That's good, right?"

Case 2: A 9-month-old male presents to clinic for a chief complaint of irritability and left-sided ear pulling for the last 2 days. On examination, his tympanic membrane is erythematous with poor landmarks and reduced mobility, and he has a fever of

[a] Department of Pediatrics, New York University Grossman School of Medicine / Bellevue Hospital Center, 550 First Avenue, NBV 8S4-11, New York, NY 10016, USA; [b] Department of Pediatrics, Johns Hopkins School of Medicine / School of Nursing, 200 North Wolfe Street, Rubenstein Building 2071, Baltimore, MD 21287, USA; [c] Department of Population Health, New York University Grossman School of Medicine, New York, NY, USA
* Corresponding author. Department of Pediatrics, New York University Grossman School of Medicine, 550 First Avenue, NBV 8S4-11, New York, NY 10016.
E-mail address: yinh02@med.nyu.edu

0031-3955/23/© 2023 Elsevier Inc. All rights reserved.
pediatric.theclinics.com

101F. He is diagnosed with acute otitis media and is prescribed Amoxicillin. Two days later, he returns to clinic with worsened irritability, ear pulling, and persistent fevers. His examination now shows a bulging drum. The mother shares that she has been administering Amoxicillin in the child's ear rather than in the child's mouth. The prescription label she had received was written in English and not her primary language, Spanish. She also had not been counseled on the route of medication administration by her child's doctor or at the pharmacy. She remembered having medicine put inside her ear as a young child with an ear infection.

HEALTH LITERACY – A HIGHLY IMPORTANT AND PREVALENT ISSUE IMPACTING CHILD HEALTH

The National Academy of Medicine, Joint Commission, Agency for Healthcare Research and Quality (AHRQ), and other organizations have cited health literacy as a critical health care quality and safety issue.[1–7] Health literacy is defined as "the degree to which individuals have the capacity to obtain, process and understand basic health information and services needed to make appropriate health decisions."[8] Recognition of the importance of addressing health literacy builds from a large body of research that has documented strong associations between low health literacy and poorer health knowledge, suboptimal health behaviors, and worse health outcomes.[9]

According to the National Assessment of Adult Literacy [NAAL] about 1 in 4 U.S. parents has "Basic" or "Below Basic" health literacy,[10,11] struggling with common health-related tasks, such as interpreting dosage instructions on medication bottle labels. Importantly, only about 15% are considered to have "Proficient" health literacy, indicating that the vast majority of U.S. parents likely face health literacy challenges.[11] While the health literacy of the parent or primary caregiver is especially important during early and middle childhood (birth to 12 years), with documented impacts on child health outcomes,[12] during adolescence and young adulthood, a child's own health literacy becomes increasingly important as the child begins to rely on their own health literacy skills to manage their health.

THE BROAD SCOPE OF HEALTH LITERACY

Health literacy encompasses a broad range of skills, with far-reaching implications for those with low health literacy. The Institute of Medicine (IoM)[8] model of health literacy contains four constructs: knowledge (cultural and conceptual), print health literacy (reading and writing skills), oral health literacy (listening and speaking), and numeracy. Others have included the navigation of the health care system as well as information-seeking skills,[13] including the ability to discern which sources of health information are trustworthy. Another approach to defining health literacy is based upon how literacy can enable an individual,[14] with health literacy categorized into three levels: (1) basic/functional health literacy (i.e. skills for effective functioning in everyday situations), (2) communicative/interactive literacy (i.e. skills for extracting information deriving meaning, and applying this information to new circumstances), and (3) critical literacy (i.e. utilizing advanced cognitive skills to critically analyze and selectively apply information).

HEALTH LITERACY FRAMEWORK

For patients and their families, health care system encounters are challenging when verbal communication is not in plain language (e.g. medical jargon used), written information is not provided, or is provided at too high of a reading grade level without visuals and other elements to support clear communication, and contradictory and difficult to understand health messages are broadcasted via the news, online, and social media. An important framework for understanding the concept of health literacy places health literacy at the intersection point between the skills and abilities of individuals and the demands and complexities of tasks being placed on individuals by the health care system.[8] As such, those that are part of the health care system have a responsibility to meet individuals "where they are" in terms of their health literacy skills. When the relationship between the two sides is optimized, and the health literacy needs of individuals are adequately addressed by the health system, the health knowledge, behaviors, and outcomes can be optimized.[9] The term "organizational health literacy," adds that the responsibility for addressing health literacy challenges extends beyond individual health care providers to organizations, who can support providers and staff to create "health literate" environments (e.g. availability of training, plain language materials).[4,15,16] Focusing on upstream solutions to address structural barriers related to health literacy challenges should be the priority, while at the same time supporting individuals to obtain health literacy skills, without placing blame on individuals for experiencing health literacy challenges.

HEALTH LITERACY IS A STATE – NOT A TRAIT

For clinicians in practice, it is also important to recognize that an individual's health literacy level can vary within one individual and fluctuate over time, depending on context. For example, an individual's health literacy can be affected by emotional state (e.g. stress, fear), acute pain or illness, fatigue, vision and hearing deficits, and cognitive impairment, as well as by topic area.[17] For example, a parent who brings their sick child to the emergency department may face challenges processing information provided to them about diagnosis and treatment plan due to stress. A pediatrician may face health literacy challenges in navigating issues related to oncologic care for their aging parent because this may be an unfamiliar topic area, as well as because of stress.

HEALTH LITERACY IS AN EQUITY ISSUE

Unfortunately, low health literacy is more common in people who experience systematic disadvantage: those living in poverty, minoritized communities (e.g. Latino, Black, American Indian, and Alaskan Native populations), those who do not speak English well, and immigrants.[11,18,19] Growing evidence highlights that health literacy is an important mediator of income- and race/ethnicity-associated health disparities. This has led to recommendations for clinicians to integrate health equity-aligned principles into daily practice to address the structural barriers encountered by individuals who face health literacy challenges.[10,20–22] In addition to using health literacy-informed communication strategies, clinicians can "break the cycle" that contributes to the continued persistence of health inequities across generations by supporting the development of health literacy skills (i.e. as children become adolescents and ultimately parents who can then support their own children's health literacy).

Health Literacy and Poverty

Children from families with low socioeconomic status (SES) backgrounds are at increased risk for poor health-related outcomes.[23,24] Poverty and financial stress have long been recognized as contributors to poor health-related outcomes,[25] as disparities in economic conditions fundamentally affect the social conditions in which people live, and social conditions influence both environment and behaviors which ultimately affects health-related outcomes. Health literacy mediates the relationship between SES and health status, quality of life, specific health-related outcomes (e.g. glycemic control), health behaviors (e.g. lack of physical activity, smoking, and lack of fresh fruit/vegetable consumption), and access to/use of preventive services.[26]

Health Literacy and Race

Race/ethnicity are related to health-related disparities likely through a pathway of systemic racism, as structural, cultural, and interpersonal racism interact with and drive health and health inequities.[27] Limited health literacy is prevalent among certain racial/ethnic minority groups, with nearly 60% of Black Americans, and nearly 70% of Latinos impacted.[11] Those from racial/ethnic minority groups with limited health literacy experience greater disease burden, worse health outcomes, and reduced access to quality health care.[20,28]

Health Literacy and English Language Proficiency

Similar to health literacy, Limited English Proficiency (LEP) is a key barrier associated with poorer health outcomes.[29,30] LEP is defined as possessing limited ability to read, write, speak, and understand the English language.[31] Low health literacy disproportionately impacts those with LEP,[18] and LEP may contribute to and exacerbate the health consequences of low health literacy.[32,33] This may continue to worsen, as children in immigrant families are the fastest-growing segment of the U.S. population. In 2019, over a quarter of youth aged seventeen and under lived with an immigrant parent, up from 15 percent in 1990.[34]

IMPLICATIONS OF LOW HEALTH LITERACY ON CHILD HEALTH-RELATED OUTCOMES

Awareness of the significant impact of low health literacy on child health can inform the everyday actions of clinicians in practice who care for children.

Implications of Low Parent Health Literacy

Parents with low health literacy have less health-related knowledge, including less awareness of preventive health measures (e.g. less injury prevention knowledge, such as choking or burn management[35]), which contributes to less healthy behaviors, and poorer health outcomes.[36,37] With respect to the management of acute illnesses, low parent health literacy has been associated with decreased knowledge of medication instructions (e.g. dose, frequency),[38] difficulty interpreting OTC medication dosing charts,[10] and increased dosing errors.[38] Low parent health literacy is also associated with worse outcomes in several common chronic pediatric conditions, such as asthma, diabetes, obesity, and sickle cell disease.[9] For example, parents of children with asthma with low health literacy have ~two-fold increased rate of asthma-related ED visits, >four-fold increased rate of hospitalizations, and overall worse asthma control.[39]

Implications of Low Child Health Literacy

Lower child (e.g. adolescent) health literacy is also associated with poorer health behaviors, such as, increased rate of carrying guns, increased rate of smoking, and increased rate of physical violence.[37] However, studies connecting adolescent health literacy with other health behaviors are limited.[40]

THE DIFFICULTY OF IDENTIFYING INDIVIDUALS WITH LOW HEALTH LITERACY IN THE CLINICAL SETTING

There are many signs that suggest that an individual may have low health literacy, such as a parent asking a healthcare provider to read information with the excuse of "I forgot my glasses" or a parent returning forms that haven't been completely filled out (**Table 1**).[36] However, those with limited literacy skills may go to great lengths to hide their literacy status from others (e.g. bringing decoy reading materials).[36] Most individuals with limited literacy skills have never told anyone in the health care system, and most have never even told family members.[41] Identification of individuals with limited health literacy may thus be challenging.[7]

FORMAL ASSESSMENTS OF INDIVIDUAL-LEVEL HEALTH LITERACY ARE NOT A RECOMMENDED PART OF ROUTINE CLINICAL PRACTICE

The benefits of formally measuring health literacy have been debated, given the limitations of existing tools to measure individual-level health literacy, and unclear impact of measuring health literacy on an individual's clinical outcomes. Many tools exist that measure health literacy, and vary in terms of domains assessed (e.g. prose literacy, numeracy, navigation), language availability, topic area (e.g. general, disease-specific), target age group (e.g. adults, adolescents), and length (**Table 2**). While some health systems have integrated health literacy assessment into routine care, these tools are mainly used in research. It is not recommended that these tools be used as part of routine practice in clinical settings.[42] Assessing health literacy in a subset of individuals served can help providers gain a better understanding of the health literacy level of individuals seen at a particular clinic or site.

INTEGRATING A UNIVERSAL PRECAUTIONS APPROACH TO CLEAR COMMUNICATION IN CLINICAL CARE

The high prevalence of low health literacy, the challenges of being able to easily identify who has low health literacy, and the fluctuating nature of an individual's health literacy, have led organizations such as the American Medical Association (AMA) and the AHRQ to recommend a universal precautions approach to using health literacy-informed communication strategies.[7,36,43,44] The main goals of a universal precautions approach are to simplify communication, confirm comprehension of communication, make the clinical setting easier to navigate, and support the efforts of patients and their families to improve their health.[7] Prior research supports the use of health literacy-informed communication strategies; for example, improving use of such strategies for medication counseling (pictographic dosing diagram, demonstration, teach-back/show-back) is associated with reduced parent medication dosing errors.[45,46]

The specific strategies recommended to include as part of universal precautions include the following:

Oral Communication strategies. "Plain language," defined as "a communication style that allows listeners to understand any message the first time they hear it,"[4] is at the core of health literacy-informed communication, and considered a "basic" communication skill. Experts advocate for using "living room" language, the kind of communication one would use with family members and friends, rather than medical jargon.[4] For example, saying "doctor" instead of "physician," "by mouth" instead of "oral," or "ear infection" instead of "otitis media." Resources on how to communicate in plain language are available, including from public health agencies such as the CDC (**Table 3**).[47,48]

Limiting the scope of information presented to the "need to know" to take action, and excluding the "nice to know" information is also key.[36,49–51] Information should be limited to 2-3 key takeaway points, and information should be organized into "bite-sized" "digestible" "chunks."[36,49–51] Provision of "explicit" information and instructions is also beneficial; for example, asking parents of a child with asthma to

Table 1
Warning signs that may indicate that a parent or patient has limited health literacy

Behaviors of Patients	Responses to Receiving Written Information	Responses to Questions About Medication Regimens
• Patient registration forms that are incomplete or inaccurately completed • Frequently missing appointments • Non-adherence with medication regimens • Lack of follow-through with laboratory tests, imaging tests, or referrals to consultants • Patients/families reporting medication adherence; however, laboratory tests or physiological parameters do not change in the expected fashion	• "Let me bring this home so I can discuss it with my family." • "I forgot my glasses. I'll read this when I get home." • "I forgot my glasses. Can you read this to me?"	• Unable to name current prescribed medications • Unable to explain need of current prescribed medications • Unable to explain timing of medication administration

Table 2
Examples of health literacy assessment tools

	Newest Vital Sign (NVS)	Rapid Estimate of Adult Literacy in Medicine (REALM)	Test of Functional Health Literacy in Adult (TOFHLA)	Short Test of Functional Health Literacy in Adults (S-TOFHLA)	Single Item Literacy Screener (SILS)	Parental Health Literacy Activities Test (PHLAT-10)
Measurement	Numeracy skills, Prose and document literacy [objective assessment]	Word recognition and pronunciation [objective assessment]	Reading comprehension and numeracy skills [objective assessment]	Reading comprehension and numeracy skills [objective assessment]	Self-assessed health literacy skill [subjective assessment]	Prose and document literacy, numeracy skills [objective assessment]
Administration time	2–6 minutes	3 minutes	22 minutes	12 minutes	1–2 minutes	No time limit (but average time 15-20 minutes)
Number of items	6 questions based upon a Nutrition Facts label	66 medical terms to be read aloud	50 questions based upon 3 prose passages, plus 17 numeracy questions	36 questions based upon 2 prose passages, plus 4 numeracy questions	1 question: How often do you need to have someone help you when you read instructions, pamphlets, or other written material from your doctor or pharmacy?	10 questions (7 items focused on nutrition, 1 item on understanding a growth chart, and 2 items on medication dosing)
Languages measure originally validated in	English, Spanish	English only	English, Spanish	English, Spanish	English only	English, Spanish

Table 3
Helpful resources to support provider use of health literacy strategies

Resource Type	Details
Resources to support providers in integrating health literacy principles into practice	AHRQ Health Literacy resources. https://www.ahrq.gov/health-literacy/index.html AHRQ Universal Precautions Toolkit (includes strategies related to verbal and written communication) https://www.ahrq.gov/professionals/quality-patient-safety/quality-resources/tools/literacy-toolkit/index.html https://www.ahrq.gov/sites/default/files/publications/files/healthlittoolkit2_3.pdf Plainlanguage.gov website https://www.plainlanguage.gov/ CDC Plain Language Materials and Resources https://www.cdc.gov/healthliteracy/developmaterials/plainlanguage.html Plain language at NIH. https://www.nih.gov/institutes-nih/nih-office-director/office-communications-public-liaison/clear-communication/plain-language/ NIH. Plain Language: Getting Started or Brushing Up https://www.nih.gov/institutes-nih/nih-office-director/office-communications-public-liaison/clear-communication/plain-language/plain-language-getting-started-or-brushing World Health Organization (WHO) Tactics to apply to make your communications understandable https://www.who.int/about/communications/understandable/plain-language
Plain language glossaries	CDC Everyday Words for Public Health Communication https://tools.cdc.gov/ewapi/termsearch.html National Center for Health Marketing - DHHS, CDC. Plain Language Thesaurus for Health Communications. https://www.plainlanguage.gov/media/Thesaurus_V-10.doc
Tools to support development and assessment of written materials	Readability formulas (assessment of reading grade level) https://readabilityformulas.com/free-readability-formula-tests.php The Patient Education Materials Assessment Tool (PEMAT) and User's Guide. https://www.ahrq.gov/health-literacy/patient-education/pemat.html Doak and Doak. Suitability Assessment of Materials (SAM) http://aspiruslibrary.org/literacy/sam.pdf CDC Clear Communication Index. https://www.cdc.gov/ccindex/index.html
Health literacy-informed materials to support provider medication counseling	AHRQ How to Create a Pill Card https://www.ahrq.gov/patients-consumers/diagnosis-treatment/treatments/pillcard/index.html HELPix Pictographic Medication Instruction Sheets https://med.nyu.edu/helpix/helpix-intervention/instructions-providers

look for "ribs showing when breathing" is more effective than having them look for "difficulty breathing."[52] In alignment with cognitive load theory, integrating such strategies helps promote understanding by decreasing cognitive demand.[53]

Teach-back is a more advanced communication technique where a health provider asks a patient or family member to say in their own words, what they understood of the information that was just discussed.[45] Teach-back is promoted by the American Academy of Pediatrics, AMA, and Joint Commission as a critical communication strategy for improving adherence to treatment plans and promoting patient safety.[36,50,54] Unfortunately, a survey of pediatricians indicated that the technique is used less than 25% of the time.[49] Providers should take responsibility by stating: "I want to make sure I did a good job explaining how much medication to give Christopher. Can you say in your own words how much medication you plan to give?"[9]

The phrase "chunk and check," is an easy way for providers to remember to provide information that is limited to a small number of topics, and to check for comprehension before discussing subsequent topics.[7]

Written communication. Health care providers should optimize written communication to help patients and families overcome structural barriers to understanding health information. Available health information is often written at too high of a reading grade level, lack features that promote actionability, and is often only available in English.[55–57] Providers should supplement verbal counseling with written information. Verbal counseling while referring to printed instructions, or writing down instructions for families to take home, can be especially effective (dual code theory).[58] Written materials should be at a 6th-8th grade reading level for the average patient/family (4th-5th grade level for a low literacy population).[59] Document readability and level statistics can be easily accessed in everyday word processing programs (e.g. Microsoft Word; note that the Flesh-Kincaid grade level shown may underestimate grade level).[60] Providers should also include images to support text (e.g.pictograms, infographics) and use written materials that have sufficient white space and have summaries at the end.[59] Tools are available to providers to help them assess how optimal written materials are in terms of understandability/actionability, as well as guide providers in developing written materials (**Table 3**).[59,61]

Electronic communication. The rapid adoption of mobile phones and smartphones, and use of text-messaging, apps, and other electronic modes of communication, presents a tremendous opportunity for improving access to health information and tools to promote health.[62] "eHealth" literacy refers to the practice of using the Internet and telecommunication technology as modalities for the provision of health communication and services.[63] Promotion of eHealth literacy is considered a promising way to support the diffusion of health information to audiences with low health literacy. Tailored strategies are likely to be needed; populations with low health literacy are especially likely to rely on a smartphone to access the Internet.[64]

SPECIAL CONSIDERATIONS FOR MITIGATING HEALTH LITERACY CHALLENGES BY PRACTICE SETTING
Well-Child Care in the Outpatient Primary Care Setting

The primary care setting is an important venue for the communication of anticipatory guidance that supports optimal child growth and development, spanning a wide range of topics. Providers should be aware of health literacy challenges even for routine tasks such as reviewing a child's weight trajectory using growth charts. As illustrated in *Case 1*, low health literacy/numeracy skills may lead parents to confuse rapid crossing of weight percentiles in weight, or achieving a 95th or 99th percentile BMI, as being good, when these may be concerning for obesity risk. The use of color-coded growth charts can help providers communicate about growth trajectories in a more understandable way.[65]

Health care providers have a unique opportunity to optimize the communication of preventive health recommendations and support families in the first two years of a child's life, taking advantage of the frequency of well-child visits and the trusted relationship that develops between providers and parents.[66] For example, Greenlight, a primary care-based obesity prevention intervention was designed to address disparities in obesity for Black/African-American and Latino families from low SES backgrounds. Greenlight includes booklets designed using health literacy principles, along with provider training in health communication strategies (e.g. teach-back, goal-setting), and has been associated with lower BMI-z scores through 15-18 months of age, among children whose parents received Greenlight compared to an active comparator group that received an injury prevention intervention.[66,67] The booklets are meant to be integrated into verbal counseling, helping providers to more effectively discuss 2-3 key evidence based age-specific recommendations with parents, using plain language and visuals (e.g. sample menus showing appropriate portion sizes, photographs to support the recognition of satiety cues, red-green-yellow motif for drinks that are good for the baby vs. drinks to avoid); teach-back and setting of SMART goals (specific, measurable, action-oriented, relevant, time-bound) is also recommended.[59,68]

Management of Chronic Illnesses in the Outpatient Specialty Setting

Communication is especially important for families managing chronic illness symptoms. For example, parents of children with asthma must learn to be aware of specific symptoms that indicate that an escalation of care is needed (e.g. "rescue" medication, need for emergency care). Patients with persistent asthma should be given a written asthma action plan to supplement verbal counseling.[69] Use of a low literacy, pictographic action plan for persistent asthma can improve the quality of provider communication, as well as parent knowledge of the importance of taking everyday preventive medicine even when sick, and knowledge of the importance of spacer use, without increased time burden for providers.[52,70]

Urgent and Emergency Room Care

Health literacy skills of parents are especially critical when a child is sick, and caregivers must assess whether an urgent visit to the primary care office or to the emergency room is needed. Low health literacy is associated with non-urgent emergency department visits.[71] The health literacy skills of caregivers is critical for communicating disease course and symptoms. Providers in this setting should be aware that health literacy skills are often compromised,[9,17] and that clear communication strategies, including to confirm disease history and symptoms, is needed. In addition, because urgent visits tend to be rushed, verbal counseling of discharge instructions needs to accompany the provision of discharge materials written in plain language. Providers can write out instructions or draw out visual depictions of concepts to support understanding of instructions, such as medication administration.[46] Administration of medication to children in the outpatient setting can be challenging for parents and caregivers; studies have documented that >40% make dosing errors.[38,46,72] Case 2 illustrates how confusion can occur not only with regard to dose, but also with regard to route of delivery; giving medicine for otitis media in the ear instead of orally. "Teach-back" should be used to assure understanding before leaving urgent care settings, to prevent burden of families from prolonged/unresolved symptoms, and unnecessary utilization of medical services, including hospital revisits.[73]

Inpatient Setting

Within the inpatient setting, providers should be aware of numerous health literacy challenges that impact communication at all stages from getting an accurate history of the present illness, getting to a shared understanding of the diagnosis and plan, participation of families as true partners in decision-making with the medical team, to the communication of instructions at the time of hospital discharge.[74] Errors in the comprehension of, and adherence to, discharge instructions for parents of hospitalized children are common, especially when discharge plans are complex; the impact of plan complexity on comprehension errors is greatest for parents with low health literacy.[74] A key driver of poor adherence to discharge instructions is poor comprehension.[75]

Special Considerations for Mitigating Health Literacy Challenges Outside of the Clinical Encounter (i.e. Navigating Healthcare Systems)

As healthcare systems become more complex, the demands on parents to navigate healthcare systems increase. Parents must be able to identify a sufficient entry point to the healthcare system, orient themselves within an organization, and maneuver through the system to meet the needs of their children.[36] For example, a patient may need to determine health care costs and insurance coverage, to understand insurance rights and responsibilities, to review the explanation of benefits, and understand how to pay and/or appeal a medical bill. Caregivers with limited health literacy face greater navigation difficulties, often leading to uncertainty and discontinuities in health care.[76] Health literacy environmental scans can be conducted to identify institutional or agency-centric interventions that can be leveraged to improve navigation, including review of accessibility, signage, navigation, and written/spoken communications.[77]

THE FUTURE OF ADDRESSING HEALTH LITERACY IN PRACTICE - ESSENTIAL FOR ACHIEVING HEALTH EQUITY

By taking action to address health literacy in their clinical practices, health care providers can begin to help patients and their families overcome structural barriers that have contributed to longstanding disparities in health outcomes that disproportionately impact individuals from low SES backgrounds, as well as those from racial/ethnic minority groups, those who don't speak English, and immigrants.[36,45,49–51,58] To fully tackle the problem of health literacy and impact health disparities, a multi-pronged and multi-disciplinary and systems-level approach is needed, leveraging health system redesign as a way to decrease demands placed on individuals, such that health literacy-informed best practices are woven throughout the fabric of the health care system.

CLINICS CARE POINTS

- Health literacy is a highly prevalent issue impacting child health, which can be impacted by contextual factors, including stress.
- Low health literacy has been linked to poor health knowledge, less optimal health behaviors, and worse child health-related outcomes across domains of preventive health, acute care as well as chronic disease management.
- Health literacy is a health equity issue. Providers can use health literacy-informed communication best practices as a strategy to ameliorate health disparities.

- While it is difficult to identify patient and families who face low health literacy challenges when they present at a clinical visit, "warning signs" may be helpful.
- A universal precautions approach to utilizing health literacy-informed communication strategies is recommended.
- Key basic communication strategies include: using plain language and avoiding medical jargon, limiting counseling to 2–3 (need to know vs. nice to know) main concepts, and "chunking" of information into small digestible components. Advanced counseling strategies include: the use of teach-back/show-back, leveraging drawings/pictures, and supplementing verbal counseling with plain language written information.
- Health literacy challenges exist across clinical settings with special considerations for each.
- Health care providers should change individual-level communication practices by choosing from a menu of recommended health literacy-informed best practices, and also make changes more widely at the setting level. A multi-disciplinary approach is likely needed for all team members who play a role in communicating with families.

DISCLOSURE

The authors have no financial disclosures to report.

ACKNOWLEDGMENTS

We would like to acknowledge Divya Konduru, a undergraduate student at Johns Hopkins University, for her assistance in literature review.

REFERENCES

1. Schwartzberg JG, VanGeest J, Wang C. Understanding health literacy : implications for medicine and public health, xv. American Medical Association; 2005. p. 253.
2. Roundtable on Health Literacy. Board on Population Health and Public Health Practice. Institute of Medicine. Facilitating Patient Understanding of Discharge Instructions: Workshop Summary. Washington (DC): National Academy Press (US); 2014.
3. Joint Commission Resources Inc. Addressing patients' health literacy needs. unspecified. Joint Commission Resources,; 2009.
4. U.S. Department of Health and Human Services. Healthy People 2030: building a healthier future for all. 2020. Available at: https://health.gov/healthypeople. Accessed October 11, 2022.
5. U.S. Department of Health and Human Services. Office of Disease Prevention and Health Promotion. National Action Plan to Improve Health Literacy. 2010. Available at: https://health.gov/sites/default/files/2019-09/Health_Literacy_Action_Plan.pdf. Accessed October 13, 2022.
6. Kiechle ES, Bailey SC, Hedlund LA, et al. Different Measures, Different Outcomes? A Systematic Review of Performance-Based versus Self-Reported Measures of Health Literacy and Numeracy. J Gen Intern Med 2015;30(10):1538–46.
7. DeWalt D, Callahan L, Hawk V. Agency for Healthcare Research and Quality: Health Literacy Universal Precautions Toolkit. Available at: http://www.ahrq.gov/professionals/quality-patient-safety/quality-resources/tools/literacy-toolkit/index.html. Accessed August 8, 2022.
8. Institute of Medicine. Health literacy: a prescription to end confusion. Washington, DC: National Academies Press; 2004.

9. Morrison AK, Glick A, Yin HS. Health Literacy: Implications for Child Health. Pediatr Rev 2019;40(6):263–77.

10. Yin HS, Johnson M, Mendelsohn AL, et al. The health literacy of parents in the United States: a nationally representative study. Pediatrics 2009;124(Suppl 3): S289–98.

11. Doak LG, Doak CC, Kutner MA, United States. Department of Education., National Center for Education Statistics. The health literacy of America's adults : results from the 2003 National Assessment of Adult Literacy. NCES (Series). United States Department of Education, National Center for Education Statistics; 2006. p. 60, xiv.

12. Scotten M. Parental health literacy and its impact on patient care. Prim Care 2015;42(1):1–16.

13. World Health Organization. *WHO Global Strategy on People-Centred and Integrated Health Services, Interim report.* Geneva, Switzerland: World Health Organization; 2015.

14. Freebody P, Luke A. Literacies' programs: debates and demands in cultural context. Prospect: An Australian Journal of TESOL 1990;5:7–16.

15. Brach C, Keller D, Hernandez L, et al. Ten Attributes of Health Literate Health Care Organizations. *NAM Perspectives.* Discussion Paper. Washington, DC: National Academy of Medicine; 2012.

16. Institute of Medicine (U.S.). Roundtable on Health Literacy. Implications of health literacy for public health: workshop summary. Washington (DC): National Academies Press (US); 2014. p. 160, xvi.

17. Baker DW, Gazmararian JA, Sudano J, et al. The association between age and health literacy among elderly persons. J Gerontol B Psychol Sci Soc Sci 2000; 55(6):S368–74.

18. Sentell T, Braun KL. Low health literacy, limited English proficiency, and health status in Asians, Latinos, and other racial/ethnic groups in California. J Health Commun 2012;17(Suppl 3):82–99.

19. Berkman ND, Dewalt DA, Pignone MP, et al. Literacy and health outcomes. Evid Rep Technol Assess 2004;(87):1–8.

20. Paasche-Orlow MK, Wolf MS. Promoting health literacy research to reduce health disparities. J Health Commun 2010;15(Suppl 2):34–41.

21. Sentell TL, Halpin HA. Importance of adult literacy in understanding health disparities. J Gen Intern Med 2006;21(8):862–6.

22. Gwynn KB, Winter MR, Cabral HJ, et al. Racial disparities in patient activation: Evaluating the mediating role of health literacy with path analyses. Patient Educ Couns 2016;99(6):1033–7.

23. Najman JM, Hayatbakhsh MR, Heron MA, et al. The impact of episodic and chronic poverty on child cognitive development. J Pediatr 2009;154(2):284–9.

24. Walker SP, Wachs TD, Grantham-McGregor S, et al. Inequality in early childhood: risk and protective factors for early child development. Lancet 2011;378(9799): 1325–38.

25. Marmot M. and Wilkinson R. *Social determinants of health.* 2005. United Kingdom: OUP Oxford.

26. Stormacq C, Van den Broucke S, Wosinski J. Does health literacy mediate the relationship between socioeconomic status and health disparities? Integrative review. Health Promot Int 2018;34(5):e1–17.

27. Williams DR, Lawrence JA, Davis BA. Racism and Health: Evidence and Needed Research. Annu Rev Public Health 2019;40:105–25.

28. Berkman ND, Sheridan SL, Donahue KE, et al. Low health literacy and health outcomes: an updated systematic review. Ann Intern Med 2011;155(2):97–107.

29. Shi L, Lebrun LA, Tsai J. The influence of English proficiency on access to care. Ethn Health 2009;14(6):625–42.

30. Wilson E, Chen AH, Grumbach K, et al. Effects of limited English proficiency and physician language on health care comprehension. J Gen Intern Med 2005;20(9): 800–6.

31. Office for Civil Rights. U.S. Department of Health and Human Services. Guidance to Federal Financial Assistance Recipients Regarding Title VI Prohibition Against National Origin Discrimination Affecting Limited English Proficient Persons. 2004. Available at: https://www.hhs.gov/civil-rights/for-individuals/special-topics/limited-english-proficiency/guidance-federal-financial-assistance-recipients-title-vi/index.html. Accessed October 11, 2022.

32. Shaw SJ, Huebner C, Armin J, et al. The role of culture in health literacy and chronic disease screening and management. J Immigr Minor Health 2009; 11(6):460–7.

33. Leyva M, Sharif I, Ozuah PO. Health literacy among Spanish-speaking Latino parents with limited English proficiency. Ambul Pediatr 2005;5(1):56–9.

34. Passel J, Taylor P. Undocumented immigrants and their U.S.-Born Children. Washington (DC): Pew Research Center; 2010.

35. Cheng ER, Bauer NS, Downs SM, et al. Parent Health Literacy, Depression, and Risk for Pediatric Injury. Pediatrics 2016;138(1). https://doi.org/10.1542/peds. 2016-0025.

36. Weiss BD. Health literacy and patient safety: help patients understand. Manual for Clinicians. Chicago, IL: AMA Foundation; 2007.

37. DeWalt DA, Hink A. Health literacy and child health outcomes: a systematic review of the literature. Pediatrics 2009;124(Suppl 3):S265–74.

38. Yin HS, Mendelsohn AL, Wolf MS, et al. Parents' medication administration errors: role of dosing instruments and health literacy. Arch Pediatr Adolesc Med 2010; 164(2):181–6.

39. DeWalt DA, Dilling MH, Rosenthal MS, et al. Low parental literacy is associated with worse asthma care measures in children. Ambul Pediatr 2007;7(1):25–31.

40. Fleary SA, Joseph P, Pappagianopoulos JE. Adolescent health literacy and health behaviors: A systematic review. J Adolesc 2018;62:116–27.

41. Parikh NS, Parker RM, Nurss JR, et al. Shame and health literacy: the unspoken connection. Patient Educ Couns 1996;27(1):33–9.

42. Paasche-Orlow MK, Wolf MS. Evidence does not support clinical screening of literacy. J Gen Intern Med 2008;23(1):100–2.

43. Weiss BD. How to bridge the health literacy gap. Fam Pract Manag 2014; 21(1):14–8.

44. DeWalt DA, Broucksou KA, Hawk V, et al. Developing and testing the health literacy universal precautions toolkit. Nurs Outlook 2011;59(2):85–94.

45. Paasche-Orlow MK, Schillinger D, Greene SM, et al. How Health Care Systems Can Begin to Address the Challenge of Limited Literacy. J Gen Intern Med 2006;21(8):884–7.

46. Yin H, Dreyer B, van Schaick L, et al. Randomized controlled trial of a pictogram-based intervention to reduce liquid medication dosing errors and improve adherence among caregivers of young children. Arch Pediatr Adolesc Med 2008; 162(9):814–22.

47. Center for Disease Control and Prevention. Plain Language Communication. Available at: https://www.cdc.gov/healthliteracy/developmaterials/plain-language-communication.html. Accessed October 11, 2022.
48. World Health Organization. Use plain language. Available at: https://www.who.int/about/communications/understandable/plain-language. Accessed October 11, 2022.
49. Turner T, Cull WL, Bayldon B, et al. Pediatricians and health literacy: descriptive results from a national survey. Pediatrics 2009;124(Suppl 3):S299–305.
50. Abrams MA and Dreyer BP. American Academy of Pediatrics. *Plain language pediatrics: health literacy strategies and communication resources for common pediatric topics*.2009. Elk Grove Village, IL: American Academy of Pediatrics. 337, xi.
51. Schwartzberg JG, Cowett A, VanGeest J, et al. Communication techniques for patients with low health literacy: a survey of physicians, nurses, and pharmacists. Am J Health Behav 2007;31(Suppl 1):S96–104.
52. Yin HS, Gupta RS, Tomopoulos S, et al. A Low-Literacy Asthma Action Plan to Improve Provider Asthma Counseling: A Randomized Study. Pediatrics 2016; 137(1). https://doi.org/10.1542/peds.2015-0468.
53. Chandler P, Sweller J. Cognitive Load Theory and the Format of Instruction. Cognit InStruct 1991;8(4):293–332.
54. Joint Commission (Oakbrook Terrace Ill.). What did the doctor say? : improving health literacy to protect patient safety. Joint Commission on Accreditation of Healthcare Organizations; 2007. p. 61.
55. Chhabra R, Chisolm DJ, Bayldon B, et al. Evaluation of Pediatric Human Papillomavirus Vaccination Provider Counseling Written Materials: A Health Literacy Perspective. Acad Pediatr 2018;18(2S):S28–36.
56. Unaka N, Statile A, Jerardi K, et al. Improving the Readability of Pediatric Hospital Medicine Discharge Instructions. J Hosp Med 2017;12(7):551–7.
57. Kuo DZ, O'Connor KG, Flores G, et al. Pediatricians' use of language services for families with limited English proficiency. Pediatrics 2007;119(4):e920–7.
58. Pusic MV, Ching K, Yin HS, et al. Seven practical principles for improving patient education: Evidence-based ideas from cognition science. Paediatr Child Health 2014;19(3):119–22.
59. Doak CC, Doak LG, Root JH. *2nd edition. Teaching patients with low literacy skills*, 212. Philadelphia, PA: J.B. Lippincott; 1995. p. xii.
60. Sharma N, Tridimas A, Fitzsimmons PR. A readability assessment of online stroke information. J Stroke Cerebrovasc Dis 2014;23(6):1362–7.
61. Agency for Healthcare Research and Quality. The Patient Education Materials Assessment Tool (PEMAT) and User's Guide. Accessed October 11, 2022. Available at: https://www.ahrq.gov/health-literacy/patient-education/pemat.html.
62. Mackert M, Love B, Whitten P. Patient education on mobile devices: an e-health intervention for low health literate audiences. J Inf Sci 2008;35(1):82–93.
63. Eysenbach G. What is e-health? J Med Internet Res 2001;3(2):E20.
64. Smith A. U.S. Smartphone Use in 2015. Pew Research Center. Available at: https://www.pewinternet.org/2015/04/01/us-smartphone-use-in-2015. Accessed September 4, 2022.
65. Oettinger MD, Finkle JP, Esserman D, et al. Color-coding improves parental understanding of body mass index charting. Acad Pediatr 2009;9(5):330–8.
66. Sanders LM, Perrin EM, Yin HS, et al. Greenlight study": a controlled trial of low-literacy, early childhood obesity prevention. Pediatrics 2014;133(6):e1724–37.

67. Sanders LM, Perrin EM, Yin HS, et al. A Health-Literacy Intervention for Early Childhood Obesity Prevention: A Cluster-Randomized Controlled Trial. Pediatrics 2021;(5):147. https://doi.org/10.1542/peds.2020-049866.

68. Bovend'Eerdt TJ, Botell RE, Wade DT. Writing SMART rehabilitation goals and achieving goal attainment scaling: a practical guide. Clin Rehabil 2009;23(4): 352–61.

69. Cloutier MM, Baptist AP, Blake KV, et al. 2020 Focused Updates to the Asthma Management Guidelines: A Report from the National Asthma Education and Prevention Program Coordinating Committee Expert Panel Working Group. J Allergy Clin Immunol 2020;146(6):1217–70.

70. Yin HS, Gupta RS, Tomopoulos S, et al. Readability, suitability, and characteristics of asthma action plans: examination of factors that may impair understanding. Pediatrics 2013;131(1):e116–26.

71. Morrison AK, Schapira MM, Gorelick MH, et al. Low caregiver health literacy is associated with higher pediatric emergency department use and nonurgent visits. Acad Pediatr 2014;14(3):309–14.

72. Davis TC, Wolf MS, Bass PF, et al. Literacy and misunderstanding prescription drug labels. Ann Intern Med 2006;145(12):887–94.

73. Hesselink G, Sir Ö, Koster N, et al. Teach-back of discharge instructions in the emergency department: a pre-post pilot evaluation. Emerg Med J 2022;39(2): 139–46.

74. Glick AF, Farkas JS, Mendelsohn AL, et al. Discharge Instruction Comprehension and Adherence Errors: Interrelationship Between Plan Complexity and Parent Health Literacy. J Pediatr 2019;214:193–200.e3.

75. Zuckerman KE, Perrin JM, Hobrecker K, et al. Barriers to specialty care and specialty referral completion in the community health center setting. J Pediatr 2013; 162(2):409–14.e1.

76. Griese L, Berens EM, Nowak P, et al. Challenges in Navigating the Health Care System: Development of an Instrument Measuring Navigation Health Literacy. Int J Environ Res Public Health 2020;17(16). https://doi.org/10.3390/ijerph17 165731.

77. Rudd R, Oelschlegel S, Grabeel K, et al. The HLE2 assessment tool. Harvard TH. Boston, MA: Chan School of Public Health 2019.

Health Care Anchors' Responsibilities and Approaches to Achieving Child Health Equity

Desiree Yeboah, MD[a],*, Alicia Tieder, MSW, LICSW[b],
Ashley Durkin, MPH, PMP[b], Leslie R. Walker-Harding, MD, FSAHM[c]

KEYWORDS

- Determinants of health • Anchor institution • Community partnership • Equity
- Anti-racism • Workforce planning • Quality improvement

KEY POINTS

- Anchor institutions are placed-based, mission-driven institutions that play an integral role in addressing upstream determinants of health by leveraging their economic assets, spending power, and social capital.
- Anchor institutions should invest in cultural competency, equity, diversity, and inclusion education, and equity-focused quality improvement to help eliminate disparities in patient outcomes.
- An intentional anchor mission approach involves institutional leadership alignment on vision and goals, development of clear metrics, and strategic planning and accountability with community partnerships.

INTRODUCTION

There is growing recognition that social, economic, and environmental conditions have a significantly greater impact on an individual's health outcomes than medical care alone.[1–5] Economic and housing instability, educational disparities, inadequate nutrition, and environmental risks contribute to numerous health inequities in the United States.[1,5] The World Health Organization(WHO) defines social determinants of health (SDOH) as "the conditions in which people are born, grow, live, work, and

[a] University of Washington/Seattle Children's Hospital, 4800 Sand Point Way Northeast, M/S OC.7830 PO Box 5371, Seattle, WA 98145-5005, USA; [b] Seattle Children's Center for Diversity and Health Equity, 4800 Sand Point Way Northeast, M/S RB.2.419, Seattle, WA 98105, USA; [c] University of Washington/Seattle Children's Hospital, 4800 Sand Point Way Northeast, Seattle, WA 98105, USA
* Corresponding author.
E-mail address: Desiree.yeboah@seattlechildrens.org

Pediatr Clin N Am 70 (2023) 761–774
https://doi.org/10.1016/j.pcl.2023.04.002   **pediatric.theclinics.com**
0031-3955/23/© 2023 Elsevier Inc. All rights reserved.

age; these conditions are shaped by the availability of resources and distribution of power at the global, national, and local levels."[1,2,4,5] As awareness of SDOH becomes increasingly prevalent, health care institutions are recognizing their role in implementing strategies to improve population health and reduce disparities. More health care systems are working to identify individuals' immediate social needs such as food insecurity or transportation access. Although efforts to address social needs have proven to be beneficial, more is required at the community level to address the upstream structural factors, policies, and practices which disproportionately affect health outcomes.[1–5] As a result, health care systems across the United States have developed an anchor mission approach to help allocate economic assets and intellectual resources toward tackling SDOH.[1–3]

THE ANCHOR MISSION

Anchor institutions are defined as large, spatially immobile, usually non-profit institutions with a social-purpose mission rooted in equity, social and racial justice, and community.[3,6] The anchor institution concept emerged in the 1960s during a period when American cities were facing disinvestment, leading to poverty-stricken neighborhoods with massive unemployment, poor schooling, and decaying infrastructure.[1,2,6] In this climate, institutions of higher education and academic medical centers ("eds and meds") stepped forward as the anchors of their communities.[1,2] Anchor institutions gained prominence in the late 1990s as policymakers and university leaders contemplated innovative ways to reinvest in their communities.[1,2,6] They adopted an "anchor mission" described as "a commitment to leveraging hiring, purchasing, and investing assets along with human capital, in partnership with their communities to mutually benefit the long-term well-being of both."[7] Through this mission, the community itself is recognized as the primary driver for health outcomes.[1,5]

The anchor mission concept is not unique to health care systems. Many non-profit or public placed entities such as universities, municipal governments, and faith-based foundations have an established anchor mission approach to addressing economic and racial inequities in their communities. Health care systems have the largest impact of any nongovernmental anchor institution in the United States[2,8] According to a recently published report by the Democracy Collaborative at the University of Maryland, hospitals employ more than 5.4 million individuals and spend more than $340 billion per year on goods and services.[2] Specifically, pediatric health care institutions have a considerable impact on reducing health disparities through their engagement with local community health needs. Two studies led by Franz highlight that children's hospitals tend to be in larger geographic regions with disproportionate social needs than the national average. Therefore, children's hospitals are uniquely poised to improve health disparities for both children and adults.[4,9]

Anchor institutions have a vested interest in ensuring that the communities in which they are based remain healthy and well resourced. In addition to the profound impact on community health outcomes, the US hospitals are also embracing an anchor mission for financial and political interests. Businesses generated through community partnerships and investments yield economic returns for both communities and hospitals while also fulfilling community benefit requirements for tax exemptions (**Fig. 1**).[8,9] As hospitals have increased their efforts in community engagement and development, networks have emerged to help support this work. The Health Care Anchor Network (HAN) has been the most notable since its creation in 2017.[1,7] HAN, a collaborative of over 50 health care systems, comprising over 700 hospitals, aids institutions in initiating, implementing, and institutionalizing anchor mission strategies.[1,7]

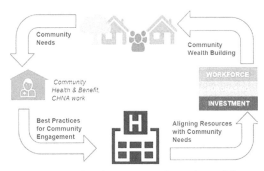

Fig. 1. Anchor institutions impact local economics through workforce, purchasing, and investment strategies. This economic strategy has a multiplier effect within the local community, increasing economic activity, while also addressing community health needs. The work of rebuilding local communities has a direct impact on the longstanding success of anchor institutions. (Credit: Original Figure, Source Seattle Children's Hospital, External Affairs Department- Community Health.)

HAN members can engage in structured learning opportunities such as peer-to-peer initiative workgroups, educational webinars, and conferences where strategies are shared, discussed, and challenged. The network is supported through its backbone organization called the Democracy Collaborative, an entity responsible for providing example initiatives, successful roadmaps, and other advisory services to establish an anchor mission. Partnerships with community-based organizations and collaborative networks can help scale up the impact of anchor mission work.

CASE STUDY: ODESSA BROWN CHILDREN'S CLINIC IN SEATTLE, WASHINGTON

Seattle Children's Odessa Brown Children's Clinic (OBCC), based in Seattle, Washington, has a rich heritage that began with African American women including Mrs. Odessa Brown and Dr. Blanche Lavizzo in the community making a commitment to integrating medical care and social services for African American underserved children in Central Seattle.[10] Since the foundation of the first clinic in 1970, Seattle Children's Hospital (SCH) has been a founding partner for OBCC's vision, execution, and resource support which allowed OBCC to serve the last 52 years as a medical home and community partner dedicated to addressing root causes of illnesses.[10] As SCH's only primary care clinic, it remains committed to quality health care delivery and community development. In March 2022, OBCC opened a new clinic site in Southeast Seattle, a location that brings its longstanding mission closer to communities most in need.[10,11] Seattle Children's multi-million-dollar investment supported the completion of this pediatric clinic.[10] Throughout the years, prominent leaders in the African American community have established business partnerships with OBCC medical directors. SCH serves as the anchoring institution consisting of an equally strong hospital system, board of trustees, and executive leadership committed to delivering excellent care to all who come to OBCC looking for equitable, appropriate, quality care for their children. It remains a beloved pillar of the community 52 years since it opened.

OBCC has integrated services to address both individual social needs and upstream determinants of health in the local community. Families can receive assistance with accessing food, fitness, and legal aid services, among other needs impacting their overall health and wellness.[10,11] This clinic site is part of the Othello Square

---

Box 1
Key strategies for inclusive, local purchasing

Key Strategies.

- Hiring a supplier diversity consultant to help lead a supplier diversity program that aligns internal operations to promote inclusive, local purchasing
- Develop specific supplier diversity initiatives with spending goals and reporting mechanisms to track diversity activity spending
- Commit to contracting with local businesses owned by residents of color, women, or veterans, with an aim to procure 10% to 15% of total purchasing from these diverse vendors
- Foster long-term relationships with local businesses and diverse vendors
- Build the capacity of small, locally owned businesses by offering training and support in navigating purchasing programs and policies

---

neighborhood redevelopment, which includes a charter school and affordable housing units.[12] SCH has partnered with other investors to develop housing units for middle-income households in the community.[12] Additionally, through the Measurement and Innovation Hub in OBCC, pediatric professionals can partner with community members to research prevention and intervention strategies that tackle the root causes of childhood diseases.[10,11] OBCC has committed to establishing long-term partnerships with community health members to improve community engagement and prioritize community needs.[11]

ANCHOR MISSION STRATEGIES FOR LEVERAGING ECONOMIC ASSETS

Hospitals and integrated health care systems have tremendous assets to disrupt upstream social, economic, and environmental factors that contribute to poor health outcomes. They have significant economic assets related to the procurement of goods and services and place-based investments. This section highlights key strategic economic avenues such as purchasing and investing initiatives, and how they impact local communities surrounding health care anchors.

Purchasing Power

Income inequality and the racial wealth gap are inextricably linked to differences in health outcomes. Local purchasing is one avenue hospitals can use to leverage their economic resources to eliminate these inequities and also grow vibrant economies. Procuring goods and services locally has a multiplier effect on the local economy.[13–15] The money spent on local businesses will recirculate in the community in the form of salaries paid to employees or tax revenue collected and spent by the municipality.[13–15] The money that is circulated within the community alleviates economic insecurity, particularly for communities most impacted by structural racism in the United States. Anchor institutions should develop procurement strategies that prioritize contracting with local businesses owned by residents of color, women, and veterans.[2] Shifting the spending to historically marginalized individuals contributes to more equitable supply chains and supports community wealth building. See **Box 1** for some key strategies for inclusive and local purchasing. Intentional procurement of goods and services can have long-term impacts on community health. Local procurement initiatives can connect existing local and diverse vendors to contracting opportunities that help facilitate job stability and access to health care benefits.[15,16] Health care anchor institutions which desire to initiate local and diverse spending initiatives should implement strategies with clear goals and metrics to track progress.

Anchor institutions can leverage their purchasing power to reduce their carbon footprint and increase sustainability. Approximately 70% of hospital emissions come from their supply chain.[17] Hospitals should implement sustainable procurement guidelines with measurable goals specific to environment-friendly practices. These practices should identify suppliers with a similar mission of low-impact, environment-friendly practices, that limit utilization of non-recycled goods when possible.[16,17] Sustainable procurement practices can reduce supply chain waste and bolster revenue growth while concurrently improving environmental health in communities. In recent years, SCH has been recognized for its sustainable practices and environmental stewardship, receiving external Environmental Excellence Awards and high rankings for Greenest Hospitals in America according to Becker Hospital Review.[18] In 2022, SCH joined other institutions in the health care sector by pledging to reduce greenhouse gas emissions and build more climate-resilient infrastructure under the Department of Health and Human Services' (HSS) Health Care Sector Pledge.[18,19] SCH hospital campus aims to be carbon neutral by 2025, eventually reducing greenhouse emissions by 50% by 2030, and eventually to net zero by 2050.[18]

One of the most direct connections between sustainable practices and community health is in food purchasing.[2] Anchor institutions have a significant influence on the local economy around food services. Purchasing from local food vendors provides greater market access and job stability for producers.[2] The widespread impact of sustainable food purchasing includes the reduction of environmental waste and the increased circulation of high-quality, healthy food within the community.[2,16,17] Anchor institutions embracing an anchor mission should leverage their economic assets to increase access to locally produced foods and help eliminate health disparities related to food access.

Place-Based Investing

Structural and racist systemic factors have resulted in considerable disparities in neighborhood investments and subsequently poor health outcomes for Black, Indigenous, and Latine[1] communities. Research has shown that severely impoverished neighborhoods have deleterious effects on child health outcomes.[2,20,21] Children living in low-income and low-resourced communities are more likely to be exposed to environmental toxins, crime, and other physical hazards.[20] Anchor institutions can contribute their investment assets toward addressing economic and environmental disparities in local communities; this concept is referred to as place-based investing.[20] These investments can result in energy-efficient projects, economic development around arts and culture, and transit-oriented development.[20] A unifying theme to these projects requires establishing trusting partnerships with community members and assessing which infrastructure needs must be prioritized. It is vital that place-based investment strategies are discussed and planned with community members and leaders to ensure that projects align with their community health and economic needs.

Rush University Medical Center, a national leader of the anchor mission strategy, has leveraged its financial resources and social capital to improve health in numerous neighborhoods in the West Side of Chicago. Social impact investing is one of Rush's broader anchor efforts that provides financial investments which yield both economic and social returns for the community. The first of Rush's social impact investments in 2017 was a $1.08 million loan to the community development financial institutions (CDFI) Chicago Community Loan Fund, which contributed to Chicago's Neighborhood

---

Box 2
Key strategies for place-based investing

Key Strategies

- Establish a place-based investment program in the anchor institution, and have community members serve on advisory boards for workgroup initiatives and planning
- Prioritize investment projects that align with community health needs
- Allocate a fixed amount annually from an investment portfolio to target investments in different sectors
- Collect health data landscape to identify and then direct funding to highest-risk neighborhoods
- Invest in the revitalization of urban and rural areas, agriculture, and renewable energy projects in the community
- Partner with local housing organizations to rehabilitate abandoned properties, transforming properties into housing for low-income families, and hospital employees

---

Rebuild Training Pilot Program.[22] The program not only helped rebuild 50 homes in the West Side of Chicago but also created job opportunities for youth and former incarcerated individuals.[22] Since 2017, Rush has invested an additional $2 million to help rehabilitate homes in Chicago neighborhoods, increasing high-quality and affordable housing units in some of the hardest hit neighborhoods in the city.[22]

Place-based investing creates healthy and thriving communities by addressing housing affordability, supporting local and diverse business developments, and empowering low-income individuals to create and own enterprises.[21] Anchor institutions can engage in place-based investing across various assets and sectors. Investment strategies can include shifting cash or cash equivalents to local banks, investing in financial intermediaries such as CDFI, and investing in local housing and infrastructure.[21] Anchor institutions should consider engaging with local social service agencies already involved in community development projects.[20,21] There should be a focus on investments in local, sustainable, and minority owned businesses. As anchor institutions, hospitals must view affordable housing and infrastructure as integral to healthy, safe, and thriving communities. See **Box 2** for key strategies for place-based investing.

ANCHOR MISSION STRATEGIES TO ADDRESS SYSTEMIC INEQUITIES

Anchor institutions also can utilize their social capital and intellectual resources to advance health equity. This section highlights anchor institution approaches to addressing systemic inequities through education, research, quality improvement (QI), and employment.

Equity, Diversity, Inclusion (EDI) and Cultural Competency Education

To prioritize strategies related to equity, diversity, inclusion, health equity, and anti-racism, anchor institutions must invest resources for education and training in these areas. A department dedicated to learning and organizational development can help facilitate change and a shared mental model. Utilization of the Awareness, Desire, Knowledge, Ability, Reinforcement model is one approach leaders and organizations can utilize to drive individual change and achieve organizational results.[23]

Anchor institutions should focus on connecting to knowledge and ability in core content, and in connecting to day-to-day operations through required core annual

> **Box 3**
> **Key strategies for EDI and culturally responsive education**
>
> *Key Strategies*
>
> - Mandatory annual e-learning on EDI, cultural competency, and anti-racism for all employees
> - Ongoing learning events (eg, Grand Rounds, guest speakers)
> - Accessible resources and tools
> - Interactive scenarios with discussion tools

training requirements and new staff onboarding. Some examples include mandatory annual e-learning, ongoing learning events, and resources such as Grand Rounds, conversation series, and just-in-time resources that promote cultural responsiveness (eg, CultureVision).[23] See **Box 3** for key strategies for EDI and culturally responsive education.

Equitable Outcomes Through Equity-Focused Quality Improvement

Anchor institutions should prioritize achieving equitable outcomes by reducing, and ultimately, eliminating disparities in health outcomes. Several approaches should be utilized by anchor institutions to advance equity, including within the QI space. The first is stratifying outcome measures by race, ethnicity, and language (REaL).[24] Typically, these metrics are collected at patient registration and can be utilized to look at outcome measures in a more granular way. A simple first step for an equity-focused QI project would be to eliminate any disparities found upon REaL stratification. Other ways to stratify are by the payor, sex assigned at birth, gender, etc. After metrics have been stratified by REaL, an Equity Impact Assessment (EIA), or similar tool, is helpful to ensure interventions, policies, guidelines of care, or other efforts are equitable in their development and implementation.[25] The EIA serves as a critical thought exercise introduced at the beginning of work to ensure equity is embedded throughout.

Anchor institutions must also foster a close working relationship between their equity and diversity team and their patient quality and safety colleagues. This may include the development of microsystems, or small groups within units focused on small tests of change and QI; sponsorship of staff development through QI training and mentoring programs; engagement of advanced practice providers in EDI QI through an equity-focused Maintenance of Certification project; development of visualizations of annual quality goals, stratified by REaL; and methodology to identify and address equity concerns through internal safety event reporting.

Recruitment and Retention of a Diverse Workforce

To achieve and sustain a diverse and inclusive workforce, anchor institutions must prioritize inclusive and equitable recruitment and retention practices in both clinical and non-clinical areas. Having clear strategies and initiatives with clear oversight and accountability measures can benefit the teams responsible for supporting this work. Anchor institutions should have a robust recruitment and talent acquisition department that can successfully implement strategies such as mandatory equitable recruitment training for all hiring managers, establishing strong sourcing and diversity outreach, as well as prioritizing diverse candidate slates in the recruitment process.[26] Focusing on leaders and hiring managers is a very important leadership diversity tactic. Expanding inclusive and equitable recruitment training can help to sustain diversity in the workplace and enhance opportunities for strong pipeline development and

---

Box 4
Key strategies for recruitment and retention of a diverse workforce

Key Strategies

• Redesigning career pages with intentional equity, diversity, inclusion, and anti-racist focus
• Highlighting employee testimonials and photos
• Displaying diversity dashboards and data
• Celebrating diversity milestones

---

internal mobility. Leaders should be provided tools to conduct interviews and hiring practices that are aligned with values, leadership principles, diversity, and anti-racism. Ensuring diverse candidate slates requires demographic data collection from candidates that are protected and confidential by the hiring manager. These data are secured and displayed in the aggregate to the hiring manager once the pool of candidates reaches a target goal (eg, 20% diverse candidate slate), then the hiring manager can proceed with screening and interviews.

Recruitment and talent acquisition departments in anchor institutions should prioritize strong community partnerships with a targeted focus and investment in diverse sourcing and outreach at local and national levels. This includes alignment with community-based organizations, resourcing for relocation, as well as investments in historically diverse colleges and universities.[26] Anchor institutions must invest in the workforce by offering competitive compensation and benefits. For example, supportive parental leave, ensuring minimum wage, emergency employee assessment funds, and tuition assistance. At Seattle Children's, tuition assistance recipients have a higher retention rate and estimated savings of $420,000 over 5 years. See **Box 4** for key strategies for recruitment and retention of a diverse workforce. Anchor institutions should be transparent and strengthen their employer brand by showcasing commitments to equity, diversity, inclusion, and anti-racism.

Prioritization of diversity does not stop at recruitment and hiring. Anchor institutions must invest in retention, career pathways development as well as internal mobility, with a focus on diversity. Specific practices include, but are not limited to, support for nurse residency diversity recruitment efforts, tuition assistance programs, expanding labor pool outside of state boundaries, employee resource groups, and creating pathways to enhance opportunities for diverse staff.[27,28]

Research Recruitment and Retention

The development of a diverse workforce must be imperative for anchor institutions, not only to show a commitment to the community in which it serves but also to develop a workforce that is reflective of this community. A variety of different pathway programs can be leveraged to foster an interest and ability to pursue a career in health sciences.

Science exploration and discovery may begin as early as kindergarten and foster an interest in science. High school summer programs may provide training and job skill development. As students advance through their schooling, more robust summer programs for college students are essential to give students whose race and ethnicity are historically underrepresented in biomedical and health sciences the opportunity to be exposed to research and develop professional skills beneficial to pursuing careers in the health sciences.[27,28] Seattle Children's Research Institute (SCRI) created the SCRI Summer Scholars Program to provide a unique experience for students that combines

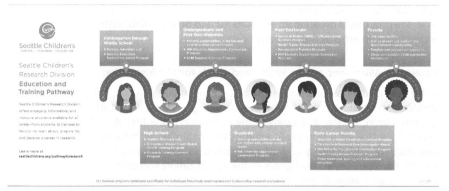

Fig. 2. Seattle Children's Research Division Education and Training Pathway offers engaging, informative, and inclusive programs available for all levels to learn about, prepare for, and develop a career in research. (Credit: From Seattle Children's Research Division.)

exposure and engagement in basic science laboratory experiences, community-based research opportunities, and professional development.[28] The program is dedicated to removing any kind of financial barriers to participation by funding transportation to and from Seattle, housing accommodation, and food stipends.[28] Approximately 20% to 30% of participants are retained each year as either paid employees or as for-credit research students or volunteers, with a high percentage reporting feelings of belonging in the biomedical and health sciences after participating.[28]

The next juncture in the pathway is supporting students as they graduate from college and look to bridge the next step of their career. At this stage, opportunities such as the National Institutes of Health (NIH) Diversity Supplements should be facilitated by anchor institutions.[28] These supplements provide additional funding to support the research and training of trainees, ranging from high school to early career faculty, through lab experience, career mentorship, and development.[28] A Diversity Supplements Connection Program works to match candidates for potential NIH Diversity Supplement awards with principal investigators who hold NIH grants eligible for a diversity supplement, offer grant writing services and support to applicants, and share resources to help outline tasks, timelines, and due dates (**Fig. 2**).

Additional streams of funding are essential for supporting and retaining early career research staff within the institution. Funding should focus on advancing health equity, reducing disparities, providing mentorship, and expanding career pathways for trainees.[23–28] Awards available to residents, post-doctoral fellows, and early career faculty allow for an expanded pool of candidates to better create links in the career development pathway. Integration and alignment of professional development opportunities and community building from kindergarten through early career is a critical avenue for anchor institutions to funnel their investments. Streamlining processes can increase efficiency and capacity, allowing for greater impact and increased diversity of the workforce.

DEVELOPING AN ANCHOR MISSION: STRATEGIES FOR IMPLEMENTATION, CHALLENGES, AND CONSIDERATIONS

This article has discussed what an anchor institution is, how it can be impactful in the community and institution, and what types of strategies can be employed by anchor institutions to address inequities and social injustice. This section highlights how to begin the process of creating an infrastructure to be an anchor institution and the challenges that can arise in the process.

Leadership Alignment on the Vision and Goals for the Institution

At the start of the development as an anchor institution mission, the leadership of the organization must be not only aligned but engaged and committed. Reevaluating the mission, vision, values, and goals of the institution is the first step. This new lens acknowledges that as a non-profit established institution with roots in the community, sustainability and thriving of that community is essential to the anchor institution and the mission, vision, and goals of the organization and community. Once leaders are aware and clear about the importance of becoming an anchor institution then they must be empowered to motivate others in the institution to invest in the vision. Identifying a champion to take the lead in the next steps will help to ensure continued progress and attention to metrics.

Developing Clear Metrics, Strategic Planning and Accountability

Once it is established that the will and commitment are sufficient to form an anchor mission, the next step is to develop a process to realize the goals of that mission. It is important at this stage to have a team that includes those with lived community experience as well as institution leaders and process managers.[29] Together developing measurable goals based on community needs and institution resources is a first step. A plan to achieve those goals and who will be accountable for each goal is the next step. In identifying areas to focus on in addition to community partners, the Community Health Needs Assessment (CHNA) can be helpful. The CHNA is a required process that non-profit health organizations must gather. It is the global needs assessment of the local community and/or catchment area where patients and families will reside.[29] Area demographics, health metrics, resources available, and focus groups of community residents, young and older, give input in identifying what gaps and challenges are present. The data are analyzed by the community engagement team of the health organization and recommendations are made showing where the anchor institution can focus its resources and planning.

Starting with Structure

To create a multipronged, well-integrated, and effective anchor mission and intervention, structure and process are essential. This structure can come out of the community benefit assessment team that creates the CHNA, or it can be a new structure set up to manage multiple goals for community organizations to partner with the anchor institution. One example is the University of Pennsylvania's anchor mission for improving health by creating a University Assisted Community School site that gives health services to high school students, their families, and community residents (**Fig. 3**).[29] This was accomplished by the Penn's Netter Center for Community Partnerships and a number of Penn's health institutions all working together.[29] To develop these types of community partnerships, the key to success is collaboration and co-design with local partners, developing relationships that lead to building deep community connections and relationships. With established relationships and mutual understanding, anchor institutions and communities can work together to address community needs and build a lasting foundation for continued success.

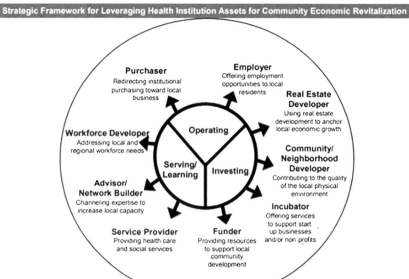

Fig. 3. A Strategic Framework for Leveraging Health Institution Assets for Community Revitalization. Anchor Institutions Toolkit: A guide for neighborhood revitalization. (Credit: Netter Center for Community Partnerships (2008). Anchor Institutions toolkit. Philadelphia, PA: University of Pennsylvania. www.nettercenter.upenn.edu. This figured was adapted from "Leveraging Colleges and Universities for Urban Economic Revitalization: An Action Agenda" A Joint Study by Initiative for a Competitive Inner City and CEOs for Cities, 2003.)

CHALLENGES AND CONSIDERATIONS

In initiating and solidifying lasting effective relationships, the anchor institution must work to remove any barriers to the community's interest and motivation to work with the institution. Some challenges that large medical or health institutions have include a history of mistrust, particularly within Black, Indigenous, and Latine communities. There can even be specific transgressions with the institution that caused clear and remembered harm to a community in the past.[30] It is important to look for ways to reestablish trust, working through a restorative justice framework may be helpful.[30] Patience and consistency will also be important in the repair and in centering the community as the catalyst for change rather than the anchor institution. Restorative justice is rooted in Indigenous traditions and is a process that gives voice to those harmed so that the perpetrator of the harm can gain a better understanding of the harm caused with the goal of addressing and repairing the relationship and preventing further harm.[30] There are three phases to the process and a facilitator with expertise in restorative justice is essential so that further harm or division is not created from the process itself.

Once stable relationships are formed between the community and the anchor institution, they must be maintained and cultivated. Caring for this codesigned and action-oriented relationship takes bidirectional intentionality. Continuing to keep a focus on equity and inclusion will help to balance the power dynamics within an institution and community. It is not enough to declare that the relationship will work from an anti-racist, diverse, inclusive, and equitable framework. It is important to collaborate to develop clear action plans and measurable metrics that continually assess whether

> **Box 5**
> **Key strategies for implementing an anchor mission**
>
> *Key Strategies*
>
> - Start with research and mapping to identify local areas with immediate needs and to gather information about existing community anchor organizations or initiatives for potential collaboration
> - Identify institutional leadership and process managers to ensure that the mission of the anchor institution aligns at all levels of the organization and has shared values with community members
> - Leadership should clearly define decision-making processes and accountability for each team role
> - Define initiative goals and key metrics to track progress; hold monthly meetings with key stakeholders from the institution and community to report progress

their relationship is on the continuum to achieve the highest level of a power-sharing partnership. This type of relationship development and power sharing can be challenging for academic institutions and for communities that have not been included in the past. Executive sponsorship and community leadership will be instrumental to its success. See **Box 5** for key strategies for implementing an anchor mission.

SUMMARY

Health equity starts and is sustained in economically stable, socially cohesive, and environmentally friendly communities. Anchor institutions, particularly health care anchors, can play a leading role in alleviating drivers of poor health outcomes. Implementing an anchor mission requires an intentional approach and commitment to leveraging economic, intellectual, and social resources to address the root causes of disease. This approach calls for redefining the institution's culture to reflect an anchor mission centered on equity, diversity, inclusion, and anti-racism. Successful anchor institutions are sustained by organizational leadership, accountability, and collaborative relationships with the local community.

CLINICS CARE POINTS

> - When measuring treatment outcomes, include patient's REaL demographics to help identify and track outcome disparities.
> - Remember to involve community members in the beginning stages of program development and in the design and delivery of clinical services.
> - Assure adequate language services are available for every patient encounter.

DISCLOSURE

There are no conflicts of interest to disclose.

REFERENCES

1. Sarkar S. Health System Investments to Address Social and Economic Determinants of Health. Healthcare Anchor Model 2020;1:208.

2. Zuckerman D. Hospitals Building Healthier Communities: Embracing the anchor mission. Healthcare Anchor Network. 2019. Available at: https://healthcareanchor.network/2019/12/hospitals-building-healthier-communities-embracing-the-anchor-mission/. Accessed 9 September, 2022.

3. Porter J, Fisher-Bruns D, Pham BH. Anchor collaboratives: Building Bridges with place-based partnerships and Anchor Institutions. Healthcare Anchor Network. 2022. Available at: https://healthcareanchor.network/2019/05/anchor-collaboratives-building-bridges-with-place-based-partnerships-and-anchor-institutions/. Accessed 7 August, 2022.

4. Franz B, Flint J, Cronin CE. Assessing the strategies that children's Hospitals adopt to engage the social determinants of health in US cities. J Publ Health Manag Pract 2020;28(1). https://doi.org/10.1097/phh.0000000000001227.

5. Castrucci BC, Auerbach J. Meeting individual social needs falls short of addressing social determinants of health. Health Affairs Forefront. 2019. Available at: https://www.healthaffairs.org/do/10.1377/forefront.20190115.234942/. Accessed 9 October, 2022.

6. Luter G, Taylor HL. Anchor institutions: An interpretive review essay. Netter Center for Community Partnerships. 2017. Available at: https://www.nettercenter.upenn.edu/anchor-institutions-interpretive-review-essay-now-available. Accessed 15 September, 2022.

7. About the healthcare anchor network. Healthcare Anchor Network. 2022. Available at: https://healthcareanchor.network/about-the-healthcare-anchor-network/. Accessed 24 August, 2022.

8. Cronin CE, Franz B, Choyke K, et al. For-profit hospitals have a unique opportunity to serve as anchor institutions in the U.S. Preventive Medicine Reports 2021; 22:101372.

9. Franz B, Cronin CE. Are children's hospitals unique in the community benefits they provide? exploring decisions to prioritize community health needs among U.S. children's and General Hospitals. Front Public Health 2020;8. https://doi.org/10.3389/fpubh.2020.00047.

10. About Odessa Brown Children's Clinic - Seattle Children's. Seattle Children's Hospital. Available at: https://www.seattlechildrens.org/clinics/odessa-brown/about/. Accessed October 30, 2022.

11. Report highlight: Odessa Brown Children's Clinic. Seattle Children's Hospital. Available at: https://www.seattlechildrens.org/about/commitment-anti-racism/report-highlight-odessa-brown-childrens-clinic/. Accessed 30 October, 2022.

12. Speller A. Uniting to innovate early learning in Seattle's Othello Square. On the Pulse. 2022. Available at: https://pulse.seattlechildrens.org/uniting-to-innovate-early-learning-in-seattles-othello-square/. Accessed 29 October, 2022.

13. Zuckerman, D., Parker, K. Resources for the Anchor Mission: Inclusive, Local Sourcing. 2016. Available at: https://healthcareanchor.network/2019/11/inclusive-local-sourcing/. Accessed 2 September, 2022.

14. Anchor Institutions Task Force Health Professionals' Subgroup. Value Added: Adopting a 'Social Determinants of Health' Lens. March 2019.

15. Serang, F., Thompson, J., Howard, T. The Anchor Mission: Leveraging the Power of Anchor Institutions to Build Community Wealth. A Case Study of University Hospitals Vision 2010 Program. Democracy Collborative. 2013. Available at: https://www.colab.mit.edu/resources-1/2013/2/1/the-anchor-mission-leveraging-the-power-of-anchor-institutions-to-build-community-wealth-a-case-study-of-university-hospitals-vision-2010-program-cleveland-ohio. Accessed 2 September, 2022.

16. Rubin V, Rose K. Strategies for strengthening anchor institutions' community impact. PolicyLink. 2015. Available at: https://www.policylink.org/resources-tools/strategies-for-strengthening-anchor-institutions. Accessed 29 August, 2022.

17. Burmahl B. Hospitals reduce their carbon footprints with Sustainable Solutions. Health Facilities Management. Available at: https://www.hfmmagazine.com/articles/4274-hospitals-reduce-their-carbon-footprints-with-sustainable-solutions. Published August 31, 2021. Accessed 22 September, 2022.

18. Seattle Children's commitment to sustainability strengthens with signing of HHS Health Care Sector Pledge. Available at https://www.seattlechildrens.org/media/press-releases/Seattle-childrens-commitment-to-sustainability-strengthens-with-signing-of-hhs-health-care-sector-pledge/. Accessed 18 December, 2022.

19. Office of the Assistant Secretary for Health (OASH). HHS launches pledge initiative to mobilize health care sector to reduce emissions. Available at: https://www.hhs.gov/about/news/2022/04/22/hhs-launches-pledge-initiative-mobilize-health-care-sector-reduce-emissions.html. April 22 2022. Accessed 18 December, 2022.

20. Kelleher K, Reece J, Sandel M. The Healthy Neighborhood, healthy families initiative. Pediatrics 2018;142(3). https://doi.org/10.1542/peds.2018-0261.

21. Zuckerman, D., Parker, K. Resources for the Anchor Mission: Place-based Investing. 2017. Available at: https://healthcareanchor.network/2019/11/place-based-investing/. Accessed 2 September, 2022.

22. Rush makes First Impact Investment. Available at: https://www.rush.edu/news/rush-makes-first-impact-investment September 19 2017. Accessed 18 December, 2022.

23. Our commitment to anti-racism - Seattle Children's. Seattle Children's Hospital. Available at: https://www.seattlechildrens.org/about/commitment-anti-racism/. Accessed 1 November, 2022.

24. Olszewski AE, Adiele A, Patneaude A, et al. The Health Equity Impact Assessment: A Case Study in covid-19 visitor policy. Hosp Pediatr 2021. https://doi.org/10.1542/hpeds.2021-006128.

25. Equity Impact Review Tool-University of Washington. Available at: equity-impact-assessment.pdf (seattlechildrens.org). Accessed 1 October, 2022.

26. Careers - Seattle children's. Seattle Children's Hospital. Available at: https://www.seattlechildrens.org/careers/. Accessed 1 October, 2022.

27. Center for Diversity and Health Equity (CDHE) - Seattle Children's. Seattle Children's Hospital. Available at: https://www.seattlechildrens.org/clinics/diversity-health-equity/. Accessed 1 October, 2022.

28. Careers, Educational and Training Opportunities at Seattle Children's Research Institute. Seattle Children's Hospital. https://www.seattlechildrens.org/research/research-institute/careers/. Accessed 2 October, 2022.

29. A Guide for Neighborhood Revitalization - Netter Center for Community. 2008. Available at: http://www.nettercenter.upenn.edu/sites/default/files/Anchor_Toolkit6_09.pdf. Accessed 2 September7, 2022.

30. Eniasivam A, Pereira L, Dzeng E. A call for restorative and transformative justice approaches to anti-racism in medicine. J Gen Intern Med 2022;37(10):2335–6. https://doi.org/10.1007/s11606-022-07605-2.

Special Topics

Pediatric Primary-Care Integrated Behavioral Health

A Framework for Reducing Inequities in Behavioral Health Care and Outcomes for Children

Maria J. Arrojo, MA[a,b], Jonas Bromberg, PsyD[a,b,c],
Heather J. Walter, MD, MPH[a,b,c], Louis Vernacchio, MD, MSc[a,b,c],*

KEYWORDS

- Behavioral health • Primary care • Pediatrics • Health disparities

KEY POINTS

- Behavioral health (BH) disorders are common among children and adolescents, with a substantially greater risk among racial/ethnic minorities, LGBTQ+ youth, and socio-economically disadvantaged children.
- The current specialty pediatric BH workforce is inadequate to meet the need and is mal-distributed, leading to further disparities in access to care.
- Integrating BH care into the pediatric primary care medical home has the potential to reduce disparities in BH care and outcomes for vulnerable children through a preventive focus, universal screening, and early intervention.
- Integrating BH care into pediatric primary care will require overcoming barriers such as clinician training, organization of primary care practices, and funding but early experiences are demonstrating integration to be feasible and fruitful.

CASE PRESENTATION

Keysha, a 6-year-old Black girl of Puerto Rican descent presents along with her single mother to her pediatrician for a well-child visit in a busy suburban practice.[a] After the

[a] Pediatric Physicians' Organization at Children's, 112 Worcester Street, Suite 300, Wellesley, MA 02481, USA; [b] Boston Children's Hospital, 300 Longwood Avenue, Boston, MA 02115, USA; [c] Harvard Medical School, 25 Shattuck Street, Boston, MA 02115, USA
* Corresponding author. 112 Worcester Street, Suite 300, Wellesley, MA 02481.
E-mail address: louis.vernacchio@childrens.harvard.edu

[a] Actual case used with permission; names and other specific clinical details have been modified to protect patient confidentiality.

Pediatr Clin N Am 70 (2023) 775–789
https://doi.org/10.1016/j.pcl.2023.04.004
0031-3955/23/© 2023 Elsevier Inc. All rights reserved.

pediatric.theclinics.com

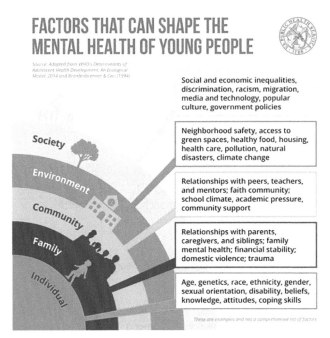

Fig. 1. Factors that can shape the mental health of young people. (*From Protecting Youth Mental Health: The U.S. Surgeon General's Advisory.* https://pubmed.ncbi.nlm.nih.gov/34982518/.)

pediatrician addresses the child's general health, medical issues, immunizations, and routine screenings, the mother mentions that Keysha has been very worried about school, experiencing frequent abdominal pain and headaches, and sneaking into the mother's bed in the middle of the night. The pediatrician feels that the child's symptoms are most likely manifestations of anxiety and suggests that the child could benefit from counseling. She provides the mother with a list of child therapists in the area and instructs her to call their offices to see if they are accepting new patients and if they take the family's health insurance. An appointment is made for next year's annual checkup and the pediatrician tells the mother to return sooner if the child is not doing well. *How could a pediatric primary care clinician (PCC) be equipped to respond more effectively to this mother's concerns?*

THE YOUTH BEHAVIORAL HEALTH CRISIS AND ITS DISPARITIES

According to the US Centers for Disease Control and Prevention, optimal behavioral health (BH) in childhood is characterized by the achievement of developmental and emotional milestones, healthy social development, and effective coping skills allowing children and adolescents to have a positive quality of life and function well at home, in school, and in their communities (**Fig. 1**).[1] BH disorders are characterized by significant changes in the way children typically learn, behave, or handle their emotions, which cause distress and affect daily functioning. Such disorders are associated with health risks throughout the life course.[2,3]

It has been estimated that 1 in 5 children and adolescents experience a BH disorder each year, 2 in 5 by the age of 18 years; one-half of BH disorders have an onset before the age of 14 years.[2,4] During the past 2 decades, data have indicated that the prevalence of youth BH disorders has been increasing, including severe presentations leading to emergency department visits and suicide attempts.[5,6]

Although children in all sociodemographic groups are affected by BH disorders, studies show increased rates of BH disorders and poorer outcomes for racial/ethnic minorities,[2,7] lesbian, gay, transgender, queer (LGBTQ+) youth,[8–10] poor children,[11] and those with developmental disabilities.[12] Rates of suicide among Black youth have increased faster than in any other racial/ethnic group in the past 2 decades, with suicide rates in Black males aged 10 to 19 years increasing by 60%. Early adolescent Black youth are twice as likely to die by suicide as compared with their White counterparts, with those belonging to more than one minoritized group significantly increasing suicide risk.[13]

Reasons for these disparities are complex and occur at many levels ranging from individual factors to broad societal constructs. Some of the most important factors emerging from recent research are the effects of adverse childhood experiences, including exposure to violence, lack of supportive community resources, and individual and structural racism and other forms of bias.[14–16] For example, BH disorders in Black youth are often under recognized and/or undertreated; when they do come to clinical attention, Black youth are more often diagnosed with behavioral problems rather than other diagnosable BH conditions, and they are less likely to receive follow-up care after discharge from crisis or hospital services.[13]

CORONAVIRUS DISEASE 2019 AND YOUTH MENTAL HEALTH

Since early 2020, the coronavirus disease 2019 pandemic has had additional negative effects on youth mental health, especially on those with preexisting vulnerabilities. Reports indicate a general deterioration,[17] with increases in anxiety and depression symptoms[18] and suicidality.[19,20] The pandemic seems to have taken a disproportionate toll on children with developmental disabilities,[21] minority communities,[22] and LGBTQ+ youth,[23] with the longer term effects still to be determined. For example, nearly 1 in 5 transgender and nonbinary youth attempted suicide in the past year, with LGBTQ+ youth of color reporting higher rates than their White peers and Native/Indigenous youth reporting the highest rates.[24]

Recognizing these trends, the American Academy of Pediatrics (AAP), American Academy of Child and Adolescent Psychiatry (AACAP), and Children's Hospital Association jointly declared a national emergency in children's mental health[25] and the US Surgeon General issued a call to action,[26] together outlining the long-standing challenges and the unprecedented impacts the pandemic has had on the mental health of America's youth.

KEY DRIVERS OF DISPARITIES IN BEHAVIORAL HEALTH CARE

Within this context, there is a broad recognition that the current BH workforce (primarily child and adolescent psychiatrists [CAP] and therapists trained to treat young people) is inadequate to address the needs of affected children and adolescents; indeed, fewer than one-half of children diagnosed with BH disorders currently receive care.[4,27] Lack of access is a key factor in the disparities in BH care and outcomes. For example, minority children have significantly lower BH utilization compared with their White counterparts despite suffering greater burden of BH disorders.[2,7,28] Similarly, LGBTQ+ youth are less frequently able to access needed BH services.[24] Furthermore, the uneven distribution of BH specialists ensures that children living in poverty and in rural areas are significantly disadvantaged.[29–31]

In addition, structural aspects such as racism, bias, and discrimination result in worse BH and lack of effective care among disadvantaged youth.[32–34] Socio-cultural factors, particularly stigma associated with seeking BH care, health literacy, not perceiving the need for BH treatment, and not knowing where to seek treatment, may also play a role in some vulnerable children not receiving needed BH care.[35] Finally, a range of institutional factors including insurance coverage, cost, transportation, childcare availability, openings for services at specialty BH centers, ability to attend appointments during working hours, and cultural mismatch with caregivers, may provide barriers to care for youth with BH needs.[36] As an example, Latinx youth as a group have lower incomes, less insurance coverage, and less years of formal education than non-Latinx Whites, resulting in increased structural barriers to care. They also perceive greater barriers to engage in specialty BH care than non-Latinx White patients.[36]

RATIONALE FOR INTEGRATION OF BEHAVIORAL HEALTH CARE INTO PEDIATRIC PRIMARY CARE

Given the high prevalence of youth BH disorders, the inadequacy of the specialty workforce, and the disparities in access to care for disadvantaged youth, providing BH care in the primary care medical home has been proposed as a solution for several decades.[37–39] Although the pace of change had been slow, largely due to lack of training, time, and reimbursement,[40] there are signs that momentum is being gained.[41–43] With progress, there is hope that such integration could help mitigate disparities in BH care for more vulnerable children for a variety of reasons.

First, approximately 95% of US children currently have health insurance—the highest proportion in US history—and the gap in insurance coverage between minority and nonminority individuals is closing.[44,45] Preventive health-care services are covered without copays by the Affordable Care Act. As a result, most children have at least one visit to their PCC annually,[46] and many have a long-term trusting relationship with their PCC, providing an opportunity to detect and treat BH problems earlier in their course. Indeed, PCCs are often the first access point for children with BH concerns.[47]

Moreover, although the specialty BH system is focused largely on diagnosis and management of symptomatic BH disorders, PCCs are in a unique position to detect subclinical signs of BH problems through screening, an activity which has always been fundamental to pediatric primary care. PCCs are accustomed to screening for a variety of conditions (eg, developmental disorders, vision/hearing problems, lead poisoning, and so forth), so incorporating the processes of universal BH screening is a natural fit. Indeed, current projects support the feasibility of this approach (**Box 1**).[48,49] Universality of screening is critical to disparity reduction as more vulnerable patients/families may be less apt to volunteer BH concerns; selective screening has the potential to be restigmatizing and to reinforce biases. Screening should also incorporate knowledge about the effects of adverse childhood experiences and trauma—including trauma experienced within the health-care system—and protective childhood experiences as well which may mitigate the effects of trauma.[26] An emerging specific area of screening relates to suicide, a leading cause of death among adolescents, with substantially higher rates among minority and LGTBQ+ youth.[50] Although not currently recommended by the US Preventive Services Task Force because of insufficient evidence,[51] the AAP,[52] AACAP,[53] and the American

---

Box 1
Examples of behavioral health screening instruments commonly used in pediatric primary care settings (acronyms)

Postnatal Period
  Edinburgh Post-Natal Depression Scale (EPDS)
  Patient Health Questionnaire-2 or Patient Health Questionnaire-9 for parents (PHQ-2, PHQ-9)

Infants and Young Children
  Ages and Stages: Social-Emotional (ASQ:SE)
  Parents' Evaluation of Developmental Status (PEDS)
  Pediatric Symptom Checklist (PSC)
  Survey of Well-being of Young Children (SWYC)

Adolescents and Young Adults
  Ask Suicide Screening Questions (ASQ)
  Generalized Anxiety Disorder-7 (GAD-7)
  Patient Health Questionnaire-4 (PHQ-4)
  Patient Health Questionnaire-9 (PHQ-9)
  Pediatric Symptom Checklist (PSC)

Psychological Association[54] have all advocated for universal suicide screening for youth. The effect of universal screening on suicide disparities remains to be studied.

For screening to be of value, a path to further evaluation and treatment needs to be in place. Traditionally, PCCs who identified BH problems would attempt to refer patients to the specialty BH setting; however, many never received care, with disadvantaged children even less likely to do so.[55–57] Thus has emerged the clear imperative for integrating BH services into the primary care setting and for developing models for successful integration.

Additionally, understanding racial/ethnic and cultural considerations around administering and addressing screenings, and discussing preferences for services, is crucial to implement effective screening processes. There are limited studies available validating standard BH screening instruments within minority samples, and patients and families from diverse backgrounds might experience screening practices in different ways. Factors that influence provider–patient communication such as language, acculturation, and trust have been found to influence patient preferences for addressing BH concerns in primary care,[58] suggesting there is need for more studies that examine BH screening tools and practices within diverse populations.

THE CONTINUUM OF INTEGRATED BEHAVIORAL HEALTH CARE

Successful integration of BH services into pediatric primary care and, with it, the hope of mitigating disparities in BH care and outcomes for vulnerable children, requires a model of collaborative care between PCCs and BH specialists. The most widely adopted conceptual model describing this activity come from the Substance Abuse and Mental Health Services Administration's (SAMHSA) collaborative care spectrum (**Fig. 2**).[59] Although not proven, it seems likely that higher levels of integration hold the greatest promise for minimizing disparities in care as lower levels would not fully ameliorate the barriers to care and undesirable outcomes described earlier.

HOW INTEGRATED CARE CAN REDUCE BEHAVIORAL HEALTH DISPARITIES

Despite guidance and tools provided by the AAP and AACAP, PCCs continue to experience considerable challenges managing BH problems in the primary care setting, consistently citing lack of training, lack of confidence in their knowledge and skills,

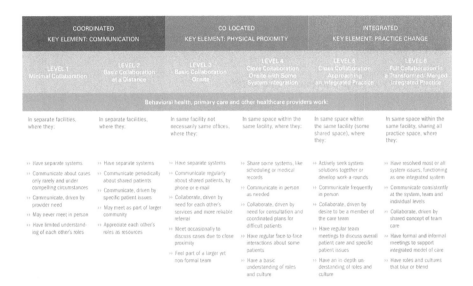

Fig. 2. Continuum of integrated behavioral health care. (*From* Standard Framework for Levels of Integrated Care - National Council for Mental Wellbeing. https://www. thenationalcouncil.org/resources/standard-framework-for-levels-of-integrated-care/.)

and administrative barriers (eg, time, space, and inadequate reimbursement).[40] Enhancing PCC expertise and confidence to identify and manage BH conditions will require substantial retraining of the current pediatric clinician workforce, which is largely not trained in BH care. Although the AAP has published specific mental health competencies for pediatric practice[60] and the American Board of Pediatrics has delineated a specific training milestone pertaining to BH,[61] surveys demonstrate ongoing gaps in PCCs BH preparedness.[62]

Besides training, access to psychiatric consultation with CAPs is also key to enhancing the ability of PCCs to provide BH care. Consultation includes advice about diagnosis, medication management, and level of care, and sometimes may involve face-to-face consultation with the patient, whether virtually or in-person. It is important to highlight, however, that significant disparities exist in access to virtual care. Therefore, flexibility for families and expanding access to BH care in all forms is necessary to eliminate disparities especially for rural, and underresourced urban communities, and immigrants, among others.[63,64]

Integrating behavioral health clinicians (BHCs; typically psychologists, licensed clinical social workers, licensed mental health counselors, and licensed marriage and family therapists) directly into primary care also has the potential to better manage BH problems in the primary care setting by providing PCCs with the support needed to deliver BH services and by substantially extending the BH workforce (**Fig. 3**).[65] Integrated BHCs can provide timely access to BH care in a "one-stop shop," without delays or external referrals, thereby making BH interventions more readily available to the largest number of children. They can also help reduce mental health stigma, enhance care coordination, improve communication between patients and providers, and increase sensitivity in addressing the health needs of diverse patients, thereby reaching individuals with BH needs who otherwise may not receive care.[36,65] Integrated BHCs can use population health approaches, tailor evidenced-based

IBH Roles, Conceptualized

BCH (Behavioral Health Clinician)	• Master Social Work, Doctor Philosophy/Doctor Psychology, Mental Health Counselor, Marriage Family Therapist, Substance Abuse Counselor
CPC (Consulting Psychiatric Clinician)	• Psychiatric Medical Doctor/Osteopathic Doctor, Psychiatric Nurse Practitioner, Psychiatric Advanced Practice Nurse, Psychiatric Physician Assistant
CE (Care Enhancer)	• Bachelor Social Work, Medical Assistant, Care Manager, Care Coordinator, Health Coach, Community Health Worker, Patient Educator, Patient Advocate, Navigator, Registered Nurse, Bachelor Science Nurse

Fig. 3. Integrated behavioral health roles. (Alexander Blount, EdD, Who Will Provide Integrated Care: Assessing The Workforce For The Integration Of Behavioral Health And Primary Care In Nh, 10/2016. Retrieved from: https://www.nhpcbhworkforce.org/resources.)

interventions to a variety of presentations and acuity levels, and support parents in providing a nurturing environment for children to thrive while minimizing the stigma often associated with seeking BH care.[66]

BARRIERS TO INTEGRATED BEHAVIORAL HEALTH CARE

Despite the value of integrating BH care into the primary care setting, integrated care faces significant barriers to implementation including financial, operational, and clinical issues. For example, although the current medical reimbursement system has allowed the integration of BHCs into pediatric primary care to be financially sustainable in at least some instances,[49] start-up costs and infrastructural support outside practices (eg, at the health system or organizational level) still pose financial barriers to integrating BHCs into practice more widely. Pediatricians wishing to integrate BH care into their practices who do not have the support of an integrated network may seek support from local pediatric academic medical centers or their local chapter of the AAP. Continued advocacy is also needed for true reimbursement parity for BH care compared with traditional medical care.

Another key barrier has been difficulty in developing successful interprofessional collaboration,[67] which is not supported by the current organizational structure of most primary care practices and not aligned with the way mental health treatment is traditionally delivered.[47,68] Furthermore, professional education is typically siloed, with medical and BH professionals having little interaction. Interprofessional education, especially when delivered early in both the PCC and BHC professional careers, has the potential to break down those siloes and build team-based skills that transcend models and practice sites, and prepare the workforce to deliver culturally effective care.[69] There is evidence that professionals who are educated in collaborative care approaches can improve access and quality of care for children with BH needs,[65] with positive patient satisfaction.[70]

Effectively expanding the scope of pediatric primary care to include BH care that reduces disparities would also include diversifying the workforce, using strategies to attract individuals from diverse gender, cultural, and linguistic backgrounds representative of the communities in which patients live. Ensuring diversity in the workforce is important to enhancing trust between providers and individuals from underserved populations, such as individuals with disabilities, communities of color, and LGBTQ+ individuals, and is essential to promoting delivery of culturally competent care. To generate a more diverse workforce initiatives are needed early in the pipeline; to this end, SAMHSA has developed the Minority Fellowship Program open to those pursuing master's or doctoral degrees in BH fields.[71]

The effort to diversify the workforce could include the use of care enhancers, nonclinical primary care staff who augment care and communication between patients and providers.[72] Care enhancers can improve patient engagement and adherence, address health literacy, enhance communication with the health-care team, and increase capacity to meet the social needs of patients, while contributing to lower clinician burn-out.[67] Care enhancers can also help patients navigate the health system, overcome structural barriers to care, and help bridge care to the community.[73] When performed by individuals with similar cultural backgrounds and/or lived experiences to patients and families, these roles can further improve engagement and reduce disparities.[73] Unfortunately, there is currently no clear pathway for financial sustainability of care enhancers in pediatric primary care, an area for future policy consideration and research.

ADDRESSING STRUCTURAL CAUSES OF BEHAVIORAL HEALTH DISPARITIES

Although integrating BH care into pediatric primary care holds great promise to mitigate disparities in BH care and outcomes for disadvantage children and adolescents, the larger societal causes of inequality remain powerful drivers of disparities. Moreover, although governmental policy, social action, and other levels of effort are necessary to address such issues, health care organizations can play an important role in larger equity efforts. To this end, The Institute for Health Improvement has provided guidance on how health care organizations can help reduce overall health disparities, including suggestions to measure disparities, select outcomes to track, and educate staff on key equity issues.[74]

Furthermore, addressing individual and institutional bias with health care institutions, whether implicit or explicit, is essential to advancing health equity.[75] The AACAP, among others, has acknowledged the role of medicine, psychiatry, and psychology in dismantling racism and advancing health equity in education, science, and health and have developed antiracism resources for health professionals.[76] Organizations can develop processes to assess bias in care delivery, such as reviewing procedural barriers to care (eg, inconvenient office hours for working parents, written materials not suited for patients' languages and literacy levels), and can also assess patient and family perspectives of care. Additionally, health-care institutions can partner with community organizations that focus on social determinants of health and reducing disparities. Such partnerships can help deploy specific strategies through which health care organizations can have a direct impact[74] and could facilitate developing a culturally representative health care workforce.[67]

A VISION FOR THE FUTURE OF PEDIATRIC INTEGRATED BEHAVIORAL HEALTH CARE

If the vision of BH integration highlighted in this article were to come to fuller fruition, BH care would be experienced as integral to all of pediatric health care in a way that infuses all care with BH principles.[68] BH issues would be treated in the same way as "physical health" issues, normalizing them and removing the stigma often associated with them.

With truly integrated BH care, during routine well-child visits starting from infancy, preventive BH services in the form of parenting support and resilience building would be part of anticipatory guidance, along with screening for and responding to parental BH issues and adverse childhood experiences. As children mature, anticipatory guidance would include coaching on stress management, risk reduction, and healthy lifestyle choices to support optimal BH, focusing especially on key touchpoints during which the developing mind is particularly vulnerable to factors such as poverty and adversity. Implementing a team-based approach to well-child care that adds nonclinical roles such as care enhancers to the team and takes advantage of services in the community setting could provide culturally relevant supports and better meet the needs of families living at the intersection of poverty, racism, and discrimination.[77]

At routine well-child visits and other key life moments such as after health events or family disruptions, culturally responsive, nonstigmatizing, and trauma-informed screening for BH concerns would be conducted with special attention to the crucial issue of depression and suicidality in teens and young adults.

When screens are positive for BH concerns, they would be immediately addressed by PCCs in concert with integrated BHCs without requiring additional visits and with minimal barriers to follow-up care. When more significant concerns are discovered through screening or volunteered by patient/families, PCCs would be comfortable conducting focused assessments, making provisional diagnoses, and initiating treatment, both in the form of psychological support in conjunction with integrated BHCs and through basic psychopharmacology. Patients and families would also be connected with appropriate community resources to assist in their care. When more severe BH issues develop, PCCs would have access to prompt CAP consultation with the choice to manage patients themselves with CAP support or refer patients to specialty care when necessary. Patients receiving specialty BH care would be transitioned back to primary care with excellent two-way communication when conditions are stabilized, permitting access for other patients to the specialty BH system.

This approach can only be possible under a whole-person, integrated care system with appropriate organization and financial support that does not discriminate between physical health and BH and adds social care into the equation. It requires a committed team trained to provide interprofessional high-quality care free of bias and discrimination, working effectively together to provide *the right care, at the right time, at the right place* equitably to all children.

CASE PRESENTATION, CONTINUED

Fortunately, Keysha was a patient of a pediatrician who had integrated BH within her practice. In response to the identified concerns, the pediatrician explained to Keysha and her mother that an integrated BHC could provide an immediate BH consultation and follow-up care within the primary care practice under the same insurance coverage the child has for her routine medical care. The pediatrician introduced Keysha and her mother to one of the practice's integrated BHCs with a warm handoff. While the pediatrician moved on to her next patient visit, the BHC began a focused BH assessment, and once assured that there were no immediate safety concerns, reviewed some coping strategies for Keysha and her mother and offered a follow-up visit to further evaluate and treat the child's anxiety. After a few visits with the BHC, the mother reported: "I think it is amazing that they have a BHC available in the doctor's office. Many different factors play like being in one location, transportation, familiarity. It is just a lot more comfortable in this setting. I was allowed to ask questions to get familiar with it. And the BHC was introduced by the doctor so it was way more comfortable. I appreciated being able to communicate with both the pediatrician and the BHC at the same time instead of waiting for an appointment. It was continuous care, very convenient; it is about the convenience of timing and the comfortability. There was no time lapse. I think it is definitely a benefit to have a BHC in the doctor's office. My daughter definitely looks forward to come to the doctor's office!"

CLINICS CARE POINTS

Get support
- Investigate what education, resources, and assistance your local academic medical center or professional organizations offer

Understand the scope of what you can accomplish for your patients and care team
- Survey your patients and care team about what they need
- Prioritize which population needs to address first
- Be mindful that every care team member starts in a different place when it comes to comfort and expertise

Start small
- Understand what BH resources already exist in your community and build collaborations
- Hire a care enhancer or peer support specialist

Build a team
- Hire a BHC; seed funding may be available through your integrated network or local grants
- Identify a PCC to serve as BH champion and drive transformation
- Form a BH integration team from all the roles in the practice and hold regular integration team meetings to design and implement integrated workflows

Measure success
- Select process and outcome measures to track; include equity measures
- Assess patient and team satisfaction
- Commit to continuous process improvement

Take care of your team
- Engage with others doing similar work for education, ideas, and support
- Show appreciation to your team; build reward system for achieving benchmarks

DISCLOSURE

The authors have nothing to disclose.

REFERENCES

1. Centers for Disease Control and Prevention. What is Children's Mental Health? Available at: https://www.cdc.gov/childrensmentalhealth/basics.html. Accessed April 30, 2023.
2. Bitsko RH, Claussen AH, Lichstein J, et al. Mental Health Surveillance Among Children - United States, 2013-2019. MMWR Suppl 2022;71(2). https://doi.org/10.15585/mmwr.su7102a1.
3. Copeland WE, Wolke D, Shanahan L, et al. Adult functional outcomes of common childhood psychiatric problems a prospective, longitudinal study. JAMA Psychiatr 2015. https://doi.org/10.1001/jamapsychiatry.2015.0730.
4. Whitney DG, Peterson MD. US National and State-Level Prevalence of Mental Health Disorders and Disparities of Mental Health Care Use in Children. JAMA Pediatr 2019;173(4):389–91.

5. Kalb LG, Stapp EK, Ballard ED, et al. Trends in Psychiatric Emergency Department Visits Among Youth and Young Adults in the US. Pediatrics 2019;143(4). https://doi.org/10.1542/PEDS.2018-2192.
6. Garnett MF, Curtin SC, Stone DM. Suicide Mortality in the United States, 2000-2020. NCHS Data Brief. 2022;(433):1-8. Available at: https://pubmed.ncbi.nlm.nih.gov/35312475/. Accessed September 23, 2022.
7. Cummings JR, Ji X, Lally C, et al. Racial and Ethnic Differences in Minimally Adequate Depression Care Among Medicaid-Enrolled Youth. J Am Acad Child Adolesc Psychiatry 2019;58(1):128–38.
8. Fox KR, Choukas-Bradley S, Salk RH, et al. Mental health among sexual and gender minority adolescents: Examining interactions with race and ethnicity. J Consult Clin Psychol 2020;88(5). https://doi.org/10.1037/CCP0000486.
9. Raifman J, Charlton BM, Arrington-Sanders R, et al. Sexual Orientation and Suicide Attempt Disparities Among US Adolescents: 2009-2017. Pediatrics 2020;(3): 145. https://doi.org/10.1542/PEDS.2019-1658.
10. di Giacomo E, Krausz M, Colmegna F, et al. Estimating the Risk of Attempted Suicide Among Sexual Minority Youths: A Systematic Review and Meta-analysis. JAMA Pediatr 2018;172(12):1145–52.
11. Reiss F. Socioeconomic inequalities and mental health problems in children and adolescents: A systematic review. Soc Sci Med 2013;90. https://doi.org/10.1016/j.socscimed.2013.04.026.
12. Einfeld SL, Ellis LA, Emerson E. Comorbidity of intellectual disability and mental disorder in children and adolescents: a systematic review. J Intellect Dev Disabil 2011;36(2):137–43.
13. AACAP Policy Statement on Increased Suicide Among Black Youth in the U.S. Available at: https://www.aacap.org/AACAP/Policy_Statements/2022/AACAP_Policy_Statement_Increased_Suicide_Among_Black_Youth_US.aspx. Accessed November 27, 2022.
14. Shonkoff JP, Garner AS, Siegel BS, et al. The lifelong effects of early childhood adversity and toxic stress. Pediatrics 2012;129(1). https://doi.org/10.1542/peds.2011-2663.
15. Shonkoff JP, Slopen N, Williams DR. Early Childhood Adversity, Toxic Stress, and the Impacts of Racism on the Foundations of Health. Annu Rev Public Health 2021;42:115–34.
16. Hughes K, Bellis MA, Hardcastle KA, et al. The effect of multiple adverse childhood experiences on health: a systematic review and meta-analysis. Lancet Public Health 2017;2(8). https://doi.org/10.1016/S2468-2667(17)30118-4.
17. Hawke LD, Barbic S, Voineskos A, et al. Impacts of COVID-19 on Youth Mental Health, Substance Use, and Wellbeing: A Rapid Survey of Clinical and Community Samples. SSRN Electron J 2020. https://doi.org/10.2139/ssrn.3586702.
18. Racine N, McArthur BA, Cooke JE, et al. Global Prevalence of Depressive and Anxiety Symptoms in Children and Adolescents during COVID-19: A Meta-analysis. JAMA Pediatr 2021;175(11). https://doi.org/10.1001/jamapediatrics.2021.2482.
19. Zima BT, Bussing R. THE EARLY IMPACT OF THE COVID-19 PANDEMIC ON CHILD MENTAL HEALTH SERVICE UTILIZATION AND DISPARITIES IN CARE. J Am Acad Child Adolesc Psychiatry 2021;60(10). https://doi.org/10.1016/j.jaac.2021.07.694.
20. Yard E, Radhakrishnan L, Ballesteros MF, et al. Emergency Department Visits for Suspected Suicide Attempts Among Persons Aged 12-25 Years Before and During the COVID-19 Pandemic — United States, January 2019-May 2021. MMWR

Recomm Rep (Morb Mortal Wkly Rep) 2021;70(24). https://doi.org/10.15585/mmwr.mm7024e1.

21. 2021 Progress Report: The Impact of COVID-19 on People with Disabilities | NCD.gov. Available at: https://ncd.gov/progressreport/2021/2021-progress-report. Accessed September 23, 2022.

22. Hillis SD, Blenkinsop A, Villaveces A, et al. COVID-19-Associated Orphanhood and Caregiver Death in the United States. Pediatrics 2021;148(6). https://doi.org/10.1542/peds.2021-053760.

23. Perl L, Oren A, Klein Z, et al. Effects of the COVID19 Pandemic on Transgender and Gender Non-Conforming Adolescents' Mental Health. Psychiatry Res 2021;302. https://doi.org/10.1016/j.psychres.2021.114042.

24. The Trevor Project: 2022 National Survey on LGBTQ Youth Mental Health. Available at: https://www.thetrevorproject.org/survey-2022/. Accessed September 24, 2022.

25. AAP-AACAP-CHA Declaration of a National Emergency in Child and Adolescent Mental Health. Available at: https://www.aap.org/en/advocacy/child-and-adolescent-healthy-mental-development/aap-aacap-cha-declaration-of-a-national-emergency-in-child-and-adolescent-mental-health/. Accessed September 23, 2022.

26. Office of the Surgeon General. Protecting Youth Mental Health: The U.S. Surgeon General's Advisory. 2021.

27. Ghandour RM, Sherman LJ, Vladutiu CJ, et al. Prevalence and Treatment of Depression, Anxiety, and Conduct Problems in US Children. J Pediatr 2019; 206:256–67.e3.

28. Marrast L, Himmelstein DU, Woolhandler S. Racial and Ethnic Disparities in Mental Health Care for Children and Young Adults: A National Study. Int J Health Serv 2016;46(4):810–24.

29. Health Resources and Services Administration. State-Level Projections of Supply and Demand for Behavioral Health Occupations: 2016-2030. Published online 2016. Available at: https://bhw.hrsa.gov/national-center-health-workforce-analysis. Accessed September 24, 2022.

30. Severe Shortage of Child and Adolescent Psychiatrists Illustrated in AACAP Workforce Maps. Available at: https://www.aacap.org/AACAP/zLatest_News/Severe_Shortage_Child_Adolescent_Psychiatrists_Illustrated_AACAP_Workforce_Maps.aspx. Accessed September 24, 2022.

31. McBain RK, Cantor JH, Kofner A, et al. Ongoing Disparities in Digital and In-Person Access to Child Psychiatric Services in the United States. J Am Acad Child Adolesc Psychiatry 2022;61(7):926–33.

32. Bernard DL, Calhoun CD, Banks DE, et al. Making the "C-ACE" for a Culturally-Informed Adverse Childhood Experiences Framework to Understand the Pervasive Mental Health Impact of Racism on Black Youth. J Child Adolesc Trauma 2020;14(2):233–47.

33. Bailey ZD, Feldman JM, Bassett MT. How Structural Racism Works — Racist Policies as a Root Cause of U.S. Racial Health Inequities. N Engl J Med 2021;384(8):768–73.

34. Hatzenbuehler ML, Pachankis JE. Stigma and Minority Stress as Social Determinants of Health Among Lesbian, Gay, Bisexual, and Transgender Youth: Research Evidence and Clinical Implications. Pediatr Clin North Am 2016; 63(6):985–97.

35. Abdullah T, Brown TL. Mental illness stigma and ethnocultural beliefs, values, and norms: an integrative review. Clin Psychol Rev 2011;31(6):934–48.

36. Anastasia EA, Guzman LE, Bridges AJ. Barriers to Integrated Primary Care and Specialty Mental Health Services: Perspectives From Latinx and Non-Latinx White Primary Care Patients. Psychol Serv 2022. https://doi.org/10.1037/ser0000639.
37. Green M, Brazelton TB, Friedman DB, et al. Pediatrics and the Psychosocial Aspects of Child and Family Health. Pediatrics 1982;70(1):126–7.
38. American Academy of Pediatrics Committee on Psychosocial Aspects of Child and Family Health. The pediatrician and the "new morbidity". Pediatrics 1993; 92(5):731–3.
39. Foy JM, Carmichael T, Duncan P, et al. Improving mental health services in primary care: reducing administrative and financial barriers to access and collaboration. Pediatrics 2009;123(4):1248–51.
40. Horwitz SMC, Storfer-Isser A, Kerker BD, et al. Barriers to the Identification and Management of Psychosocial Problems: Changes From 2004 to 2013. Acad Pediatr 2015;15(6):613–20.
41. Asarnow JR, Rozenman M, Wiblin J, et al. Integrated Medical-Behavioral Care Compared With Usual Primary Care for Child and Adolescent Behavioral Health: A Meta-analysis. JAMA Pediatr 2015;169(10):929–37.
42. Richardson LP, McCarty CA, Radovic A, et al. Research in the Integration of Behavioral Health for Adolescents and Young Adults in Primary Care Settings: A Systematic Review. J Adolesc Health 2017;60(3):261–9.
43. Yonek J, Lee CM, Harrison A, et al. Key Components of Effective Pediatric Integrated Mental Health Care Models: A Systematic Review. JAMA Pediatr 2020; 174(5):487–98.
44. Keisler-Starkey K, Bunch LN. Health Insurance Coverage in the United States: 2021 Current Population Reports Acknowledgments.
45. Baumgartner JC, Collins SR, Radley DC. Racial and Ethnic Inequities in Health Care Coverage and Access, 2013-2019.
46. QuickStats. Percentage of Children Aged 18 Years Who Received a Well-Child Checkup in the Past 12 Months, by Age Group and Year — National Health Interview Survey, United States, 2008 and 2018. MMWR Morb Mortal Wkly Rep 2020; 69(8):222.
47. Brino KAS. Pediatric Mental Health and the Power of Primary Care: Practical Approaches and Validating Challenges. J Pediatr Health Care 2020;34(2):e12–20.
48. Savageau JA, Keller D, Willis G, et al. Behavioral Health Screening among Massachusetts Children Receiving Medicaid. J Pediatr 2016;178:261–7.
49. Walter HJ, Vernacchio L, Correa ET, et al. Five-phase replication of behavioral health integration in pediatric primary care. Pediatrics 2021;148(2).
50. Disparities in Suicide | CDC. Available at: https://www.cdc.gov/suicide/facts/disparities-in-suicide.html. Accessed September 25, 2022.
51. U.S. Preventive Services Task Force. Draft Recommendation Statement. Depression and Suicide Risk in Children and Adolescents: Screening. April 12, 2022. . Available at: https://www.uspreventiveservicestaskforce.org/uspstf/draft-recommendation/screening-depression-suicide-risk-children-adolescents#fullrecommendationstart. Accessed April 30, 2023.
52. Screening for Suicide Risk in Clinical Practice. Available at: https://www.aap.org/en/patient-care/blueprint-for-youth-suicide-prevention/strategies-for-clinical-settings-for-youth-suicide-prevention/screening-for-suicide-risk-in-clinical-practice/. Accessed September 25, 2022.
53. American Academy of Child and Adolescent Psychiatry. American Academy of Child and Adolescent Psychiatry. Policy Statement on Suicide Prevention. June 2019. . Available at: https://www.aacap.org/AACAP/Policy_Statements/2019/

AACAP_Policy_Statement_on_Suicide_Prevention.aspx. Accessed April 30, 2023.

54. American Psychological Association. Mental and Behavioral Health. Responding to the US Preventive Services Task Force recommendations on screening for depression and suicide risk in children and adolescents. May 14, 2022. Available at: https://www.apaservices.org/advocacy/news/preventive-depression-suicide-children-adolescents.

55. Bridges AJ, Andrews AR Iii, Villalobos BT, et al. Does Integrated Behavioral Health Care Reduce Mental Health Disparities for Latinos? Initial Findings. J Lat Psychol 2013. https://doi.org/10.1037/lat0000009.

56. Fehr KK, Leraas BC, Littles MMD. Behavioral Health Needs, Barriers, and Parent Preferences in Rural Pediatric Primary Care. J Pediatr Psychol 2020. https://doi.org/10.1093/jpepsy/jsaa057.

57. Ogbeide SA, Landoll RR, Nielsen MK, et al. To go or not go: Patient preference in seeking specialty mental health versus behavioral consultation within the primary care behavioral health consultation model. Fam Syst Health 2018;36(4):513–7.

58. Lewis FJ, Rappleyea D, Didericksen K, et al. Bringing Inclusion Into Pediatric Primary Health Care: A Systematic Review of the Behavioral Health Treatment of Racial and Ethnic Minority Youth. J Pediatr Health Care 2021;35(6):e32–42.

59. Standard Framework for Levels of Integrated Care - National Council for Mental Wellbeing. Available at: https://www.thenationalcouncil.org/resources/standard-framework-for-levels-of-integrated-care/. Accessed September 26, 2022.

60. Foy JM, Green CM, Earls MF. POLICY STATEMENT Organizational Principles to Guide and Define the Child Health Mental Health Competencies for Pediatric Practice. Available at: http://publications.aap.org/pediatrics/article-pdf/144/5/e20192757/1078399/peds_20192757.pdf.

61. Entrustable Professional Activities for General Pediatrics | The American Board of Pediatrics. Available at: https://www.abp.org/content/entrustable-professional-activities-general-pediatrics. Accessed October 10, 2022.

62. Green C, Leyenaar JK, Turner AL, et al. Competency of future pediatricians caring for children with behavioral and mental health problems. Pediatrics 2020;146(1). https://doi.org/10.1542/peds.2019-2884.

63. Egan JE, Corey SL, Henderson ER, et al. Feasibility of a Web-Accessible Game-Based Intervention Aimed at Improving Help Seeking and Coping Among Sexual and Gender Minority Youth: Results From a Randomized Controlled Trial. J Adolesc Health 2021;69(4):604–14.

64. Cates K, Soares N. Need for Integrated Behavior Health Model in Primary Care. Pediatr Clin North Am 2021;68(3):533–40.

65. American Academy of Child and Adolescent Psychiatry (AACAP) Committee on Collaborative and Integrated Care and AACAP Committee on Quality Issues. Clinical update: collaborative mental health care for children and adolescents in pediatric primary care. J Am Acad Child Adolesc Psychiatry 2023;62(2):91–119.

66. Pediatric Group Details the Ways Integrated Care is Poised to Meet the Mental Health Crisis - Collaborative Family Healthcare Association. https://www.cfha.net/pediatric-group-details-the-ways-integrated-care-is-poised-to-meet-the-mental-health-crisis/. [Accessed 2 October 2022]. Accessed.

67. Blount A, Fauth J, Nordstrom A, et al. Assessing the workforce for the integration of behavioral health and primary care in New Hampshire who will provide integrated care? Underwritten by the Endowment for health.

68. Wissow LS, van Ginneken N, Chandna J, et al. Integrating Children's Mental Health into Primary Care. Pediatr Clin North Am 2016;63(1):97–113.
69. Cordes CC. Leveraging interprofessional education to build high functioning teams. Fam Syst Health 2022;40(1):144–6.
70. Petts RA, Lewis RK, Keyondra Brooks M, et al. Examining Patient and Provider Experiences with Integrated Care at a Community Health Clinic. J Behav Health Serv Res 2021;2022–54. https://doi.org/10.1007/s11414-021-09764-2.
71. HHS Roadmap for Behavioral Health Integration | ASPE. Available at: https://aspe.hhs.gov/reports/hhs-roadmap-behavioral-health-integration. Accessed December 2, 2022.
72. Health Equity and Behavioral Health Integration | The Academy. Available at: https://integrationacademy.ahrq.gov/about/integrated-behavioral-health/health-equity. Accessed October 2, 2022.
73. Godoy L, Hodgkinson S, Robertson HA, et al. Increasing mental health engagement from primary care: The potential role of family navigation. Pediatrics 2019;143(4). https://doi.org/10.1542/peds.2018-2418.
74. Wyatt R, Laderman M, Botwinick L, et al. Achieving health equity: a guide for health care organizations. IHI white paper. Cambridge, Massachusetts: Institute for Healthcare Improvement; 2016 (Available at ihi.org).
75. Lavizzo-Mourey RJ, Besser RE, Williams DR. Understanding and Mitigating Health Inequities — Past, Current, and Future Directions. N Engl J Med 2021; 384(18):1681–4.
76. Anti Racism Resource Library. Available at: https://www.aacap.org/AACAP/Families_and_Youth/Resource_Libraries/Racism_Resource_Library.aspx. Accessed December 2, 2022.
77. Liljenquist K, Coker TR. Transforming Well-Child Care to Meet the Needs of Families at the Intersection of Racism and Poverty. Acad Pediatr 2021;21(8):S102–7.

Health Care for Children in Immigrant Families

Key Considerations and Addressing Barriers

Keith J. Martin, DO, MS[a,b], Sarah Polk, MD, ScM[a,b],
Janine Young, MD[c,d], Lisa Ross DeCamp, MD, MSPH[e,f,g,h],*

KEYWORDS

- Immigrants • Limited English proficiency • Health care disparities • Medical home
- Social determinants of health

KEY POINTS

- One in four US children is a child in an immigrant family and children in immigrant families (CIF) have distinct health and health care needs.
- Promoting access to health insurance is fundamental to providing services to CIF.
- The National Standards for Culturally and Linguistically Appropriate Services in Health Care (CLAS standards) issued by the US Department of Health and Human Services stipulate that health care organizations must provide language interpretation and translated documents (eg, consent forms) (**Fig. 1**).
- There are many example programs of expanded medical home services and community-partnerships that address the unmet social determinants of health needs of immigrant families.
- Policy change holds the promise of reducing health and health care disparities experienced by CIF. The 2 leading policy changes that would benefit the health and well-being of children in immigrant families are immigration reform and Medicaid/Medicare for All.

[a] Department of Pediatrics, Johns Hopkins University School of Medicine, Baltimore, MD, USA;
[b] Centro SOL-Center for Salud/Health and Opportunity for Latinos, Johns Hopkins University School of Medicine; [c] Department of Pediatrics University of California San Diego School of Medicine; [d] Rady Children's Hospital San Diego; [e] Children's Hospital Colorado, Aurora, CO, USA; [f] Department of Pediatrics, University of Colorado School of Medicine, Aurora, CO, USA; [g] Adult and Child Center for Outcomes Research and Delivery Science, Aurora, CO, USA; [h] Latino Research and Policy Center, Denver, CO, USA
* Corresponding author. ACCORDS (Adult and Child Center for Health Outcomes Research and Delivery Science) Department of Pediatrics, University of Colorado School of Medicine and Children's Hospital Colorado, 1890 N Revere Ct Third Floor, Mail Stop F443 Aurora, CO 80045, USA.
E-mail address: lisa.decamp@childrenscolorado.org

Pediatr Clin N Am 70 (2023) 791–811
https://doi.org/10.1016/j.pcl.2023.03.011
0031-3955/23/© 2023 Elsevier Inc. All rights reserved.
pediatric.theclinics.com

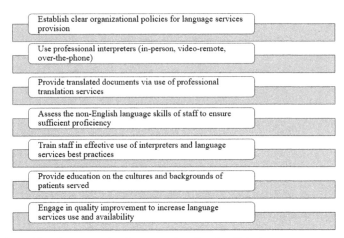

Establish clear organizational policies for language services provision

Use professional interpreters (in-person, video-remote, over-the-phone)

Provide translated documents via use of professional translation services

Assess the non-English language skills of staff to ensure sufficient proficiency

Train staff in effective use of interpreters and language services best practices

Provide education on the cultures and backgrounds of patients served

Engage in quality improvement to increase language services use and availability

Fig. 1. Best practices for managing language barriers in clinical care.

CASE STUDY

Ms M brings her 6- and 9-year-old children to see you for their well-child visit. Ms M has a preferred health care language of Spanish. You communicate with her in Spanish via your status as qualified Spanish/English bilingual provider. Ms M has no pressing concerns today. Both children gained a great deal of weight during the pandemic and now qualify as obese. Mom shares your concern about their weight status, as her mother suffers from type 2 diabetes mellitus. Mom believes that everything is fine at school with the exception that may be her 9-year-old is not reading as well as he should be. Mom reports little contact with school due to language barriers.

On review of social situation, you hear that there are 3 children living at home. You only know the 6- and the 9-year-olds. Mom shares that her 16-year-old son joined the household 3 months ago having traveled to the United States with mom's cousin. The 16-year-old has not shared much about the journey but has been waking up with nightmares and does not want to stay at home alone. The 16-year-old had remained in the care of mom's parents when mom migrated from Honduras to the United States 12 years ago. She and the 16-year-old are very happy to be together again, but there is a lot to figure out—school, health care, mental health support, parenting an adolescent, and establishing a new family dynamic. Mom has been trying to call a local free clinic, as your clinic requires insurance and he is ineligible, but so far efforts to make an appointment have been unsuccessful. Ms M has not been able to reach anyone who speaks Spanish.

At the end of the visit, you connect mom with a community outreach specialist who can enroll the 6- and 9-year-olds in a community-based program to treat childhood obesity and with an English/Spanish bilingual social worker who will help mom connect the 16-year-old to health care and to an after-school program for recently arrived immigrant youth.

INTRODUCTION

One in every four children (more than 18.4 million) in the United States is an immigrant or has at least one immigrant parent. These children have distinct health care needs from other children but there is no formal required clinical training on what many would argue is the field of Immigrant Health. When Immigrant Health topics are covered in medical student or residency curricula at all, they most often are presented under the auspices of "Global Health" or "local Global health," both of which imply that the care of immigrant children and children with immigrant parents is somehow *outside* of the United States and not, in fact, something that is part of the United States, inherently needs to be addressed by the US health care system, and is essential for the promotion of the well-being for children, families, and the community. In this article the authors review the demographics of this population, health trends, recommendations for the care of newly arrived immigrant children, and the care of children in immigrant families over time and review promising practices that provide comprehensive care that meets the sociocultural needs of immigrant families and addresses their social determinants of health needs. This article helps practicing pediatricians adopt practices that address the unique needs of immigrant families and promote health equity for this population.

Section 1: Defining Immigrant Children and Demographic Overview

Defining immigrant children

Immigrant children are those children born outside the United States to non-US citizen parents.[1] Children in immigrant families (CIF) include immigrant children *and* US-born children who have at least 1 parent who is foreign born (**Table 1**).[2] Nonrefugee legal immigrants include lawful permanent residents or "green card" holders who have permission to live and work permanently in the United States. Immigrants who are refugees obtain legal status before arrival to the United States, whereas asylees obtain legal status after arrival. Both refugees and asylees must have a well-founded fear of persecution based on nationality, membership in a particular social group, political opinion, race, religion, or sexual/gender orientation.[3] Undocumented immigrants do not have a federally recognized citizenship or refugee status.[4]

Demographic distribution of immigrants in the United States

In 1850, the United States had 2.2 million immigrants, representing nearly 10% of the total US population (**Fig. 2**).[5] Between 1860 and 1920, the immigrant proportion of the population (vs US native nonimmigrants) was ~14%, peaking at 14.8% in 1890, largely due to high levels of immigration from Europe. Restrictive immigration laws in 1921 and 1924 limited immigration almost exclusively to western and northern Europe. These laws as well as the Great Depression and World War II led to a sharp drop in the number of immigrants. The US proportion of immigrants steadily declined, hitting a record low of 4.7% (or 9.6 million immigrants) in 1970. Since 1970, the proportion of immigrants has increased rapidly, mainly because of increased immigration from Asia and Latin America. Important shifts in US immigration law were responsible for this change in the flow of immigrants to the US. Other factors were US economic ties with southern neighbors, for example, Mexico, as well as growing US military presence in both Latin America and Asia.

In 2019, the median age of US immigrants was 45.7 years, with 7% of immigrants aged 5 to 17 years and less than 1% of immigrants aged less than 5 years.[5] That year, ~45 million immigrants lived in the United States and 26% (17.8 million) of the nearly 70 million US children younger than 18 years were CIF. Of the ~18 million CIF, 88% (15.6 million) were second-generation immigrant children born in the United States to at least one foreign-born parent. Of these, 5.3 million children had at least one undocumented parent.[6] The remaining CIF (2.2 million) were born outside the United States; 2017 data of CIF in the United States indicates that 38% (7 million) of CIF have a parent from Mexico, 19% (3.5 million) from Central or South America, and 43% (8 million) from other countries.[7]

Table 1
Immigrant classifications

Term	Description
Children in immigrant families (CIF)	Children who are foreign born and those who are born in the United States and have at least 1 parent who was foreign born
Immigrant children	Children born outside the United States
Lawful permanent residents (LPR)	Immigrants with permission to live and work permanently in the United States
Refugee	Children or adults who fled persecution in their home countries and legally entered the United States after being screened and approved by US agencies abroad
Asylum	Status that can be granted to people already in the United States who have a well-founded fear of persecution by or permitted by their government based on 1 of 5 grounds and who satisfy the requirements for refugee status
T nonimmigrant status ("T visa")	Victims of severe forms of trafficking who can demonstrate that they would suffer extreme hardship involving unusual or severe harm if removed from the United States
U nonimmigrant status ("U visa")	Victims of certain serious crimes who have cooperated with law enforcement in the investigation or prosecution of the crime
Special immigrant juvenile status (SIJS)	Noncitizen minors who were abused, neglected, or abandoned by 1 or both parents
Temporary protected status (TPS)	Status granted to individuals physically present in the United States who are from countries designated by the Secretary of the US Department of Homeland Security as unsafe to accept their return
J-1 classification (exchange visitors)	Status granted to those who intend to participate in an approved program for the purposes of teaching, instructing or lecturing, studying, observing, conducting research, consulting, demonstrating special skills, receiving training, or receiving graduate medical education or training
Deferred Action for Childhood Arrivals (DACA)	Temporary relief from deportation with strict criteria based on age of arrival to United States, whether the individual is in school or working, and whether the individual has no criminal offenses or threats
Deferred Action for Parents of Americans and Lawful Permanent Residents	Temporary relief from deportation for parents of children who are US citizens or have LPR that was never implemented

Reprinted with permission from Linton et al.[2]

Although 62% of CIF live in the 6 traditional immigrant destination states (California, Florida, Illinois, New Jersey, New York, and Texas), 77% of net population growth is in other states.[8] In other words, states with the largest growth in the proportion of CIF are nontraditional migration areas, that is, new destination states, regions, or cities with

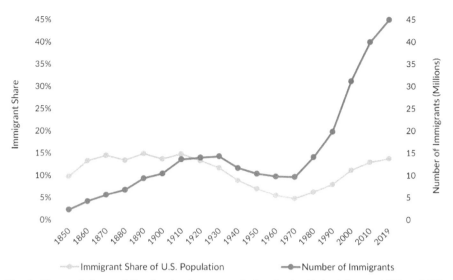

Fig. 2. Size and share of the foreign-born population in the United States, 1850 to 2019. (This figure was originally published in Nicole Ward and Jeanne Batalova, "Frequently Requested Statistics on Immigrants and Immigration in the United States," Migration Information Source, March 14, 2023, https://www.migrationpolicy.org/article/frequently-requested-statistics-immigrants-and-immigration-united-states. Reprinted with permission.)

previously low immigrant populations.[7] For example, between 2006 and 2017 the CIF proportion in North Carolina increased from 12% to 19%—these data suggest that immigration policy changes are important in all US states, regions, and cities, not just in areas that previously had or currently have large immigrant populations[7,8] (**Fig. 3**).

Changing migration patterns have important implications for local service delivery and promoting the health of immigrant families. Limited infrastructure as well as multilingual health, school, and social welfare support services in emerging immigrant communities can negatively affect child health, as families cannot access or use needed services.[9,10] Schools and health and social welfare services in established immigrant communities may have more capacity for meeting the needs of immigrants but codified local bureaucratic structures and cultures may decrease flexibility to adapt to changing needs of immigrant families.[9,10] In both emerging and established immigrant communities, partnerships between community clinics and immigrant-serving community agencies should be a key priority despite the particular challenges in each type of immigrant community. Immigrant-serving community organization staff often have experience addressing the needs of local immigrant populations and specialized knowledge of key barriers and challenges that may be beyond the expertise of clinical care organizations.

Section 2: Health of Immigrant Children in the United States

Health trends
Key health indicators for CIF are difficult to track, as epidemiologic or national studies may not include information on parent and child place of birth, which would allow for identification of immigrant children or US-born children with immigrant parents. If nativity information is included, public data reports may not include specific information on CIF; this results in reliance on research publications of secondary data studies from

Percentage-point change in the share of children who are children of immigrants

-0.6% 0.0% 2.5% 4.0% 5.7% 7.9% 9.6%

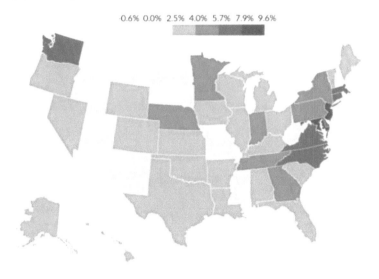

Source: Urban Institute calculations using Census Bureau American Community Survey data.   URBAN **INSTITUTE**

Fig. 3. The share of children who are children of immigrants increased substantially in some nontraditional immigrant destination states from 2006 to 2017. (*From* the The Urban Institute. Part of us: A data-driven look at children of immigrants. https://www.urban.org/features/part-us-data-driven-look-children-immigrants.)

these sources (eg, National Survey of Children's Health), which may not track trends over time or include all immigrant groups.[11–13] For specific health conditions, information on disease prevalence and severity often comes from single-site studies by researchers interested in particular populations. Because of these limitations, the authors present available information on 3 key health disparities and rely more on information on Latinx CIF. The authors believe, however, that many of the same factors that contribute to disparities in Latinx CIF apply to other immigrant groups.

Childhood overweight/obesity. Childhood obesity is a risk factor for adult cardiovascular disease (CVD), the leading cause of death in the United States.[14,15] The childhood obesity epidemic is poised to undo past gains in CVD risk reduction, and health care costs associated with CVD could triple by 2030 without intervention on childhood overweight/obesity.[16] Childhood overweight and obesity for CIF varies by country and region of origin. In general, immigrant children have lower rates of child overweight and obesity than US-born children. As immigrant children spend more time in the United States and for US-born children with immigrant parents, the general trend is increasing prevalence of child overweight[17–19]; this has been consistently demonstrated for US-born Latinx children with immigrant parents, and these children have among the highest childhood obesity rates of any children in the United States.[20–22] The reasons for increasing obesity among CIF over time relates to adoption of American norms of an obesogenic diet and increased sedentary behaviors and poverty, limiting access to healthy foods and opportunities for physical activity.[18,20,23–26]

Although obesity prevention remains an important goal, pediatric primary care providers also need options for treatment of obesity, as many CIF are already overweight or obese. The US Preventive Services Task Force recommends referral of all obese children to an intensive weight management program to prompt behavior changes to decrease body mass index.[27] Intensive programs are mainly found in clinical settings, are limited in number, and are frequently not feasible for immigrant families due to language, transportation, financial, trust, and other barriers to frequent engagement with health care systems.[28,29] Community-based delivery may address immigrant families' barriers to frequent engagement with health care systems and allow them to access services in trusted spaces. Delivery in a community setting is also more consistent with immigrant family views of obesity as a multifaceted issue that reflects the complexities of family life and the influences of social determinants of health.[30,31] Unfortunately, existing intensive community-based programs also have limitations for CIF as non-English home language has been associated with program dropout.[32] There is a clear need to develop child obesity treatment programs that are tailored to the sociocultural needs of immigrant families.

Mental health. Mental health disorders affect 1 in 5 children every year.[33] The American Academy of Pediatrics advocates for mental health competencies in both subspeciality and primary care pediatrics.[34] Among CIF, those who are undocumented immigrants, refugees, or unaccompanied minors are at higher risk of mental health disorders.[35] In addition, CIF with undocumented parents may have significant caregiving responsibilities to support the medical, emotional, and financial well-being of their parents, contributing to their own mental health challenges.[36] Multivariate analysis of the mental health of CIF and non-CIF in US public middle schools demonstrates that whether CIF fare better, the same, or worse than non-CIF depends on a given child's race/ethnicity and their specific mental health challenges—for example, although European American CIF and non-CIF are found to have equivalent depression and disruptive behavior scores, Asian American and Latinx CIF demonstrate higher depression scores than non-CIF.[37] There are gaps in knowledge about mental health needs and subsequent service use for CIF. For example, Latinx CIF experience a higher rate of unmet needs and mental health underutilization compared with White children, but the reasons behind this disparity have not been fully explored.[38]

We do know that cultural stigma surrounding mental health conditions is an important contributor to underuse of mental health care utilization for CIF—there are also many barriers to use of mental health services for immigrant families that desire these services. These barriers can be addressed more easily by the health care system and could also reduce the impact of cultural stigma if more members of an immigrant community begin to use services. Finally, a key limitation in addressing the mental health needs of CIF is the lack of tools available and validated in languages other than English. Few mental health screening tools have even been validated in the United States for Latinx immigrants, thus pediatric primary care providers often lack options for culturally appropriate and validated mental health screening.[39]

Developmental disorders. A core function of pediatric primary care is to identify abnormal development among children. Many pediatric primary care practices conduct developmental screening to aid in the identification of developmental delay. CIF may have higher neurodevelopmental risks than non-CIF.[40] Data from Los Angeles County in California, a racially diverse area with a high proportion of recent immigrants, demonstrate that compared with children born to White mothers born in the United States, children of non–US-born black, Filipino, and Vietnamese mothers had higher risks of both developing or being diagnosed with developmental delay.[41] Delays in developmental screening may contribute to worse outcomes for CIF with developmental disorders. Disparities in developmental screening are critically important, as they may lead to delays in autism spectrum disorder (ASD) diagnoses.[42]

Prompt ASD diagnosis and treatment improves long-term developmental outcomes.[43] Developmental screening in immigrant families is complicated by language barriers, and children in families who communicate in languages other than English are less likely to have developmental screening, particularly families that communicate in non-English, non-Spanish languages.[44,45] Similar to mental health conditions, once a diagnosis of a developmental disorder is made, immigrant families face challenges to accessing and using developmental services as well as cultural barriers to acceptance of diagnoses and services.[46–48]

Healthy immigrant paradox
Although we have discussed several key health concerns for CIF, there is expansive literature demonstrating a healthy immigrant paradox. The healthy immigrant paradox refers to better than expected health outcomes among immigrants despite facing increased health risk factors such as lower socioeconomic status, lower educational attainment, exposure to discrimination, and health care access barriers. This healthy immigrant paradox has been demonstrated across countries of origin and varied health outcomes, including cardiovascular disease and infant mortality.[49–51] Some studies, however, have documented variations in outcomes among immigrant subgroups and that the burden of trauma, stigma/discrimination, migration stress, and concentrated poverty negatively affects immigrant health.[50,52,53] The better-than-expected health outcomes for immigrants also have been shown to decrease with increasing time in the United States. A trend toward worsening health outcomes has been shown to be related to acculturation.[54] Acculturation is defined as the process by which immigrants adapt to their new home country and potentially adopt its norms, values, and practices.[55] In the United States this may mean eating more processed food and convenience foods, thus increasing the risk of child obesity as seen for US-born Latinx children with immigrant parents.[20,21] However, acculturation is a dynamic process and can lead to both positive and negative health benefits.[55] Assessing acculturation is not recommended in clinical care, as there is no consensus on how to best measure acculturation nor its health impact. Similarly, the epidemiologic evidence of a healthy immigrant paradox should not change clinical care decision-making given the significant variation in health conditions and risks for individuals.

Section 3: Health Care Considerations

Care of recently arrived immigrant children
At present, what has been well studied is disease prevalence of multiple neglected tropical diseases in US refugee arrivals, a small subpopulation of newcomers for whom well-established screening protocols exist, both overseas as part of predeparture medical screening as well as on arrival to the United States.[56] What is currently lacking is systematic evaluation of disease prevalence in nonrefugee immigrant children. Despite this fact, expert opinion suggests that many nonrefugee immigrant children may have similar exposure risks for issues including infectious diseases, environmental hazards, malnutrition, micronutrient deficiencies, and toxic stress.

Until there is more evidence-based data addressing disease and exposure risks for other pediatric immigrant groups and subpopulations, most pediatric immigrant health experts recommend following guidelines used for screening newly arrived refugee children—these can be found in the user-friendly, in-office screening algorithm, Care-Ref,[57] and reviewed in further depth through the CDC Domestic Refugee Screening Guidelines.[58] These tools cover approaches to screening of children and adults based on birth country, country of departure to the United States, age, and gender and include screening recommendations for issues that include *Mycobacterium*

tuberculosis, micronutrient deficiencies, elevated blood lead levels, vertically transmitted diseases (ie, human immunodeficiency virus [HIV], hepatitis B and C, and syphilis), soil-transmitted helminth infections, strongyloidiasis, schistosomiasis, newborn
screening, and congenital or iodine-deficiency hypothyroidism. Also included in these
resources are evidence-based approaches to screening for mental health needs.

Another not-so-straightforward issue is how to define which immigrant children
need to be screened as well as what length of time in the United States may influence
exposure risks. For example, most immigrant health experts would recommend
screening of immigrant children born in non-Western countries (ie, *not* born in Scan-
dinavia, Canada, Australia, New Zealand, and Western Europe). Time in the United
States since immigration should also be considered when making screening decisions. For example, an immigrant child who has lived in the United States for 10 years
who has grown well and has not had any intercurrent serious infectious diseases
would not warrant testing for HIV, unless other risk factors for transmission were present. Similarly, geographic risk for specific infectious disease exposures should be
considered when performing immigrant screening, as screening is not a one-size-
fits-all approach; age of the infant or child also needs to be considered when deciding
what risks really exist for exposure as well as the interpretation of results when there is
persistent presence of maternal antibodies in infant circulation. **Fig. 4** can be used to
help guide screening decisions and resources needed for recently arrived immigrant
children cared for in your practice.

Care of children in immigrant families over time

Health insurance. Having health insurance is associated with better health outcomes
for children. Research confirms that within 12 months of obtaining public insurance
coverage, children demonstrate increased health care and dental services utilization.[59] Long-term access to public insurance coverage, from childhood to adulthood,
leads to an improvement of health outcomes in early adulthood.[60] An additional year of
public health insurance eligibility in childhood reduces the probability of health problems, asthma, and chronic conditions in early adulthood as well as improves self-rated
health.[60] National-level data reports consistently indicate that CIF are more likely to be

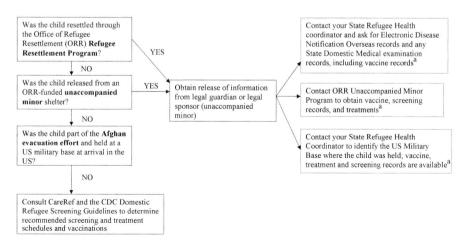

Fig. 4. Approach to screening and vaccination for immigrant children new to your practice.[57,58,78–80] [a]If concerns for current medical issues or loss to follow-up, do not delay any
relevant testing or treatment.

uninsured than other children. Although some CIF, particularly undocumented immigrant children, are ineligible for public health insurance with rare exceptions, CIF make up most of the children who are eligible but not enrolled in public health insurance.[11,61] Practical barriers to obtaining public health insurance occur at the family- and systems-level. Family-level barriers include lack of awareness of eligibility and language barriers. At a systems-level, immigrant parents who lack a social security number struggle to satisfy system requirements for proof of identity and income. Although their children may be eligible, parents themselves are ineligible, and the automated enrollment avenue is not a viable option.[62,63]

Fear also decreases public insurance enrollment of eligible CIF. The public charge rule, a provision of the Immigration and Naturalization Act that requires immigrants to demonstrate that they would not become a "public charge" in order to enter the United States or gain permanent residency, is frequently cited as disincentivizing public benefit enrollment among eligible CIF.[62,64] Changes to the public charge rule to explicitly include public health insurance among the list of programs that may result in the public charge designation were enacted in 2019.[62] Its "chilling effect" permeated immigrant communities even before final regulations were published in 2019, as many have disenrolled and forgone applying for government benefit programs in fear of jeopardizing their applications for permanence residence in the United States.[45,62–64] Although the public charge rules have since been revised to mirror the rule before the changes,[65] the fear of the public charge designation will likely still cause some immigrant families to choose not to enroll their child in public health insurance.[66] Pediatric practices should have staff or leverage community organizations to provide immigrant families with the most current guidance on the implications of use of public benefits, such as health insurance, for their children.

Language barriers. Immigrants comprise 81% of the 25.5 million people in the United States who speak English less than "very well" and thus are classified as having limited English proficiency (LEP). Forty-six percent (20.7 million) of the 44.6 million US immigrants aged 5 years and older have LEP.[5] Federal regulations stemming from Title VI of the Civil Rights mandate that health care organizations receiving federal funding (including Medicaid and Medicare) provide meaningful access to language services for patients and families with limited English proficiency.[67] Health care organizations generally ask patients/families for their preferred health care language in lieu of assessing English proficiency. There is a high level of correlation between non-English preferred health care language and LEP status.[68] The National Standards for Culturally and Linguistically Appropriate Services in Health Care (CLAS standards) issued by the US Department of Health and Human Services provide guidance on Title VI compliance and outline specific activities that health care organizations must perform for populations with LEP.[69] Key activities to adhere to CLAS standards include providing language interpretation and translated documents (eg, consent forms). There are 3 types of professional interpreters who can be used: in-person interpreters, video remote interpreters that are commonly accessed via a tablet computer, or over-the-phone interpreters. The costs and infrastructure investments, such as increasing Wi-Fi reach and capacity for video remote interpreters, vary by interpreter type. Regardless of interpretation modality, interpreters are underused.[70] Unfortunately, health care personnel commonly use patient family members, friends, or minor children as interpreters or attempt to "get by" with the patient's limited English skills or their own limited non-English skills.[71] These practices put patients at risk for worse health care outcomes and adverse patient safety events. Improving interpreter use through interventions that improve interpreter access has been more successful than provider education or provider mandates.[70] Using quality improvement approaches to increase the use of available evidence-based practices for communicating with families who communicate in languages other than English is recommended. Quality improvement efforts should also consider how immigrant families with language barriers access health care services. It is essential for providers to identify these barriers within their health systems, including addressing hospital and clinic phone trees that do not allow direct connection to an interpreter. Such barriers to phone scheduling, nurse advice lines, and pharmacy refill lines create unneeded health care barriers for immigrant families.

Specific health care organization policies for language services are also needed. Language services policies should include clear policies for use of staff non-English language skills. CLAS standards include a recommendation for ensuring competence of those providing language services; this includes staff who may provide direct patient care in languages other than English.[69] A best practice is to use commercially available, medical-focused language assessments administered via phone that have standardized cutoffs for a sufficient level of proficiency.[72] In general, these assessments are focused on direct communication with families in the target language, but some assess a staff member's skill in interpretation. Some health care organizations may choose to then use staff members who achieve threshold scores as interpreters in certain situations. Organizational policies should specify whether staff members who have passed language proficiency assessments can use their non-English skills to provide interpretation in addition to direct communication and the types of situations in which their interpretation skills can be used. It is not recommended that staff with non-English language skills replace professional interpreters, as interpretation is a distinct skillset and professional interpreters undergo extensive training to hone skills, ensure fluency in English and the target language, and understand their professional and ethical obligations. In addition, staff members have many duties, and an overreliance of noninterpreter staff members to provide interpretation can compromise their ability to fulfill their primary duties. Finally, policies must specify the type of training all health care staff receive on the types of language services available, how to access interpreters, and how to work with interpreters more effectively. Training on effectively working with interpreters and best practices in the care of patients/families with limited English proficiency is freely available from the US Department of Health and Human Services.[73]

Finally, cultural differences may also compound language barriers to negatively affect health care for immigrant children/CIF. No medical provider can be *competent* in all cultures, but every medical provider can learn how to ask about cultural practices and educate themselves about subpopulations more common in their communities. The National Resource Center for Refugees, Immigrants, and Migrants is one national resource that provides a centralized database and links in multiple languages to health education materials, toolkits, and trainings for medical providers and organizations wanting to decrease barriers to care for immigrant children and families.[74] Similarly, the CDC Domestic Refugee Screening Guidelines provide Refugee Health Profiles that include summaries of priority health conditions and historical background and cultural beliefs.[75] EthnoMed is also a helpful tool that reviews health topics and cultural practices more common in specific immigrant groups.[76]

Section 4: Health Is More than the Absence of Disease: Social Determinants of Health

CIF have twice the rate of living in poverty than children in nonimmigrant families.[77] High rates of poverty, in addition to family- and system-level challenges to accessing public benefits and other supports, leave CIF at substantial risk of unmet social needs. Consensus is building that addressing unmet social needs should be part of the provision of health care because of the ability to build on trusted, long-term relationships and because of the association between unmet social needs and worse health outcomes. **Fig. 5** shows how additional supports for CIF and their families can be layered into pediatric primary care. **Table 2** provides specific examples of initiatives of relevance to CIF that range widely in their cost and scope.

Section 5: Clinical Care Points for Child Health Providers to Promote Health Equity for Children in Immigrant Families

- Understand your local immigrant population and their health needs to inform clinic screenings, resources, and community partnerships. Needs and resources for CIF vary by immigrant/refugee status, countries of origin, and community experiences with immigrant populations *and* change over time. Even if your practice will not be serving immigrant patients and families, you can be an ally or resource if you are aware of local demographic trends.
- Promote access to health insurance, as it is fundamental to providing services to CIF. Many CIF are eligible yet unenrolled in public health insurance. Enrolling and maintaining public health insurance is especially difficult for immigrant families. Consider devoting practice resources to supporting continued enrollment or partnering with a community organization that can provide this service. Ask for data and demand accountability from local and state agencies regarding successful applications for public insurance according to parental preferred language or parental immigration status.
- Ensure language access for immigrant families who communicate in languages other than English at your practice. Have a language access plan or know what your institution's plan is. A language access plan should include ensuring that interpreters or qualified bilingual staff are available via phone and during visits to the clinic. Families should also be provided with written materials in their preferred language.

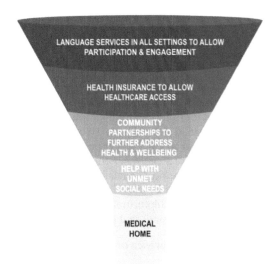

Fig. 5. Possible layers of support within and beyond the medical home to support the health and well-being of children in immigrant families.

Table 2
Sample resources to promote health of children in immigrant families in the medical home or through health system/community partnerships

Resource Category	Example Resource Name	Example Resource Description
Community Health Worker/Patient Navigators from local immigrant communities that address immigrant families' health and social needs	Denver Health Refugee, Immigrant and Migrant (RIM) Navigation Program[81] https://www.denverhealth. org/services/community-health/refugee-clinic	Provides RIM families with culturally and linguistically responsive health care navigation through multilingual navigators from RIM communities. Addresses barriers to health care such as language, transportation, bias, fear, and stigma.
	Mí Plan: Addressing Maternal Contraceptive Needs in Pediatric Primary Care[82]	Trained and supervised CHWs provide support with parents' unmet contraceptive needs within primary care pediatrics.
Health care and access to services for uninsured immigrants	The Access Partnership[83] https://www.hopkinsmedicine. org/health_care_ transformation_strategic_ planning/the-access-partnership/	Provides access to medical services; mental or behavioral health services at low or no cost for low-income immigrants ineligible for other insurance.
	Expanded School-Based Mental Health[84]	Provides school-based individual counseling to students and bills Medicaid or does not bill. Critical resource for immigrant students.
	Testimonios[85]	Free community-based support group for Latino immigrant adults with history of trauma or traumatic exposures.
	Terra Firm Medical-Legal Partnership[86] https://cccsny.org/sites/ default/files/2019-05/ 4978JF_r1_Terra_Firma_ Anniversary_Report_E_ Doc%2003.19.2019.pdf	A unique medical-legal partnership that includes integrated mental health care as well as legal representation for immigrant children seeking legal status in the United States.
Clinic-integrated program to support social determinants of health needs	Hopkins Community Connection[87] https://jhu.campusgroups. com/hl/home/	Trained and supervised college student volunteers along with paid CHWs assist patients and families to access essential resources such as food, housing, heat, and electricity in order to be healthy.
	Children's Hospital Colorado Resource Connect[88]	Social care program within a multispecialty clinic that includes on-site community partners (eg, a public benefits eligibility technician, food clinic) to address social needs on site at the time of clinical service.

(continued on next page)

Table 2
(continued)

Resource Category	Example Resource Name	Example Resource Description
Health care/ Immigrant-serving organization partnerships	UC San Diego Refugee Health Unit[89,90] https://ucsdcommunityhealth.org/work/refugee-health-unit/	The Refugee Health Unit supports and builds capacity in local ethnic-serving community–based organizations via support of the Refugee Communities Coalition in their efforts to improve the lives of refugees by serving as both an institutional and a community-minded resource hub.
	Center for Salud/Health and Opportunities for Latinos (Centro SOL)[91,92] https://www.jhcentrosol.org/	Centro SOL has initiatives in clinical innovation, research excellence, education access and exposure, and advocacy in active partnership with the Johns Hopkins Institutions and our Latino neighbors with the goal of promoting equity in health and opportunity for Latinos.
Community Resource hubs	Aurora Community Connection[93] http://www.auroracommunityconnection.com/	Provides support for immigrant families to enroll in public benefits programs; offers adult, child, and family wellness programs (eg, Parents as Teachers, tutoring, exercise/ sports programs), referrals to other community programs when need cannot be met at the center.
	Ventanilla de Salud[94] https://ventanilladesalud.org/	Mexican-consulate program in many US communities that offers health education, connections to local health services, support for obtaining public benefits.
Patient & family engagement	Latino Family Advisory Board[95]	An advisory board composed of Latino parents with limited English proficiency meets monthly to advise on procedures and initiatives of the pediatric primary care practice where they bring their children for care.
Material supports for families in the medical home	Reach Out & Read[96] https://reachoutandread.org/	Providing books to young children in pediatric primary care and modeling activities that can promote reading at home.

(continued on next page)

Table 2
(continued)

Resource Category	Example Resource Name	Example Resource Description
	Fluoride Varnish & Dental Toolkits[97,98]	Apply fluoride varnish during pediatric primary care visits for children aged 9 mo to 5 y. Provide toothbrushes, toothpaste, and sippy cups (as age appropriate) to support healthy dental hygiene practices.
	Food Pantry[99,100]	Providing emergency food supplies to families presenting for pediatric primary care and screening positive for food insecurity.
	Share Baby[101] https://www.sharebaby.org/	Providing diapers to families in pediatric primary care through partnerships with area diaper banks.

- Add programs to your clinical services that will support the health and well-being of CIF and their families. There are many example programs of expanded medical home services and community partnerships that meet the specific needs of immigrant families. Work with local colleagues and national organizations to learn more about these programs and how to establish them at your practice.
- Engage in political advocacy. The 2 leading policy changes that would benefit the health and well-being of children in immigrant families are immigration reform and Medicaid/Medicare for All. Until then, there are many opportunities for policy change at the state and local level to promote access to health insurance, other public benefits, and funding to support governmental and community services to support the health, social, and education needs of children in immigrant families.

DISCLOSURE

The authors have no conflicts of interest relevant to this article to disclose.

REFERENCES

1. Annie E. Casey Foundation. Children in immigrant families in the United States. 2020. Available at: https://datacenter.kidscount.org/. Accessed September 22, 2022.

2. Linton JM, Green A. Providing care for children in immigrant families. Pediatrics 2019;144(3).

3. United Nations Office of the High Commissioner for Refugees. 2010. Available at: www.unhcr.org/en-us/protection/basic/3b66c2aa10/convention-protocol-relating-status-refugees.html. Accessed September 22, 2022.

4. Pew Research Center. Key facts about the changing U.S. unauthorized immigrant population. 2021. Available at: https://www.pewresearch.org/fact-tank/2021/04/13/key-facts-about-the-changing-u-s-unauthorized-immigrant-population/. Accessed September 22, 2022.

5. Migration Policy Institute. Migration Information Source. Frequently requested statistics on immigrants and immigration in the United States. Available at: https://www.migrationpolicy.org/article/frequently-requested-statistics-immigrants-and-immigration-united-states#:~:text=People%20of%20working%20age%20(18,born%20in%20this%20age%20group. Published 2022. Accessed September 29, 2022.

6. Passel JS, Cohn DV, Krogstad JM, Gonzalez-Barrera A. Pew Research Hispanic Trends Project. As growth stalls, unauthorized immigrant population becomes more settled. . Available at: https://policycommons.net/artifacts/619645/as-growth-stalls-unauthorized-immigrant-population-becomes-more-settled/1600791/. Published 2014. Accessed September 22, 2022.

7. The Urban Institute. Part of us: A data-driven look at children of immigrants. Available at: https://www.urban.org/features/part-us-data-driven-look-children-immigrants. Published 2019. Accessed September 29, 2022.

8. The Urban Institute. Demographic trends of children of immigrants. Available at: https://www.urban.org/sites/default/files/publication/85071/2000971-demographic-trends-of-children-of-immigrants_1.pdf. Published 2016. Accessed September 29, 2022.

9. Turner K, Wildsmith E, Guzman L, Alvira-Hammond M. The Changing Geography of Hispanic Children and Families. National Research Center on Hispanic Children and Families, January 2016. Report No.: Contract No.: 2016-06. Available at: https://www.hispanicresearchcenter.org/wp-content/uploads/2019/08/Emerging-Communities-V21.pdf. Accessed October 26, 2022.

10. Gelatt J, Adams G, Monson W. Immigration and the Changing Landscape for Local Service Delivery: Demographic Shifts in Cities and Neighborhoods. The Urban Institute, March 2014. Report No. Available at: https://www.urban.org/research/publication/immigration-and-changing-landscape-local-service-delivery. Accessed.

11. Rosenberg J, Shabanova V, McCollum S, et al. Insurance and Health Care Outcomes in Regions Where Undocumented Children Are Medicaid-Eligible. Pediatrics 2022;150(3).

12. Zarei K, Kahle L, Buckman DW, et al. Parent-child nativity, race, ethnicity, and adverse childhood experiences among United States children. J Pediatr 2022;251. 190–195, e4.

13. Cheng TC, Lo CC. Factors Related to Use of Mental Health Services by Immigrant Children. J Child Fam Stud 2022;31(1):228–36.

14. de Ferranti SD, Steinberger J, Ameduri R, et al. Cardiovascular Risk Reduction in High-Risk Pediatric Patients: A Scientific Statement From the American Heart Association. Circulation 2019;139(13):e603–34.

15. Kochanek KD, Murphy SL, Xu J, et al. Deaths: Final Data for 2017. Natl Vital Stat Rep 2019;68(9):1–77.

16. Heidenreich PA, Trogdon JG, Khavjou OA, et al. Forecasting the future of cardiovascular disease in the United States: a policy statement from the American Heart Association. Circulation 2011;123(8):933–44.

17. Singh GK, Kogan MD, Yu SM. Disparities in obesity and overweight prevalence among US immigrant children and adolescents by generational status. J Community Health 2009;34(4):271–81.

18. MIgration Policy Institute. Moving to the Land of Milk and Cookies: Obesity among the Children of Immigrants. Available at: https://www.migrationpolicy.org/article/moving-land-milk-and-cookies-obesity-among-children-immigrants. Published 2009. Accessed November 2, 2022.

19. Singh GK, Siahpush M, Hiatt RA, et al. Dramatic increases in obesity and over-weight prevalence and body mass index among ethnic-immigrant and social class groups in the United States, 1976-2008. J Community Health 2011; 36(1):94–110.

20. Gordon-Larsen P, Harris KM, Ward DS, et al. Acculturation and overweight-related behaviors among Hispanic immigrants to the US: the National Longitu-dinal Study of Adolescent Health. Soc Sci Med 2003;57(11):2023–34.

21. Mather M, Foxen P. Toward A More Equitable Future: The Trends and Chal-lenges Facing America's Latino Children. Washington, DC: National Council of La Raza, 2016. Available at: https://www.unidosus.org/publications/1627-toward-a-more-equitable-future-the-trends-and-challenges-facing-americas-latino-children/. Accessed October 26, 2022.

22. Vilar-Compte M, Bustamante AV, López-Olmedo N, et al. Migration as a determi-nant of childhood obesity in the United States and Latin America. Obes Rev 2021;22(Suppl 3):e13240.

23. Isasi CR, Rastogi D, Molina K. Health Issues in Hispanic/Latino Youth. J Lat Psy-chol 2016;4(2):67–82.

24. Zilanawala A, Davis-Kean P, Nazroo J, et al. Race/ethnic disparities in early childhood BMI, obesity and overweight in the United Kingdom and United States. Int J Obes 2015;39(3):520–9.

25. National Center for Children in Poverty, Mailman School of Public Health, Columbia University, Basic Facts about Low-Income Children: Children under 18 Years, 2014. Jiang Y, Ekono M, Skinner C. New York: February 2016. Avail-able at: https://www.nccp.org/wp-content/uploads/2016/02/text_1145.pdf. Ac-cessed November 2, 2022.

26. Lee H, Andrew M, Gebremariam A, et al. Longitudinal associations between poverty and obesity from birth through adolescence. Am J Public Health 2014;104(5):e70–6.

27. Grossman DC, Bibbins-Domingo K, Curry SJ, et al. Screening for Obesity in Children and Adolescents: US Preventive Services Task Force Recommenda-tion Statement. JAMA 2017;317(23):2417–26.

28. Thornton RLJ, Hernandez RG, Cheng TL. Putting the US Preventive Services Task Force Recommendation for Childhood Obesity Screening in Context. JAMA 2017;317(23):2378–80.

29. American Psychological Association CPGP. Clinical practice guideline for multi-component behavioral treatment of obesity and overweight in children and ad-olescents: Current state of the evidence and research needs. Washington, DC: March 2018. Available at: https://www.apa.org/obesity-guideline/clinical-practice-guideline.pdf. Accessed November 2, 2022.

30. Martinez SM, Rhee KE, Blanco E, et al. Latino mothers' beliefs about child weight and family health. Public Health Nutr 2017;20(6):1099–106.

31. Corty EW, Charite J, Ugochukwu A, et al. The First Step to Changing Some-thing": Addressing Latinx Childhood Obesity through Photovoice. Prog Commu-nity Health Partnersh 2022;16(3):307–20.

32. Sacher PM, Kolotourou M, Poupakis S, et al. Addressing childhood obesity in low-income, ethnically diverse families: outcomes and peer effects of MEND 7-13 when delivered at scale in US communities. Int J Obes 2019;43(1):91–102.

33. Perou R, Bitsko R, Blumberg S, et al. Mental health surveillance among children-United States, 2005–2011. MMWR (Morb Mortal Wkly Rep) 2013;62(2):1–35.

34. Green CM, Foy JM, Earls MF. Achieving the Pediatric Mental Health Compe-tencies. Pediatrics 2019;144(5).

35. Kim SY, Schwartz SJ, Perreira KM, et al. Culture's Influence on Stressors, Parental Socialization, and Developmental Processes in the Mental Health of Children of Immigrants. Annu Rev Clin Psychol 2018;14:343–70.

36. Think Global Health. Children of Immigrants and Their Mental Health Needs. Available at: https://www.thinkglobalhealth.org/article/children-immigrants-and-their-mental-health-needs. Published 2020. Accessed October 30, 2022.

37. Kim J, Nicodimos S, Kushner SE, et al. Comparing Mental Health of US Children of Immigrants and Non-Immigrants in 4 Racial/Ethnic Groups. J Sch Health 2018;88(2):167–75.

38. Lopez C, Bergren MD, Painter SG. Latino disparities in child mental health services. J Child Adolesc Psychiatr Nurs 2008;21(3):137–45.

39. Caballero TM, DeCamp LR, Platt RE, et al. Addressing the Mental Health Needs of Latino Children in Immigrant Families. Clin Pediatr 2017;56(7):648–58.

40. Schmengler H, Cohen D, Tordjman S, et al. Autism Spectrum and Other Neurodevelopmental Disorders in Children of Immigrants: A Brief Review of Current Evidence and Implications for Clinical Practice. Front Psychiatry 2021;12: 566368.

41. Becerra TA, von Ehrenstein OS, Heck JE, et al. Autism spectrum disorders and race, ethnicity, and nativity: a population-based study. Pediatrics 2014;134(1): e63–71.

42. Maenner MJ, Shaw KA, Baio J, et al. Prevalence of Autism Spectrum Disorder Among Children Aged 8 Years - Autism and Developmental Disabilities Monitoring Network, 11 Sites, United States, 2016. MMWR Surveill Summ 2020; 69(4):1–12.

43. Elder JH, Kreider CM, Brasher SN, et al. Clinical impact of early diagnosis of autism on the prognosis and parent-child relationships. Psychol Res Behav Manag 2017;10:283–92.

44. Knuti Rodrigues K, Hambidge SJ, Dickinson M, et al. Developmental Screening Disparities for Languages Other than English and Spanish. Academic Pediatrics 2016;16(7):653–9.

45. Children Now. The 2022 California Children's Report Card. Available at: https://www.childrennow.org/portfolio-posts/2022-california-childrens-report-card/. Accessed November 1, 2022.

46. Guerrero MGB, Sobotka SA. Understanding the Barriers to Receiving Autism Diagnoses for Hispanic and Latinx Families. Pediatr Ann 2022;51(4):e167–71.

47. Xu Y, Zeng W, Wang Y, et al. Barriers to Service Access for Immigrant Families of Children With Developmental Disabilities: A Scoping Review. Intellect Dev Disabil 2022;60(5):382–404.

48. Sritharan B, Koola MM. Barriers faced by immigrant families of children with autism: A program to address the challenges. Asian J Psychiatr 2019;39:53–7.

49. Medina-Inojosa J, Jean N, Cortes-Bergoderi M, et al. The Hispanic paradox in cardiovascular disease and total mortality. Prog Cardiovasc Dis 2014;57(3): 286–92.

50. Montoya-Williams D, Williamson VG, Cardel M, et al. The Hispanic/Latinx Perinatal Paradox in the United States: A Scoping Review and Recommendations to Guide Future Research. J Immigr Minor Health 2021;23(5):1078–91.

51. Oh H, Goehring J, Jacob L, et al. Revisiting the Immigrant Epidemiological Paradox: Findings from the American Panel of Life 2019. Int J Environ Res Public Health 2021;18(9).

52. Sarraju A, Ngo S, Ashland M, et al. Trends in national and county-level Hispanic mortality in the United States, 2011-2020. Sci Rep 2022;12(1):11812.

53. DeCamp LR, Choi H, Fuentes-Afflick E, et al. Immigrant Latino neighborhoods and mortality among infants born to Mexican-origin Latina women. Matern Child Health J 2015;19(6):1354–63.

54. Lee S, O'Neill AH, Ihara ES, et al. Change in self-reported health status among immigrants in the United States: associations with measures of acculturation. PLoS One 2013;8(10):e76494.

55. Abraído-Lanza AF, Echeverría SE, Flórez KR. Latino Immigrants, Acculturation, and Health: Promising New Directions in Research. Annu Rev Public Health 2016;37:219–36.

56. Centers for Disease Control and Prevention. Refugee Health Guidance. Available at: https://www.cdc.gov/immigrantrefugeehealth/guidelines/refugee-guidelines.html. Accessed November 1, 2022.

57. Minnesota Department of Health. CareRef Clinical Assessment for Refugees. Available at: https://careref.web.health.state.mn.us/. Accessed November 1, 2022.

58. Centers for Disease Control and Prevention. Refugee Domestic Screening Guidance: Key Considerations and Best Practices. Available at: https://www.cdc.gov/immigrantrefugeehealth/guidelines/domestic/screening-guidance.html. Accessed November 1, 2022.

59. Bailey SR, Marino M, Hoopes M, et al. Healthcare Utilization After a Children's Health Insurance Program Expansion in Oregon. Matern Child Health J 2016; 20(5):946–54.

60. Thompson O. The long-term health impacts of Medicaid and CHIP. J Health Econ 2017;51:26–40.

61. Kaiser Family Foundation. Health Coverage of Immigrants. 2022. Available at: https://www.kff.org/racial-equity-and-health-policy/fact-sheet/health-coverage-of-immigrants/. Accessed October 30, 2022.

62. Barofsky J, Vargas A, Rodriguez D, et al. Spreading Fear: The Announcement Of The Public Charge Rule Reduced Enrollment In Child Safety-Net Programs. Health affairs (Project Hope) 2020;39(10):1752–61.

63. Parmet WE. Supreme Court Allows Public Charge Rule To Take Effect While Appeals Continue | Health Affairs. Health Affairs. Published February 3, 2020. Available at: https://www.healthaffairs.org/do/10.1377/hblog20200131.845894/full/. Accessed October 26, 2022.

64. Ku L, Matani S. Left out: immigrants' access to health care and insurance. Health affairs (Project Hope) 2001;20(1):247–56.

65. New Rule Makes Clear that Noncitizens Who Receive Health or Other Benefits to which they are Entitled Will Not Suffer Harmful Immigration Consequences. Available at: https://www.hhs.gov/about/news/2022/09/08/new-rule-makes-clear-noncitizens-who-receive-health-or-other-benefits-which-they-are-entitled-will-not-suffer-harmful-immigration-consequences.html. Accessed November 1, 2022.

66. Migration Policy Institute. The Public-Charge Final Rule Is Far from the Last Word. Available at: https://www.migrationpolicy.org/news/public-charge-final-rule-far-last-word. Published 2022. Accessed November 1, 2022.

67. US Department of Health and Human Services. Guidance to federal financial assistance recipients regarding Title VI prohibition against national origin discrimination affecting limited English proficient persons. Available at: https://www.hhs.gov/civil-rights/for-individuals/special-topics/limited-english-proficiency/guidance-federal-financial-assistance-recipients-title-vi/index.html. Accessed October 26, 2022.

68. Karliner LS, Napoles-Springer AM, Schillinger D, et al. Identification of limited English proficient patients in clinical care. J Gen Intern Med 2008;23(10): 1555–60.

69. US Department of Health and Human Services Office of Minority Health. National standards for culturally and linguistically appropriate services in health care. Washington, DC; 2001. Available at: https://minorityhealth.hhs.gov/assets/pdf/checked/finalreport.pdf. Accessed October 26, 2022.

70. Taira BR, Kim K, Mody N. Hospital and Health System-Level Interventions to Improve Care for Limited English Proficiency Patients: A Systematic Review. Jt Comm J Qual Patient Saf 2019;45(6):446–58.

71. Diamond LC, Schenker Y, Curry L, et al. Getting by: underuse of interpreters by resident physicians. J Gen Intern Med 2009;24(2):256–62.

72. Altalang. Qualified Bilingual Staff Assessment. Available at: https://www.altalang.com/language-testing/qbs/. Accessed October 26, 2022.

73. U.S. Department of Health & Human Services. Think Cultural Health. Available at: https://thinkculturalhealth.hhs.gov/. Accessed November 2, 2022.

74. University of Minnesota. National Resource Center for Refugees, Immigrants, and Migrants (NRC-RIM). Available at: https://nrcrim.org/. Accessed November 1, 2022.

75. Centers for Disease Control and Prevention. Refugee Health Profiles. Available at: https://www.cdc.gov/immigrantrefugeehealth/profiles/index.html. Accessed Novermber 1, 2022.

76. EthnoMed. Available at: https://ethnomed.org/. Accessed November 1, 2022.

77. Acevedo-Garcia D, Joshi PK, Ruskin E, et al. Including Children in Immigrant Families in Policy Approaches to Reduce Child Poverty. Academic Pediatrics 2021;21(8s):S117–25.

78. Office of Refugee Resettlement. Key State Contacts. Available at: https://www.acf.hhs.gov/orr/grant-funding/key-state-contacts. Accessed November 4, 2022.

79. Centers for Disease Control and Prevention. Electronic Disease Notification System. Available at: https://www.cdc.gov/immigrantrefugeehealth/Electronic-Disease-Notification-System.html Accessed November 4, 2022.

80. Office of Refugee Resettlement. Unaccompanied Refugee Minors Program. Available at: https://www.acf.hhs.gov/orr/programs/refugees/urm. Published 2022. Accessed November 4, 2022.

81. Denver Health. Community Health Services. Available at: https://www.denverhealth.org/services/community-health. Accessed November 4, 2022.

82. Caballero TM, Miramontes-Valdes E, Polk S. Mi Plan: Using a Pediatric-Based Community Health Worker Model to Facilitate Obtainment of Contraceptives Among Latino Immigrant Parents with Contraceptive Needs. Jt Comm J Qual Patient Saf 2022;48(11):591–8.

83. Johns Hopkins Medicine. Health Care Transformation and Strategic Planning. The Access Partnership (TAP). Available at: https://www.hopkinsmedicine.org/health_care_transformation_strategic_planning/the-access-partnership/. Accessed November 4, 2022.

84. Maryland State Department of Education. School Mental Health. Available at: https://marylandpublicschools.org/about/Pages/DSFSS/SSSP/SMH/index.aspx. Accessed November 4, 2022.

85. Jalisi A, Vazquez MG, Bucay-Harari L, et al. *Testimonios*, A Mental Health Support Group for Latino Immigrants in an Emergent Latino Community. J Health Care Poor Underserved 2018;29(2):623–32.

86. Terra Firm Medical-Legal Partnership. Available at: https://www.terrafirma.nyc/. Accessed November 4, 2022.

87. Polk S, Leifheit KM, Thornton R, et al. Addressing the Social Needs of Spanish- and English-Speaking Families in Pediatric Primary Care. Academic Pediatrics 2020;20(8):1170–6.

88. DeCamp LR, Yousuf S, Peters C, et al. Assessing strengths, challenges, and equity via pragmatic evaluation of a social care program. Acad Pediatr 2023:S1876-2859(23):00135-3. https://www.childrenscolorado.org/4ace24/globalassets/community/2019-community-benefit-report-childrens-hospital-colorado.pdf.

89. UC San Diego Center for Community Health. Refugee Health Unit. Available at: https://ucsdcommunityhealth.org/work/refugee-health-unit-2/. Published 2022. Accessed November 4, 2022.

90. UC San Diego Center for Community Health. San Diego Refugee Communities Coalition. Available at: https://ucsdcommunityhealth.org/work/refugee-health-unit-2/san-diego-refugee-communities-coalition/. Accessed November 4, 2022.

91. Center for Salud/Health and Opportunities for Latinos (Centro SOL). Available at: https://www.jhcentrosol.org/. Accessed November 4, 2022.

92. Polk S, DeCamp LR, Guerrero Vázquez M, et al. Centro SOL: A Community-Academic Partnership to Care for Undocumented Immigrants in an Emerging Latino Area. Acad Med 2019;94(4):538–43.

93. Aurora Community Connection. Available at: http://www.auroracommunityconnection.com/. Published 2022. Accessed November 4, 2022.

94. Ventanillas de Salud. Available at: https://consulmex.sre.gob.mx/sanantonio/index.php/lo-mas-vistoavisos/209-ventanilla-de-salud. Accessed November 4, 2022.

95. DeCamp LR, Polk S, Chrismer MC, et al. Health care engagement of limited English proficient Latino families: Lessons learned from advisory board development. Prog Community Health Partnersh 2015;9(4):521–30.

96. Reach Out & Read. Available at: https://reachoutandread.org/. Published 2022. Accessed November 4, 2022.

97. The Pew Charitable Trusts. Inequitable Access to Oral Health Care Continues to Harm Children of Color. Available at: https://www.pewtrusts.org/en/research-and-analysis/articles/2022/03/11/inequitable-access-to-oral-health-care-continues-to-harm-children-of-color. Published 2022. Accessed November 2022.

98. Smiles for Life. Fluoride Varnish Ordering and State Specific Information. Available at: https://www.smilesforlifeoralhealth.org/resources/practice-tools-and-resources/state-specific-fluoride-varnish-information/. Published 2022. Accessed November 4, 2022.

99. Hickey E, Phan M, Beck AF, et al. A Mixed-Methods Evaluation of a Novel Food Pantry in a Pediatric Primary Care Center. Clin Pediatr 2020;59(3):278–84.

100. American Academy of Pediatrics. Food Research and Action Center (FRAC). Available at: Available at: https://frac.org/wp-content/uploads/FRAC_AAP_Toolkit_2021.pdf. Published 2021. Accessed November 4, 2022.

101. Share Baby. Available at: https://www.sharebaby.org. Published 2022. Accessed November 4, 2022.

Achieving Health Equity for Sexual and Gender-Diverse Youth

Errol L. Fields, MD, PhD, MPH, FAAP

KEYWORDS

- Adolescents • Discrimination • Health disparity • Intersectionality • Gender identity
- Primary health care • Sexuality • Stigma

KEY POINTS

- Compared to their heterosexual and cisgender peers, sexual and gender diverse (SGD) youth, especially those from minoritized racial/ethnic groups, experience significant disparities in health and social conditions that can threaten their health and well-being.
- Disparities impacting SGD youth are caused by anti-LGBT stigma and discrimination and, for SGD youth with intersecting minoritized identities, the impact of additional intersecting social inequities.
- Health care disparities including inadequate pediatric provider training and comfort with SGD care, stigma and discrimination within health care, geographic disparities in care access, and emerging legislative restrictions on the provision of evidence-based care undermine the support pediatric care settings can offer and widen rather than reduce health disparities impacting SGD youth.
- While the risk of poor health and social outcomes is incrementally higher for SGD youth compared to heterosexual and cisgender youth, it is not universal or inevitable; pediatric providers can be a critical protective factor for the SGD youth and families they care for.
- Health equity for SGD youth will only be achieved by eliminating the structural stigma and discrimination that underlie their disparities–a task that will require coordinated and consistent effort across multiple fields and stakeholders including health-related research, pediatric and adolescent medicine clinicians, medical education and training, legislative and policy advocates, and families and communities.

CASE STUDY

Kyle is a 17-year-old Black cisgender male who presents as a new patient/well adolescent visit. He is accompanied by his mother. Since his last visit with his prior pediatrician 1 year ago, he has been seen at urgent care settings several times with chest pain

Division of Adolescent/Young Adult Medicine, Department of Pediatrics Johns Hopkins School of Medicine, 200 North Wolfe Street, Room 2015, Baltimore, MD 21287, USA
E-mail address: Errol.Fields@jhmi.edu

Pediatr Clin N Am 70 (2023) 813–835
https://doi.org/10.1016/j.pcl.2023.03.009
pediatric.theclinics.com

or abdominal and other GI complaints where he has been told his symptoms are from anxiety.

When he was 14, Kyle started having crushes on other boys at school. Even though he feels fairly certain he is gay, he has always been uncomfortable with these feelings because all the negative messages he has heard about LGBTQ people from his family, friends, at church, in his community, and social media. He has not told any friends or peers about his feelings for other boys because other kids in his high school have been terrorized on social media whenever there are even rumors about them being gay. Kyles is constantly worried the same thing will happen to him. He is also worried that his mother will not accept his sexuality so he has not told her either. He has never had anyone who he felt like he could talk to about his feelings. Once he tried to talk to his last doctor, but when he mentioned being confused about his sexuality, Kyle's doctor just lectured him about the high risk of HIV in gay Black men even though he had never been sexually active.

Kyle often feels alone and isolated, while he used to do well in school and play two varsity sports (cross-country and track) and hoped to go to college after high school, lately he has had little motivation for anything and his grades have suffered.

At his visit today, he completes a previsit questionnaire including items screening behavioral and mental health concerns. His responses suggest he has significant symptoms of depression and anxiety. To avoid another lecture, he left questions about his sexual activity, gender of sex partners, and sexual orientation blank.

As you read the article that follows, consider the factors contributing to Kyle's depression, anxiety, and isolation and what his new pediatrician might do to disrupt the impact of these factors on Kyle's life.

INTRODUCTION

Compared to their heterosexual and cisgender peers, sexual and gender diverse (SGD) youth experience significant disparities in health, health care, and social conditions that can threaten their well-being and successful transition to adulthood. SGD youth's increased risks for these conditions are not due to any intrinsic difference or vulnerability specific to their sexual orientation or gender identity, but are rather due to social disadvantages and inequities these youth experience as a result of stigma and discrimination. SGD youth who are from minoritized racial/ethnic groups often carry the greatest burden of these disparities arguably because they also experience additional and intersectional social disadvantages from their membership in minoritized racial/ethnic groups.

This article describes the disparities impacting SGD youth, their differential exposure to the stigma, and discrimination that foster these disparities, and the protective factors that can mitigate or disrupt the impact of these exposures on the health and well-being of SGD youth. On the final point, the article specifically focuses on pediatric providers and inclusive, affirming, medical homes as critical protective factors for SGD youth and their families.

Definition of terms and defining the population

The term sexual and gender diverse refers to youth with a nonheterosexual sexual orientation or youth whose gender identity is incongruent with their sex assigned at birth. Sexual orientation is a multidimensional construct that encompasses sexual identity, attraction and behavior (**Box 1**). Sexual diverse youth are individuals who identify as lesbian, gay, bisexual, or another nonheterosexual identity, are attracted to the same or multiple genders, engage in sexual behavior with the same or multiple

Box 1
Sexual orientation and gender identity terminology and definitions
Sexual Orientation: Refers to an individual's pattern of physical and emotional arousal toward other persons. It is a multidimensional that includes sexual identity, attraction and behavior.
Sexual attraction: refers to the gender or genders of people to whom an individual feels physically or romantically attracted.
Sexual Behavior: refers to the gender or genders of an individual sexual partners.
Sexual Identity: conception of self, based on attraction and behavior and/or membership in social group based on shared sexual orientation.
Gender: socially constructed roles, behaviors, activities, and attributes a given society considers appropriate for the sex assigned at birth. It is comprised of gender identity, gender expression and sex assigned at birth
Gender Identity: one's internal sense of being male, female, outside the gender binary of male or female or another gender identity
Gender expression: refers to mannerisms, personal traits, clothing and hair choices and so forth that a person uses to present their gender identity
Sex assigned at birth: refers to the sex or gender given to a baby typically based on their sex phenotype–the external genitals and/or internal sex organs a person is born with
Sexual Diverse: individuals who identify as lesbian, gay, bisexual or another non-heterosexual identity, have same-sex attractions, engage in same-sex sexual behavior, or may be questioning their sexual orientation
Gender Diverse: individuals who identify as transgender, have another gender identity that differs from their sex assigned at birth, may be questioning their gender identity or identifying as nonbinary, genderfluid or agender

genders, and/or may be questioning their sexual orientation. An individual's sexual identity, attraction and behavior may or may not be aligned, so sexual diverse youth may be teenage boy who identifies as heterosexual, has only been sexually active with girls, but is physically and emotionally attracted to boys. Gender identity refers to one's internal sense of being male, female, or another gender identity. Gender-diverse youth are individuals who identify as transgender, have another gender identity that differs from their sex assigned at birth, may be questioning their gender identity or identifying as nonbinary, genderfluid or agender.[1]

Terminology used to express identity, in particular sexual and gender identity, is often fluid, evolving and changing over time. The acronym for lesbian, gay, bisexual, transgender or queer/questioning, LGBTQ, is the mostly commonly used term to describe individuals with a nonheterosexual orientation (eg, lesbian, gay, or bisexual), a gender identity incongruent with their sex assigned at birth (eg, transgender or queer) or who are questioning their sexual orientation or gender identity (eg, questioning). This term is often used as if it refers to a single population or community. However, each letter of this acronym represents distinct populations with their own health concerns and may not capture the diversity of emerging sexual or gender identities youth may experience (eg, pansexuality– a sexual identity based on sexual, romantical or emotional attraction toward people regardless of their sex or gender identity or demi-boy–a gender identity describing someone who partially identifies as male) or the differences in the terminology used to describe identity across different cultures and communities (eg, same-gender loving a term used by some Black people as a more culturally affirming term for nonheterosexual identities and Two-Spirit a

Native American term that often refers to a third gender, and may refer to nonhetero-sexual self-identification).[1] To avoid the limitations of the LGTBQ acronym, this article will primarily use the term sexual and gender diverse (SGD) when referring to youth as it is more inclusive of the diversity of nonheterosexual orientations and noncisgender identities.

Sexual and gender diversity among adolescents and young adults

The US Census does not routinely collect data on sexual orientation or gender identity, nor are these data recorded in vital statistics. Therefore, population estimates of sex-ual and gender diverse persons are not as robust as the estimates of other demo-graphic characteristics (eg, age, race, ethnicity). However, national surveillance, polling, survey, and other research data suggest several emerging changes in sexual and gender diversity in the US–particularly among youth.

Increasing prevalence of sexual and gender diverse identities: According to data from the Youth Risk Behavior Survey (YRBS) the percentage of teens ages 13 to 17 who identify as gay, lesbian, bisexual, or unsure/questioning has more than doubled from 7.3% in 2009% to 15.6% in 2019.[2–4] The largest increase was among adolescent respondents identifying as bisexual which increased from 3.9% to 8.7%. Respon-dents identifying as gay or lesbian also increased from 1.4% to 2.5% and unsure/questioning from 2.0% to 4.5%.[2] The 2017 YRBS piloted questions on transgender identity in 10 states and 9 large school districts. Using pooled data from these 19 sites, the prevalence of transgender identity among teens ages 13 to 17 was estimated at 1.8% – a prevalence more than double the prior estimates of 0.7% prevalence.[5] An estimated 1.6% of teens were unsure of their gender identity.[5] Using these YRBS data, the Williams Institute estimates there are 1.99 million adolescents ages 13 to 17 who identify as lesbian, gay, bisexual, or transgender–including 1.92 million who identify as lesbian, gay or bisexual and 149,750 who identify as transgender.[6]

The Gallup poll, which uses random digit dialing of mobile and landline phone numbers to survey adults 18 and older, has similarly shown an increasing percentage of adults who identify as lesbian, gay, bisexual, or transgender from 3.5% in 2012% to 7.1% in 2021 – including 1.0% lesbian, 1.5% gay, 4.0% bisexual, 0.7% transgender identifying persons.[7]

Greater prevalence in current compared to past age cohorts: While the Gallup poll data reflect adult rates, the increasing prevalence of LGBT identity over time has been driven in part by increasing prevalence among younger age cohorts. Most recent Gallop poll date indicate 10.5% of millennials (born between 1981 and 1996) and 20.8% of Generation Z (born between 1997 and 2002) identify as LGBT compared to only 4.2% of Generation X (born between 1965 and 1980) and 2.6% of Boomers (born between 1946 and 1964).[7] As evidence by the YRBS data described above, these trends are likely mirrored in adolescents.[7]

Earlier ages of identity development and disclosure: Recent data also suggest that SGD youth are understanding and disclosing their sexual orientation or gender identity at earlier ages than previous cohorts. The Generations Study, a longitudinal study examining health and well-being of sexual diverse persons across three age cohorts (ages 18–26, 32–43, 50–60) found a 2.5 year lag in understanding sexual identity and a 4 year lag in disclosing sexual identity across the three cohorts–with the youn-gest cohort understanding and disclosing sexual identity on average at ages 14 and 16 respectively and the oldest cohort reporting these milestones at ages 19 and 24 respectively.[8] A online cross-sectional study exploring gender identity and milestones across age cohorts, similarly found earlier ages of recognizing a transgender or other gender diverse identity, social transitioning and presenting for gender-affirming care in

Generation Z cohorts compared to Millennials, Generation X and Boomers–with generation Z reporting these milestones at ages 15, 16 and 17 respectively compared to Boomers at ages 26, 40, and 51.[9]

US estimates of sexual and gender diverse populations parallel global estimates: While global estimates are limited and vary widely by country/continent, a recent survey of 16 to 74-year-old persons across 27 countries show that the estimates of sexual and gender diverse populations in THE US are consistent with global average estimates–with approximately 10% on average identifying as lesbian, gay, bisexual, or otherwise sexual diverse and 2% on average identifying as transgender or otherwise gender diverse.[10]

SEXUAL AND GENDER DIVERSE YOUTH EXPOSURES TO DISCRIMINATION AND STIGMA

The changing patterns of identification and disclosure among sexual and gender diversity youth likely reflect the positive shift in attitudes and overall decline in bias and prejudice against sexual and gender diverse people that has occurred over the last 20 years. The cultural shift of the 2000s and 2010s-as evidenced by significant policy changes such as Marriage Equality, the repeal of "Don't Ask, Don't Tell," and Obama era Title IX protections for transgender students-made space for sexual and gender diverse people in everyday life that prior generations did not experience. However, as more recent anti-LGBTQ policy and legislative changes have illustrated, this cultural shift has not been ubiquitous. Discrimination and stigma continue to contribute to minority stress in SGD youth which–as described later in discussion –negatively impacts their health and well-being.

Minority stress is THE theoretical framework that explains how the hostile and stressful environment caused by anti-LGBTQ stigma and discrimination impacts the health of sexual and gender diverse people. While initially developed to explain the role of minority stress on mental health disparities in gay men,[11] this framework has since been applied to other health disparities including substance use, sexual health (eg, HIV/STI), and reproductive health outcomes across sexual and gender diverse populations.[12,13] The framework examines minority stress at both distal and proximal levels. Distal minority stress includes external sources of anti-LGBTQ stigma and discrimination. Proximal minority stress refers to internal processes that result from experiencing distal stressors and includes the internalization of stigma, the expectation of rejection, and concealment. This might present as a transgender female adolescent who is afraid to disclose her gender identity to her parents or isolates herself from her friends for fear of rejection or a same-gender loving cisgender male adolescent who believes he will inevitably acquire HIV because he has internalized homophobic messages that equate his sexual identity with negative sexual health outcomes.

The distal minority stressors that SGD youth may experience and subsequently internalize are rooted in attitudes, systems, and structures that are homophobic, transphobic, heterosexist, and/or cissexist (**Box 2**). Homophobia and transphobia are both types of bias based on fear, hatred, negative attitudes, discomfort with, or discriminatory treatment directed toward individuals or groups of people. Homophobia is directed against people based on their sexual orientation, and transphobia is directed against people based on their gender identity. Similar to other forms of bias or prejudice homophobia and transphobia are both assaults on an individual's personhood or self-identity. Homophobia and transphobia, however, can also be uniquely harmful, because the offenders can often be central to one's group identity

> **Box 2**
> **Forms of anti-LGBTQ + stigma and discrimination**
>
> Homophobia: fear, hatred, negative attitudes or feelings, discomfort with, or discriminatory treatment directed toward people based on an actual or perceived non-heterosexual orientation
>
> Transphobia: fear, hatred, negative attitudes or feelings, discomfort with, or discriminatory treatment directed toward people whose identity or gender presentation (or their perceived gender or gender identity) does not match in the societally expected way the sex they were assigned at birth
>
> Heterosexism: implicit or explicit bias that positions heterosexuality as the expected norm and any non-heterosexual orientation as abnormal, inferior, or inconsequential
>
> Cissexism: implicit or explicit bias that marginalizes any non-cisgender identity while positioning cisgender identity as normal or superior

(eg, members of one's racial/ethnic, religious, or community group) or otherwise important sources of social support (eg, parents, other family members, or peers). During adolescent development, affirmation and support from important others and interpersonal attachments are critical.[14] Experiencing homophobia and transphobia from these important others can be particularly isolating for SGD youth and can negatively impact developmental and health outcomes. Compared to sexual and gender-diverse youth who are affirmed by their families, youth who experience homophobic or transphobic family rejection are more likely to experience mental and behavioral health challenges (eg, depression, anxiety, suicidality, substance use) and poor sexual and reproductive health outcomes.[15,16] A study from the Family Acceptance Project demonstrated that increasing levels of family rejection was associated with increasing lifetime suicide attempts for SGD youth.[17] Family affirmation for SGD youth, however, is associated with greater social support, self-esteem and well-being and has demonstrated a protective effect against depression, suicidality, substance use and sexually transmitted infections.[15,16]

Heterosexism and cissexism are similar types of bias that can also contribute to minority stress, and through distal and proximal processes, negatively impact the well-being of SGD youth. These biases are based on the societal expectation of normality and the marginalization of sexual and gender diversity as abnormalities. Heterosexism positions heterosexuality as the expected norm and any nonheterosexual orientation as abnormal, inferior, or inconsequential. Similarly, cissexism marginalizes any non-cisgender identities while positioning cisgender identity as normal or superior. Both heterosexism and cissexism can operate at an internal or interpersonal level to demean or invalidate sexual or gender diversity, but can also operate at a structural level by informing anti-LBGT laws and policies, systemic processes, or social norms that exclude, marginalize or restrict the opportunities of sexual and gender diverse populations within institutions, communities or jurisdictions.[18] Examples of this structural anti-LGBTQ stigma include educational policy that prohibits references to sexual and gender diversity, legislation limiting access to gender-affirming care for adolescents, antidiscrimination policies that exclude protections for sexual orientation or gender identity, banning transgender adolescents from sports participation.

While there is currently limited data on the impact of recent anti-LGBTQ policy and legislation on SGD youth, prior studies have demonstrated a clear association between structural anti-LGBTQ stigma, operationalized through heterosexist and cissexist policies, and SGD youth's health and well-being–particularly their mental health.[19–22] An analysis of the association between state-level nondiscrimination policies, suicidality and inpatient mental health hospitalizations found a decrease in suicidality among gender diverse children, adolescents and adults in states implementing these policies.[19] Similarly, an analysis prior to federal marriage equality demonstrated state policies favoring same-sex marriage state policies were associated with reduced SGD adolescent suicide attempts.[21] In contrast, community or institutional environments with heterosexist and cissexist ideologies are associated with poor mental and behavioral health outcomes in SGD youth.[23–25] In a mixed methods study examining the relationship between regional variability in community attitudes about sexual and gender diversity, minority stress and mental health in SGD youth, Hammack and colleagues found that even among youth with social support and family/peer affirmation, community level anti-LGBTQ ideologies were associated with increased minority stress, internalized stigma, and depressive symptoms among SGD youth living in those communities.[26] The impact of structural stigma on the health and well-being of SGD youth is made more salient by the striking disparities in mental health between SGD and heterosexual and cisgender youth. In the 2019 YRBS data, suicidality measures were significantly higher in lesbian, gay, and bisexual (LGB) students compared to heterosexual students; 66.3% of LGB students compared to 32% of heterosexual students reported persistent feelings of sadness or hopelessness in the past year; 46.8% compared to 14.5% seriously considered suicide; 40.2% compared to 12.1% made a suicide plan; and 23.4% compared to 6.4% attempted suicide.[27] The 2017 YRBS data which reported these rates by gender identity similarly showed significantly higher percentages of transgender students compared to cisgender male and female students who reported feelings of sadness/hopelessness (53.1% vs 20.7% and 39.3%), considering suicide (43.9% vs 11.0% and 20.3%), planning suicide (39.3% vs 10.4% and 16.0%) and attempting suicide (34.6% vs 5.5% and 9.1%) in the past year.[28]

SGD youth who are from minoritized racial/ethnic groups also experience stigma and discrimination based on their race, ethnicity, or national origin. For these youth, it is important that providers be mindful of intersectionality—a framework that considers the impact multiple minoritized identities or experiences can have on health and well-being.[29] An intersectional approach considers the potential compounding effects multiple minority stressors on an individual but also the impact of intersecting structural inequalities and the consequences of multiple systems of oppression on populations defined by intersecting minoritized identities.[30] Consider the excess and disproportionate burden of HIV on young Black gay, bisexual and other men who have sex with men (GBMSM). While Black/African American people are only 12% of the US population, young Black GBMSM shouldered 51% of the new diagnoses among GBMSM ages 13 to 24.[31] The etiology of this health disparity is not racial differences in individual risk behavior but is rather racial differences in exposure to sexual networks that facilitate HIV transmission and acquisition.[32–39] These networks are dense, racially homogenous with high rates of undiagnosed and untreated HIV and co-factor sexually transmitted infections and the consequence of the intersection of anti-Black and anti-LGBTQ structural inequality, stigma and discrimination.[34]

SEXUAL AND GENDER DIVERSE YOUTH DISPARITIES AND INEQUITIES

In their 2011 report, The Health of Lesbian, Gay, Bisexual, and Transgender People: Building a Foundation for a Better Understanding, the Institute of Medicine made the following statement:

The disparities in both mental and physical health that are seen between LGBT and heterosexual and non-gender-variant youth are influenced largely by their experiences of stigma and discrimination during the development of their sexual orientation and gender identity and throughout the life course.[40]

As the disparities and inequities SGD youth experience are described later in discussion, this framework is important to consider as both an etiology of these disparities and a strategy for achieving health equity.

Health and Social Disparities

Population-level data on the health and well-being of SGD youth remains limited by the lack of inclusive questions about sexual orientation and gender identity in state and national surveys and other health and behavior surveillance systems. The YRBSS which is a significant source of adolescent health-related behaviors and risk does not uniformly ask students about their gender identity and only recently included questions about sexual identity and sex of sex partners in the national survey.[2] Nonetheless, available national and regional data as well as smaller studies with nonprobability samples have consistently demonstrated that SGD youth, especially youth from minoritized racial/ethnic groups, experience greater disparities in mental health (eg, anxiety, depression, suicidality),[1,41,42] substance use,[43] disordered eating behavior,[44–46] overweight and obesity, and poor sexual (HIV/STI risk)[31,47–49] and reproductive health (eg, unplanned pregnancy)[50] outcomes compared to their heterosexual and cisgender peers.[1,51] SGD youth also experience higher rates of runaway and homelessness,[51–53] foster care,[51] juvenile carceral system involvement,[51,54] bullying and victimization,[5,55,56] intimate partner violence[5,56] and other social-behavioral conditions that can threaten their well-being and successful transition to adulthood.[1,51]

Health Care Disparities

The major pediatric professional societies recommend that pediatric providers are trained in clinical, cultural, and structural competencies specific to the care needs of SGD youth. Recommendations from the Society of Adolescent Health and Medicine state that all physicians caring for adolescents and young adults "be trained to provide competent and nonjudgmental care for LGBT youth."[57] Similarly, the American Academy of Pediatrics (AAP) states that pediatricians must understand sexual orientation, behavior, and gender identity and are responsible for helping to reduce health disparities by providing culturally competent care to SGD youth and youth from other minoritized groups.[58] However, inadequate pediatric provider training and comfort with SGD care, stigma and discrimination within health care settings and systems, geographic disparities in care access, and emerging legislative restrictions on the provision of evidence-based care-undermine the potential support pediatric care settings can offer and contribute to health care disparities that widen rather than reduce health and social disparities impacting SGD youth.

Inadequate Pediatric Provider Training: In a recent AAP survey of primary care pediatricians, only 18% report routinely discussing sexual orientation and gender identity (SOGI) with their patients and families.[59] Although content specifications for the American Board of Pediatrics and certification exam includes key aspects of SGD health including sexual orientation, gender identity, gender dysphoria, and health promotion and disease prevention specific to disease outcomes disproportionately affecting sexual and gender diverse persons, there remains a lack of consistent, formal training on SGD specific health and health care needs in undergraduate and graduate medical education.[60] Routinely asking about sexual orientation and gender identity alerts youth that it is safe to disclose their identity to their provider or otherwise discuss these issues. Without this cue or other assurances, SGD youth are not likely to initiate these discussions. Growing up LGBT in America, a 2018 Human Rights Campaign's survey of over 10,000 SGD youth ages 13 to 17 found that over half of sexual (67%) and gender (61%) diverse respondents had not disclosed their identity to their provider.[55] There are important implications of this nondisclosure including missed opportunities to provide affirmation and support for patients and families, anticipatory guidance, and care directed toward the specific health-related needs of SGD youth.

For gender-diverse youth, lack of training among pediatric providers is on the of the most significant barriers to care. Even among endocrinologists and adolescent medicine subspecialists, the pediatric providers most likely to care for these youth, a lack of training is described as a leading barrier to care.[61,62]

Stigma and Discrimination in Health Care Settings and Systems: Implicit bias, stigma, and discrimination within health care settings and systems remain a significant barrier to care for sexual and gender-diverse youth–particularly for youth from minoritized racial/ethnic groups who may experience discrimination and mistreatment based on both their sexual or gender diversity and their racial/ethnic identity. Recent reviews[63,64] of prior studies examining SGD youth health encounters identified common patterns of care that were stigmatizing to SGD youth including lack of provider knowledge and clinical skills to address SGD-related health needs, false provider assumptions about SGD youth (eg, assumption of heterosexual identity and behaviors, conflation of gender and sexuality, associating gay identity with HIV, associating transgender identity with mental illness or adolescent experimentation), denial and refusal of care, verbal or physical abuse, and negative attitudes and reactions to SGD patients resulting in poor patient engagement during clinical encounters. Several studies have described delayed care seeking or health care avoidance among SGD youth due to discomfort in clinical settings, prior negative experiences or fear of stigma, particularly among transgender and gender-diverse youth.[64–67]

SGD youth from minoritized racial/ethnic groups have faced additional barriers to care discrimination and mistreatment based on their racial/ethnic identity. In a qualitative study of young Black GBMSM, participants described how previous and anticipated homophobic and anti-Black negative interactions with physician alienated them from health care settings and created significant barriers to uptake of pre-exposure prophylaxis (PrEP) for HIV prevention.[68] Recent racial disparities in monkeypox infections and vaccine uptake have similarly been ascribed to experiences of stigma and homophobia among Black GBMSM.[69]

Geographic and Socioeconomic Inequities in Access to Care: Regional and geographic variation in the availability of affirming, inclusive health care services and other health-related resources is another barrier to care for sexual and gender-diverse youth. Differential (eg, lower) access to LGBTQ friendly, youth appropriate care and resources has been noted for sexual and gender-diverse youth living in rural areas compared to larger metropolitan areas,[70,71] in communities with higher rates of poverty or higher proportion of minoritized racial/ethnic groups,[72] and states with history of laws penalizing SGD populations and/or lower levels of legal protections and anti-discrimination statutes.[71]

Limitations in workforce capacity and the structure of how some SGD-related care is provided also creates geographic disparities in care. Because few pediatricians are trained in gender-affirming care, much of pediatric and adolescent gender-affirming care occurs in pediatric subspecialty centers in academic medical centers in major metropolitan areas which limits access for youth who do not live in close proximity to one of these centers.[62]

The spatial distribution of health care services and other resources for SGD populations within metropolitan areas also creates inequitable access to care often by race/ethnicity and socioeconomic status. These services are often concentrated where sexual and gender diverse people socialize or otherwise congregate which may limit access to these services in racially segregated cities where SGD youth from minoritized racial/ethnic groups are more likely to live outside of these areas.[71] A spatial analysis of LGBTQ human services sites in Chicago showed a disproportionate percentage of these sites in majority non-Hispanic white (71%) and upper income (63.7%) block groups, while Black, Latinx and poor to low-income residents disproportionately lived in LGBTQ service deserts.[72]

For gender-affirming care specifically, the cost of care and variation in health insurance coverage creates geographic, socioeconomic, and racial disparities in care access for gender-diverse youth. While 24 states and the District of Columbia prohibit transgender exclusions in private insurance and/or Medicaid, over half of states do not have policies protecting coverage.[73] In August 2022, Florida's Agency for Health Care Administration joined eight other states by banning Medicaid coverage of any gender-affirming care–a ruling that has since been upheld by a Federal court.[73] Similarly, Arkansas law permits insurers to refuse coverage for gender-affirming care.[73] This structural anti-LGBTQ stigma is often compounded for gender-diverse youth who are from racial/ethnic minority groups. A longitudinal study of transgender and gender diverse young adults, found that racial/ethnic minoritized youth were more likely to be uninsured and lack access to healthcare.[65]

Emerging legal challenges/barriers to care: Health care disparities have been further exacerbated by the wave of state executive and legislative restrictions on the rights of SGD youth. Legislative restrictions on medically necessary and evidence-based gender-affirming care for minor pediatric patients have most directly impact access to care for gender-diverse youth. Four states (Alabama, Arkansas, Arizona and Texas) have passed laws restricting minor's access to gender-affirming care and 15 additional states are considering 25 bills proposing similar restrictions. The existing and proposed laws vary but include provisions that penalize health professionals and parents for providing or helping youth access gender-affirming care, allow individuals to file for damages against health professions providing gender-affirming care, and limit third party reimbursement or prohibit use of state funds for gender-affirming services(eg, Florida's Medicaid ban).[74]

In addition to the bills restricting healthcare for transgender youth, there have been a number of other bills and executive orders targeting sexual and gender diverse people for discrimination. These bills include single-sex facility restrictions, restricting access to sports participation for transgender students, prohibiting content related to sexual and gender identity in school curricula, impeding access to identification with correct name and gender, religious exemptions for healthcare, adoption and foster care restrictions for SGD people, and bills pre-empting cities and other local jurisdictions from passing nondiscrimination protections for SGD people.[75] As described earlier in this article, this structural anti-LGBTQ stigma operationalized through heterosexist and cissexist policies have a negative impact on the health and well-being of SGD youth, but they also contribute to a sociopolitical environment that further stigmatizes sexual and gender diversity and compounds the health care disparities described above.

PEDIATRIC PROVIDERS AS CRITICAL PROTECTIVE FACTORS FOR SEXUAL AND GENDER DIVERSE YOUTH

The National Academies 2020 report *Understanding the Well-Being of LGBTQI + Populations*[13] notes the following:

> Early life course exposure to discrimination and stigma based on sexual orienta-
> tion, gender identity, or intersex status can have lifelong consequences [...and]
> can set trajectories of health and well-being into motion that may be exacerbated
> by subsequent exposures to discrimination or interrupted by subsequent expo-
> sures to protective factors.[1]

While their risk for poor health and social outcomes is incrementally higher it is not universal. Pediatric providers and an inclusive medical home can be a critical protective factor. As the first health care contacts for SGD youth, pediatric providers can potentially be the first source of support and affirmation. The clinical practice strategies described later in discussion can help pediatric providers develop therapeutic relationships with SGD youth and their families and provide an inclusive medical home that is protective against the stigma and discrimination that contribute to SGD youth health disparities.

Continuing medical education about health needs of SGD youth:

While practicing pediatric providers may have had limited exposure to SGD health needs during their undergraduate and graduate medical education, there is a growing body of continuing medical education content and curricula practitioners can access to increase their knowledge and skills in this area–including clinical practice guidelines, e-learning, and other online modules and live continuing medical education. This content is offered by pediatric and adolescent medicine professional societies (eg, AAP, SAHM, American Academy of Child and Adolescent Psychiatry), professional societies and organizations focused on sexual and reproductive health wellness (eg, Physicians for Reproductive Health, American Sexual health Association, Planned Parenthood) and LGBTQ specific health and medicine professional societies (eg, World Professional Association for Transgender Health, Gay and Lesbian Medical Association). The National LGBTQIA Health Education Center–a program of the Fenway Institute similarly offers comprehensive educational resources for individual providers and has partnered with many of the organizations above to support their educational initiatives (**Table 1** for provider educational resources and specific trainings).

Creating an affirming and inclusive clinical environment: The organizations referenced above are also a good resource for strategies to ensure all youth, including SGD youth, youth from minoritized racial/ethnic groups and those with intersecting identities feel safe, supported and welcomed in clinical settings. A number of studies[63,76,77] have also described attributes of affirming, inclusive, adolescent friendly clinics that pediatric providers can incorporate into their clinical practice while avoiding the heteronormative approaches described above.

- Environmental markers of affirmation and inclusion (eg, rainbow flags; posters, flyers, and pamphlets featuring SGD youth, safe space designations)
- Patient materials that avoid heteronormative assumptions and includes inclusive language (eg, clinic pamphlets, website, questionnaires)
- All staff trained in LGBTQ affirming and inclusive care–including front desk staff and all clinical staff (eg, providers, nursing, social work, and so forth)
- Electronic medical record systems that allow the designation of preferred name, pronouns and documentation of sexual orientation and gender identity

Table 1
Provider, youth and parent/family resources for support sexual and gender-diverse youth

	Resources
Providers	Medical Education, Training and Clinical Guidelines

American Academy of Pediatrics Policy Statements, Technical Reports, and Guidelines
- Office Based Care for Lesbian, Gay, Bisexual, Transgender and Questioning Youth
- Ensuring Comprehensive Care and Support for Transgender and Gender-Diverse Children and Adolescents
- A Pediatrician's Guide to an LGBTQ + Friendly Practice

Society for Adolescent Health and Medicine Position Papers
- Recommendations for Promoting the Health and Well-being of Sexual and Gender–diverse Adolescents Through Supportive Families and Affirming Support Networks
- Promoting Health Equality and Nondiscrimination for Transgender and Gender-Diverse Youth

The National LGBT Health Education Center of The Fenway Institute: https://fenwayhealth.org/the-fenway-institute/education/the-national-lgbtia-health-education-center/
- Provides educational programs, resources, and consultation to health care organizations with the goal of optimizing quality, cost-effective health care for lesbian, gay, bisexual, transgender, queer, intersex, asexual, and all sexual and gender minority (LGBTQIA+) people

Advocates for Youth – Adolescent Reproductive and Sexual Health Education Project (ARSHEP): https://www.advocatesforyouth.org/arshep-presentations-sign-up/
- A comprehensive educational tool for adolescent reproductive and sexual health.
- ARSHEP modules provide a curated set of lectures, created as PowerPoint slide decks and Case Videos that can be freely downloaded, modified, and presented to audiences of clinical providers including physicians, nurse practitioners, physician associates, and others who provide care and services to adolescent patients
- Includes specific content focused on care of SGD youth

Center for Excellent in Transgender Health: http://www.transhealth.ucsf.edu/
- Includes training modules, guidelines and toolkits for care of transgender and gender non-binary communities

Endocrine Society Clinical Practice Guidelines- Gender Dysphoria/Gender Incongruence Guideline Resources: https://www.endocrine.org/clinical-practice-guidelines/gender-dysphoria-gender-incongruence

World Professional Association for Transgender Health Global Education Institute: https://www.wpath.org/gei
- Certified training courses in Best Practices in Transgender Medical and Mental Health care
- Training Courses are offered in an interdisciplinary, interactive, live format, providing ample opportunity for networking and building referral systems.

Resources for Physician Advocacy

SIECUS Sex Ed for Social Change: https://siecus.org/
- Includes resources and information related to policy and advocacy, education and resource development and strategic communications

Human Rights Campaign: www.hrc.org
- Advocacy and research organization that promotes rights and well-being for all LGBTQ + individuals

(continued on next page)

Table 1 (continued)	
	Resources
SGD Youth	Online Crisis and Social Support Resources The Trevor Project: www.thetrevorproject.org • Leading national organization providing crisis intervention and suicide prevention services to LGBTQ young people under 25 • Resources, including a hotline, text and chat features, to support LGBTQ youth It Gets Better: www.itgetsbetter.org • Mission is to communicate to LGBTQ youth around the world that it gets better, and to create and inspire the changes needed to make it better for them • Website features a stories page of over 60,000 video messages Q Chat Space: https://www.lgbtcenters.org/QChatSpace • Professionally facilitated text-based online support groups • Gives youth safe opportunities to connect with each other in spaces moderated by trusted adults SGD Youth Affirming and Advocacy Resources The GenderCool Project: https://gendercool.org/ • The GenderCool Project is a youth-led movement bringing positive change to the world. The Champions are helping replace misinformed opinions with positive experiences meeting transgender and non-binary youth who are thriving ACLU- LGBTQ Youth & Schools Resource Library: https://www.aclu.org/library-lgbt-youth-schools-resources-and-links • Includes information and resources for youth to help them learn more about their rights and what they can do to make their school a safer, more welcoming place PFLAG Index of LGBTQ Camps for Youth: https://pflag.org/youthcamps
Parents and Families	Resources for Supporting Understanding and Acceptance and other Parenting Resources PFLAG Parents, Families, and Friends of Lesbian and Gays: www.pflag.org • Organization supporting and connecting parents, families and friends of the LGBTQ community • 400 chapters nationwide, in nearly every state • Provides information on coming out help for families, friends, and allies, including resources, terminology, and advice for families The Family Acceptance Project: http://familyproject.sfsu.edu/ • Family support module and research-based resources to help diverse families including conservative families support their SGM children in the context of their values and beliefs The AAP Parenting Website: https://www.healthychildren.org • Parenting website backed by 67,000 pediatricians committed to the attainment of optimal physical, mental, and social health and well-being for all infants, children, adolescents, and young adults • Searchable content includes specific resources for parents of SGD youth Resources for Parent/Family Advocacy PFLAG Advocacy Toolkit: https://pflag.org/AdvocacyTools Family Equality: https://www.familyequality.org/ • Founded in 1979 at the National March on Washington for Lesbian and Gay Rights, Family Equality has spent more than 40 y ensuring that everyone has the freedom to find, form, and sustain their families by advancing equality for the LGBTQ + community

(continued on next page)

| Table 1 |
| *(continued)* |

Resources
GLSEN: https://www.glsen.org/
• GLSEN works to ensure that LGBTQ students are able to learn and grow in a school environment free from bullying and harassment
• Includes resources for youth, parents and educators

- Demonstrated knowledge about and sensitivity to specific SGD youth health care needs
- Mirror patient language used to describe sexual orientation and gender identity, relationships, anatomy, sexual behavior, and so forth.
- Approach to all patients that acknowledges and normalizes the diversity of sexuality and gender identity
- Patient-provider rapport that creates a welcoming and safe environment
- Clear establishment of confidentiality (and the limits of confidentiality) for all AYA.

Assessing sexual orientation and gender identity assessment and linking to or providing appropriate affirming care:

Routine and universal conversations about sexual orientation and gender identity create an environment of support and reassurance so that children, adolescents and young adults feel safe bringing up questions and concerns. Universally engaging patients and families about sexuality and gender also provides an opportunity to model to children and families that diverse sexual and gender identities are a normal and expected aspect of human diversity. There are no specific guidelines for SOGI assessment in children and adolescents, but general recommendations have been described and are summarized in **Box 3**.[78–80] Links to SOGI assessment demonstration videos can be found in **Table 1**.

Provider-initiated SOGI discussions are associated with youth disclosure of sexual and gender diversity and lowered barriers to accessing SGD-related health care.[81–84] For example, in gender-diverse youth, earlier disclosure can lead to earlier referral to gender-affirming care services which is associated with lower rates of mental health problems.[85] Knowing and understanding a patient's gender diversity also allows providers to incorporate the gender-affirming care model (GACM) in the care of gender diverse patients. GACM is developmentally appropriate care focused on understanding and appreciating a pediatric or adolescent patient's gender experience. This care approach communicates the following affirming messages to patients and families: (1) gender diverse identities are not mental disorders, (2) gender diversity is a normal aspect of human diversity, (3) gender identity is informed by an interplay of biology, development, socialization, and culture, and (4) mental health challenges if present are the result of antitransgender stigma and discrimination (**Box 4**).[86]

Providers who are aware of a patient's sexual or gender diversity can also address potential vulnerabilities related to health and social disparities impacting SGD youth. For example, increased risk for HIV acquisition is a potential vulnerability for GBMSM and transgender women who have sex with me. In a study examining factors associated with HIV testing in adolescent GBMSM, the most significant predictors of HIV testing were providers asking about sexual orientation, same-sex behavior and HIV.[82] Mental health disparities in SGD youth represent another potential vulnerability that providers can address. Minority stressors that contribute to mental health disparities for SGD youth point to important intervention targets pediatric providers can

Box 3
Recommended guidelines for SOGI assessments in children and adolescents

Where to ask: SOGI assessments should be made in the context of a safe and supportive clinical environment, be age and developmentally appropriate and provide appropriate protections for confidentiality. Appropriate protections for confidentiality include assurances that SOGI information will not be shared without permission and clear explanation of potential for inadvertent disclosures (eg, parent/care giver access to SOGI documentation in the patient electronic health record)

How to ask: SOGI may be assessed as part of a self-administered previsit questionnaire and/or during the clinical encounter while taking a social history. SOGI assessments on previsit questionnaires can signal an inclusive environment for SGD youth and allow opportunity to initiate SOGI assessments during the clinical encounter.

When to ask: Assessment of gender identity may start at ages 3 to 5, when most children have reached the developmental stage where they can verbalize and understand their gender identity. Asking about sexual orientation may start in early adolescence (ages 11–13) the developmental stage when identity formation including sexual identity formation begins.

Who to ask: SOGI assessment should be routine and universal and both patients and parents/caregivers should be aware these questions are asked of all patients. Whether or not parents/caregivers are present and included in the assessment may be based on the typical age where providers begin collecting the social history from adolescent patients without parents/caregivers present (eg, ages 11–17).

What to ask: Gender identity assessment typically include questions about both gender identity and expression and sex assigned at birth. Sexual orientation assessments may include questions about sexual attraction, behavior and identity. Questions about attraction or romantic interests may be more appropriate for younger adolescents who have not engaged in sexual behavior or completed sexual identity formation. Additionally, sexual attraction, behavior, and identity may or may not align so asking about each component of sexual orientation separately may provide a more complete assessment of an adolescent patient's sexuality.

Box 4
Gender-affirming care model

- Developmentally appropriate care that is oriented toward understanding and appreciating the youth's gender experience.
- Based on research that suggests that valuing a child for who they are now
  ○ Rather than focusing on who they may become
  ○ Fosters secure attachment and resilience for the child and family
- This model of care conveys the following messages to patients and families:
  ○ Transgender identities and diverse gender are not a mental disorder;
  ○ Variations in gender identity and expression are normal aspects of human diversity
  ○ Gender identity evolves as an interplay of biology, development, socialization, and culture
  ○ If a mental health issue exists the etiology is most likely stigma and negative experiences rather than being intrinsic to the child
- Gender-affirming care is NOT "watchful waiting"
  ○ Child's gender-diverse assertions are held as "possibly true" until an arbitrary age (often after pubertal onset) when they can be considered valid
  ○ Does not serve the child because critical support is withheld
  ○ Based on binary notions of gender in which gender diversity and fluidity is pathologized

leverage for their SGD patients with mental health concerns. Proximate minority stressors (eg, internalization of stigma, the expectation of rejection, and concealment) that negatively impact mental health are cognitive, behavioral, and affective adaptations to distal/external minority stressors that can be addressed through mental health and other supportive services–including virtual crisis services and peer support groups specific to SGD youth (eg, Trevor Project, Q Chat) and LGBTQ affirming cognitive behavioral therapy.[51,87,88]

So, it is important the providers not only engage patients about sexual orientation and gender diversity, but also be prepared to respond to patients who disclose their sexual or gender diversity with affirmation and support-including developmentally appropriate care oriented toward understanding and appreciating the youth's experience, screening for SGD-related health needs, and providing additional resources as needed.[89]

Supporting parents and caregivers:

As discussed above, parent and family acceptance, support, and affirmation can help SGD youth successfully transition to adulthood, combat minority stress and intersectional stigma, develop resilience, and avoid significant health and social disparities. Pediatric and adolescent medicine providers should help parents and families understand they are the most critical protective factor for SGD youth and prioritize facilitating family acceptance by supporting, educating, and equipping parents with the tools needed to affirm and protect their SGD child against the negative effects of anti-LGBTQ stigma. Providers may consider incorporating the following recommended strategies for engaging and supporting parents and families.

- Create an environment that meets parents where they are and invites them to share their questions, fears, concerns, and beliefs.
- Share the evidence of the importance of parent and family support for the health and well-being of SGD youth.
- Provide parents with anticipatory guidance important for all youth-parental monitoring, parent-child communication, and expectations and limit setting-as they navigate the transition to adulthood.
- Provide resources (eg, LGBTQ support groups, educational resources, affirming individual and family mental health care resources) to assist parents and families with the acceptance and support of their SGD youth

Linking patients and families to community resources and support:In addition to parent and family acceptance described above,[16,51,90] safe and inclusive school environments,[51,91,92] and community and peer supports[93,94] can help SGD youth develop internal assets and engage external resources to help avoid risk and navigate the minority stressors many of these youth experience. Providers can also play a critical role in connecting SGD youth to these additional protective factors outside of the clinic and medical home. Community resources for SGD youth and families are summarized in **Table 1**.

ACHIEVING HEALTH EQUITY FOR SEXUAL AND GENDER-DIVERSE YOUTH

Health equity has been defined as an "ethical and human rights principle that motivates people to eliminate disparities in health and in the determinants of health that adversely affect excluded or marginalized groups"[95] It is a concept grounded in social justice and a strategy focused on removing the inequities that produce health disparities.

This article has described many of the social inequities that underlie disparities in health, health care, and well-being that SGD youth experience. The prior section describes how pediatric providers can position themselves and their clinical practice to protect and support SGD youth and their families against these inequities, increase access to care and reduce health care disparities for the patients they encounter, and foster a positive youth development approach that builds resiliency. This is a critical strategy for ensuring the SGD youth have the additional supports they need to accommodate for the social inequities they experience.

However, health equity for SGD youth will not ultimately be achieved without eliminating the structural stigma and discrimination that underlie their disparities. While addressing these inequities is not an insurmountable goal, it will require deliberate, coordinated, and consistent effort across multiple fields and stakeholders including health-related research, pediatric and adolescent medicine clinicians, medical education and training, legislative and policy advocates, and families and communities.[51]

Finally, these efforts must be aligned with efforts to dismantle structural stigma and discrimination of all forms. The Center for Intersectional Justice describes intersectionality as a strategy focused on "fighting discrimination within discrimination, tackling inequalities within inequalities, and protecting minorities within minorities."[96] The health, social, and healthcare disparities SGD youth experience are shaped by layers of social disadvantage and intersecting systems of oppression. Without an intersectional approach, any effort to achieve health equity for SGD youth, will be mired by the persistence of discrimination within discrimination, inequalities within inequalities, and the continued disparities minoritized subgroups within SGD youth will continue to experience.

CLINICS CARE POINTS

- Pediatricians and other primary care providers should be aware that they can be a valuable source of support and affirmation and a significant protective factor against the stigma and discrimination that contribute to SGD youth health disparities.

- While practicing pediatric providers may have had limited exposure to SGD health needs during their undergraduate and graduate medical education, there is a growing body of continuing medical education content and curricula practitioners can access to increase their knowledge and skills in this area–including clinical practice guidelines, e-learning modules and live continuing medical education.

- Pediatricians and other primary care providers should ensure that all youth, including SGD youth, youth from minoritized racial/ethnic groups and those with intersecting identities feel safe, supported, and welcomed in their clinical practice settings.

- Pediatricians and other primary care providers should engage in routine, universal, and developmentally appropriate conversations about sexual orientation and gender identity with patients and families and be prepared to respond to patients who disclose their sexual or gender diversity with affirmation and support including providing developmentally appropriate care and anticipatory guidance, screening for SGD-related health needs, protecting privacy and confidentiality as appropriate, and providing additional resources as needed.

- Pediatricians and other primary care providers should help parents and families understand they are the most critical protective factor for SGD youth and prioritize facilitating family acceptance by supporting, educating, and equipping parents with the tools needed to affirm and protect their SGD child against the negative effects of anti-LGBTQ stigma.

DISCLOSURE

Dr E.L. Fields has no relevant commercial or financial conflicts of interest. There are no relevant funding sources.

REFERENCES

1. National Academies of Sciences, Engineering, and Medicine. Understanding the well-being of LGBTQI+ populations. Washington, DC: The National Academies Press; 2020.
2. Underwood JM, Brener N, Thornton J, et al. Overview and methods for the youth risk behavior surveillance system—United States, 2019. MMWR supplements 2020;69(1):1.
3. Kann L, Olsen EOM, McManus T, et al. Sexual identity, sex of sexual contacts, and health-related behaviors among students in grades 9–12—United States and selected sites, 2015. MMWR Surveill Summ 2016;65(9):1–202.
4. Kann L, Olsen E, McManus T, et al. Sexual identity, sex of sexual contacts, and health-risk behaviors among students in grades 9-12–youth risk behavior surveillance, selected sites, United States, 2001-2009. MMWR Surveill Summ 2011; 60(7):1–133.
5. Johns MM, Lowry R, Andrzejewski J, et al. Transgender Identity and Experiences of Violence Victimization, Substance Use, Suicide Risk, and Sexual Risk Behaviors Among High School Students - 19 States and Large Urban School Districts, 2017. MMWR 2019;68(3):67–71. https://doi.org/10.15585/mmwr.mm6803a3.
6. Conron KJ. LGBT youth population in the United States (September 2020). The Williams Institute, UCLA 2020. Available at: https://williamsinstitute.law.ucla.edu/publications/lgbt-youth-pop-us/.
7. Jones JM. LGBT Identification in U.S. Ticks Up to 7.1%. Gallup Politics. 2022. February 17, 2022. Available at: https://news.gallup.com/poll/389792/lgbt-identification-ticks-up.aspx.
8. Bishop MD, Fish JN, Hammack PL, et al. Sexual identity development milestones in three generations of sexual minority people: A national probability sample. Dev Psychol 2020;56(11):2177–93. https://doi.org/10.1037/dev0001105.
9. Puckett JA, Tornello S, Mustanski B, et al. Gender variations, generational effects, and mental health of transgender people in relation to timing and status of gender identity milestones. Psychology of Sexual Orientation and Gender Diversity 2022; 9(2):165.
10. Ipsos. Which, if any, of the following would you identify as?. Chart. June 9, 2021. Statista. Available at: https://www.statista.com/statistics/1270143/lgbt-identification-worldwide-country/. Accessed January 19, 2023.
11. Meyer IH. Minority stress and mental health in gay men. J Health Soc Behav 1995;38–56.
12. Meyer I.H. and Frost D.M., Minority stress and the health of sexual minorities, In: Patterson C.J. and D'Augelli A.R., *Handbook of psychology and sexual orientation*, 2013, Oxford University Press, New York, 252–266.
13. Testa RJ, Habarth J, Peta J, et al. Development of the gender minority stress and resilience measure. Psychology of Sexual Orientation and Gender Diversity 2015; 2(1):65.
14. McNeely C, Blanchard J. The teen years explained: a guide to healthy adolescent development. Baltimore, MD: Johns Hopkins Bloomberg School of Public Health, Center for Adoelscent Health; 2010.

15. Russell ST, Fish JN. Mental health in lesbian, gay, bisexual, and transgender (LGBT) youth. Annu Rev Clin Psychol 2016;12:465–87.

16. Ryan C, Russell ST, Huebner D, et al. Family acceptance in adolescence and the health of LGBT young adults. J Child Adolesc Psychiatr Nurs 2010;23(4):205–13.

17. Ryan C, Huebner D, Diaz RM, et al. Family rejection as a predictor of negative health outcomes in white and Latino lesbian, gay, and bisexual young adults. Pediatrics 2009;123(1):346–52.

18. Hatzenbuehler ML. Structural stigma and Health Inequalities: Research evidence and implications for psychological science. Am Psychol. Nov 2016;71(8):742–51. https://doi.org/10.1037/amp0000068.

19. McDowell A, Raifman J, Progovac AM, et al. Association of Nondiscrimination Policies With Mental Health Among Gender Minority Individuals. JAMA Psychiatr 2020;77(9):952. https://doi.org/10.1001/jamapsychiatry.2020.0770.

20. Wanta JW, Gianakakos G, Belfort E, et al. Considering "Spheres of Influence" in the Care of Lesbian, Gay, Bisexual Transgender, and Queer-Identified Youth. Child and Adolescent Psychiatric Clinics of North America 2022;31(4):649–64. https://doi.org/10.1016/j.chc.2022.05.008.

21. Raifman J, Moscoe E, Austin SB, et al. Difference-in-differences analysis of the association between state same-sex marriage policies and adolescent suicide attempts. JAMA Pediatr 2017;171(4):350–6.

22. Woodford MR, Kulick A, Garvey JC, et al. LGBTQ policies and resources on campus and the experiences and psychological well-being of sexual minority college students: Advancing research on structural inclusion. Psychology of Sexual Orientation and Gender Diversity 2018;5(4):445.

23. Hatzenbuehler ML, Jun H-J, Corliss HL, et al. Structural stigma and sexual orientation disparities in adolescent drug use. Addict Behav 2015;46:14–8.

24. Watson RJ, Fish JN, Denary W, et al. LGBTQ state policies: A lever for reducing SGM youth substance use and bullying. Drug Alcohol Depend 2021;221:108659.

25. Price-Feeney M, Green AE, Dorison SH. Impact of Bathroom Discrimination on Mental Health Among Transgender and Nonbinary Youth. J Adolesc Health 2021;68(6):1142–7.

26. Hammack PL, Pletta DR, Hughes SD, et al. Community support for sexual and gender diversity, minority stress, and mental health: a mixed-methods study of adolescents with minoritized sexual and gender identities. Psychology of Sexual Orientation and Gender Diversity 2022.

27. Johns MM, Lowry R, Haderxhanaj LT, et al. Trends in Violence Victimization and Suicide Risk by Sexual Identity Among High School Students — Youth Risk Behavior Survey, United States, 2015–2019. MMWR Supplements 2020;69(1): 19–27. https://doi.org/10.15585/mmwr.su6901a3.

28. Johns MM, Lowry R, Andrzejewski J, et al. Transgender identity and experiences of violence victimization, substance use, suicide risk, and sexual risk behaviors among high school students—19 states and large urban school districts, 2017. MMWR (Morb Mortal Wkly Rep) 2019;68(3):67.

29. Crenshaw K. Demarginalizing the Intersection of Race and Sex: Black Feminist Critique of Antidiscrimination Doctrine, Feminist Theory and Antiracist Politics. Chicago: University of Chicago Legal Forum; 1989. p. 139–68.

30. Homan P, Brown TH, King B. Structural Intersectionality as a New Direction for Health Disparities Research. J Health Soc Behav 2021;62(3):350–70. https://doi.org/10.1177/00221465211032947.

31. Centers for Disease Control and Prevention. HIV Surveillance Report, 2019; vol.32. Available at: http://www.cdc.gov/hiv/library/reports/hiv-surveillance.html. Published May 2021. Accessed 15 September, 2022.

32. Janulis P, Phillips G, Birkett M, et al. Sexual Networks of Racially Diverse Young MSM Differ in Racial Homophily But Not Concurrency. J Acquir Immune Defic Syndr 2018;77(5):459–66. https://doi.org/10.1097/qai.0000000000001620.

33. Mustanski B, Morgan E, D'Aquila R, et al. Individual and Network Factors Associated With Racial Disparities in HIV Among Young Men Who Have Sex With Men: Results From the RADAR Cohort Study. J Acquir Immune Defic Syndr 2019;80(1): 24–30. https://doi.org/10.1097/qai.0000000000001886.

34. Millett GA, Flores SA, Peterson JL, et al. Explaining disparities in HIV infection among black and white men who have sex with men: a meta-analysis of HIV risk behaviors. Aids 2007;21(15):2083–91.

35. Kelley CF, Vaughan AS, Luisi N, et al. The effect of high rates of bacterial sexually transmitted infections on HIV incidence in a cohort of black and white men who have sex with men in Atlanta, Georgia. AIDS Res Hum Retrovir 2015;31(6): 587–92.

36. Pathela P, Braunstein SL, Blank S, et al. The high risk of an HIV diagnosis following a diagnosis of syphilis: a population-level analysis of New York City men. Clin Infect Dis 2015;61(2):281–7.

37. Tilchin C, Schumacher CM, Psoter KJ, et al. Human Immunodeficiency Virus Diagnosis After a Syphilis, Gonorrhea, or Repeat Diagnosis Among Males Including non–Men Who Have Sex With Men: What Is the Incidence? Sex Transm Dis 2019;46(4):271–7. https://doi.org/10.1097/olq.0000000000000964.

38. Agwu A, Ellen J. Rising rates of HIV infection among young US men who have sex with men. Pediatr Infect Dis J 2009;28(7):633–4.

39. Beck EC, Birkett M, Armbruster B, et al. A data-driven simulation of HIV spread among young men who have sex with men: the role of age and race mixing, and STIs. J Acquir Immune Defic Syndr 2015;70(2):186.

40. Institute of Medicine. The health of lesbian, gay, bisexual, and transgender people: building a foundation for better understanding. Washington, DC: The National Academies Press; 2011. p. 366.

41. Raifman J, Charlton BM, Arrington-Sanders R, et al. Sexual orientation and suicide attempt disparities among US adolescents: 2009–2017. Pediatrics 2020; 145(3).

42. Ivey-Stephenson AZ, Demissie Z, Crosby AE, et al. Suicidal ideation and behaviors among high school students—youth risk behavior survey, United States, 2019. MMWR supplements 2020;69(1):47.

43. Jones CM, Clayton HB, Deputy NP, et al. Prescription opioid misuse and use of alcohol and other substances among high school students—Youth Risk Behavior Survey, United States, 2019. MMWR supplements 2020;69(1):38.

44. Calzo JP, Blashill AJ, Brown TA, et al. Eating Disorders and Disordered Weight and Shape Control Behaviors in Sexual Minority Populations. Curr Psychiatr Rep 2017;19(8):49. https://doi.org/10.1007/s11920-017-0801-y.

45. Murray SB, Nagata JM, Griffiths S, et al. The enigma of male eating disorders: A critical review and synthesis. Clin Psychol Rev 2017;57:1–11.

46. Nagata JM, Ganson KT, Austin SB. Emerging trends in eating disorders among sexual and gender minorities. Curr Opin Psychiatry 2020;33(6):562–7. https://doi.org/10.1097/yco.0000000000000645.

47. Centers for Disease Control and Prevention. Sexually transmitted disease surveillance 2020. Atlanta: US Department of Health and Human Services; 2022.

48. Charlton BM, Corliss HL, Missmer SA, et al. Reproductive health screening disparities and sexual orientation in a cohort study of US adolescent and young adult females. J Adolesc Health 2011;49(5):505–10.

49. Agénor M, Muzny CA, Schick V, et al. Sexual orientation and sexual health services utilization among women in the United States. Prev Med 2017;95:74–81.

50. Charlton BM, Roberts AL, Rosario M, et al. Teen Pregnancy Risk Factors Among Young Women of Diverse Sexual Orientations. Pediatrics 2018;141(4). https://doi.org/10.1542/peds.2017-2278.

51. National Academies of Science E and Medicine. Reducing inequalities between LGBTQ adolescents and cisgender, heterosexual adolescents: proceedings of a workshop. Washington, DC: The National Academies Press.

52. Fraser B, Pierse N, Chisholm E, et al. LGBTIQ+ Homelessness: A Review of the Literature. Int J Environ Res Publ Health 2019;16(15):2677.

53. Fish JN, Baams L, Wojciak AS, et al. Are sexual minority youth overrepresented in foster care, child welfare, and out-of-home placement? Findings from nationally representative data. Child Abuse & Neglect 2019;89:203–11. https://doi.org/10.1016/j.chiabu.2019.01.005.

54. McCandless S. LGBT Homeless Youth and Policing. Public Integr 2018;20(6):558–70. https://doi.org/10.1080/10999922.2017.1402738.

55. Kahn E, Johnson A, Lee M, Miranda L. 2018 LGBTQ Youth Report. Available at: https://www.hrc.org/resources/2018-lgbtq-youth-report. Accessed 25, 2021 April, 2018.

56. Johns MM, Lowry R, Haderxhanaj LT, et al. Trends in violence victimization and suicide risk by sexual identity among high school students—Youth Risk Behavior Survey, United States, 2015–2019. MMWR supplements 2020;69(1):19.

57. Reitman DS, Austin B, Belkind U, et al. Recommendations for promoting the health and well-being of lesbian, gay, bisexual, and transgender adolescents: A position paper of the society for adolescent health and medicine. J Adolesc Health 2013;52(4):506–10.

58. Levine DA. Office-based care for lesbian, gay, bisexual, transgender, and questioning youth. Pediatrics 2013;132(1):e297–313.

59. Alexander SCFJ, Pollak KI, Bravender T, et al. Sexuality talk during adolescent health maintenance visits. JAMA Pediatr 2014;168(2):163–9.

60. Roth LT, Cooper MB, Lurie B, et al. Developing an entrustable professional activity to Improve the care of LGBTQ+ youth. Academic Pediatrics 2022. https://doi.org/10.1016/j.acap.2022.09.006.

61. Vance SR Jr, Halpern-Felsher BL, Rosenthal SM. Health Care Providers' Comfort With and Barriers to Care of Transgender Youth. J Adolesc Health 2//2015;56(2):251–3.

62. Gridley SJ, Crouch JM, Evans Y, et al. Youth and Caregiver Perspectives on Barriers to Gender-Affirming Health Care for Transgender Youth. J Adolesc Health 2016/09/01/2016;59(3):254–61.

63. Laiti M, Pakarinen A, Parisod H, et al. Encountering sexual and gender minority youth in healthcare: an integrative review. Prim Health Care Res Dev. Mar 20 2019;20:e30. https://doi.org/10.1017/s146342361900001x.

64. Ayhan CHB, Bilgin H, Uluman OT, et al. A Systematic Review of the Discrimination Against Sexual and Gender Minority in Health Care Settings. Int J Health Serv 2020;50(1):44–61. https://doi.org/10.1177/0020731419885093.

65. Macapagal K, Bhatia R, Greene GJ. Differences in healthcare access, use, and experiences within a community sample of racially diverse lesbian, gay, bisexual, transgender, and questioning emerging adults. LGBT Health 2016;3(6):434–42.

66. Rider GN, McMorris BJ, Gower AL, et al. Health and Care Utilization of Transgender and Gender Nonconforming Youth: A Population-Based Study. Pediatrics 2018;141(3). https://doi.org/10.1542/peds.2017-1683.

67. Eisenberg ME, McMorris BJ, Rider GN, et al. It's kind of hard to go to the doctor's office if you're hated there." A call for gender-affirming care from transgender and gender diverse adolescents in the United States. Health Soc Care Community 2020;28(3):1082–9.

68. Quinn K, Dickson-Gomez J, Zarwell M, et al. A Gay Man and a Doctor are Just like, a Recipe for Destruction": How Racism and Homonegativity in Healthcare Settings Influence PrEP Uptake Among Young Black MSM. AIDS Behav 2019; 23(7):1951–63. https://doi.org/10.1007/s10461-018-2375-z.

69. Bergman A, McGee K, Farley J, et al. Combating Stigma in the Era of Monkeypox—Is History Repeating Itself? J Assoc Nurses AIDS Care 2022;33(6): 668–75. https://doi.org/10.1097/jnc.0000000000000367.

70. Renner J, Blaszcyk W, Täuber L, et al. Barriers to accessing health care in rural regions by transgender, non-binary, and gender diverse people: a case-based scoping review. Front Endocrinol 2021;12.

71. Sallabank G, Chavanduka TMD, Walsh AR, et al. Mapping LGBTQ+ Youth Resource Density Across Four High HIV Prevalence Corridors in the US. Sex Res Soc Pol 2021. https://doi.org/10.1007/s13178-021-00660-0.

72. Rosentel K, Vandevusse A, Hill BJ. Racial and Socioeconomic Inequity in the Spatial Distribution of LGBTQ Human Services: an Exploratory Analysis of LGBTQ Services in Chicago. Sex Res Soc Pol 2020;17(1):87–103. https://doi.org/10.1007/s13178-019-0374-0.

73. Movement Advancement Project. "Equality maps: healthcare laws and policies."Available at: https://www.lgbtmap.org/equality-maps/healthcare_laws_and_policies. Accessed 31 October, 2022.

74. Dawson L, Kates J, Musumeci M. Youth Access to Gender Affirming Care: The Federal and State Policy Landscape. 2022. June 1, 2022Available at: https://www.kff.org/other/issue-brief/youth-access-to-gender-affirming-care-the-federal-and-state-policy-landscape/. Accessed 10 October, 2022.

75. ACLU. Legislation affecting LGBTQ Rights Across the Country, Available at: https://www.aclu.org/legislation-affecting-lgbtq-rights-across-country. Accessed 22 October, 2022.

76. Fuzzell L, Fedesco HN, Alexander SC, et al. I just think that doctors need to ask more questions": Sexual minority and majority adolescents' experiences talking about sexuality with healthcare providers. Patient Educ Counsel 2016;99(9): 1467–72.

77. O'Neill T, Wakefield J. Fifteen-minute consultation in the normal child: Challenges relating to sexuality and gender identity in children and young people. Archives of disease in childhood - Education & practice edition 2017;102(6):298–303. https://doi.org/10.1136/archdischild-2016-311449.

78. Goldhammer H, Grasso C, Katz-Wise SL, et al. Pediatric sexual orientation and gender identity data collection in the electronic health record. J Am Med Inf Assoc 2022;29(7):1303–9. https://doi.org/10.1093/jamia/ocac048.

79. Temkin D, Belford J, McDaniel T, et al. Improving measurement of sexual orientation and gender identity among middle and high school students. Child Trends 2017;22:1–64.

80. Austin SB, Conron KJ, Patel A, et al. Making Sense of Sexual Orientation Measures: Findings from a Cognitive Processing Study with Adolescents on Health

Survey Questions. J LGBT Health Res 2007;3(1):55–65. https://doi.org/10.1300/J463v03n01_07.

81. Fisher CB, Fried AL, Macapagal K, et al. Patient–Provider Communication Barriers and Facilitators to HIV and STI Preventive Services for Adolescent MSM. AIDS Behav 2018/10/01 2018;22(10):3417–28. https://doi.org/10.1007/s10461-018-2081-x.

82. Mustanski B, Moskowitz DA, Moran KO, et al. Factors Associated With HIV Testing in Teenage Men Who Have Sex With Men. Pediatrics 2020;145(3). https://doi.org/10.1542/peds.2019-2322.

83. Santelli JS, Klein JD, Song X, et al. Discussion of Potentially Sensitive Topics With Young People. Pediatrics 2019;143(2). https://doi.org/10.1542/peds.2018-1403.

84. Mehringer JE, Dowshen NL. Opportunities and challenges for previsit screening for sexual and gender identity among adolescents in primary care. J Adolesc Health 2020;66(2):133–4.

85. Sorbara JC, Chiniara LN, Thompson S, et al. Mental Health and Timing of Gender-Affirming Care. Pediatrics 2020;146(4). https://doi.org/10.1542/peds.2019-3600.

86. Rafferty J, CHILD COPAO, HEALTH F, et al. Ensuring Comprehensive Care and Support for Transgender and Gender-Diverse Children and Adolescents. Pediatrics 2018;142(4). https://doi.org/10.1542/peds.2018-2162.

87. Pachankis JE, Harkness A, Maciejewski KR, et al. LGBQ-affirmative cognitive-behavioral therapy for young gay and bisexual men's mental and sexual health: A three-arm randomized controlled trial. J Consult Clin Psychol 2022;90(6):459–77.

88. Lucassen MFG, Núñez-García A, Rimes KA, et al. Coping Strategies to Enhance the Mental Wellbeing of Sexual and Gender Minority Youths: A Scoping Review. Int J Environ Res Publ Health 2022;19(14):8738.

89. Rafferty J, CoPAo Child, Health F. Ensuring comprehensive care and support for transgender and gender-diverse children and adolescents. Pediatrics 2018;142(4).

90. Katz-Wise SL, Rosario M, Tsappis M. Lesbian, Gay, Bisexual, and Transgender Youth and Family Acceptance. Pediatr Clin 2016;63(6):1011–25.

91. Poteat VP, Fish JN, Watson RJ. Gender-sexuality alliances as a moderator of the association between victimization, depressive symptoms, and drinking behavior among LGBTQ+ youth. Drug Alcohol Depend 2021;229:109140.

92. Colvin S, Egan JE, Coulter RW. School climate & sexual and gender minority adolescent mental health. J Youth Adolesc 2019;48(10):1938–51.

93. Eisenberg ME, Mehus CJ, Saewyc EM, et al. Helping Young People Stay Afloat: A Qualitative Study of Community Resources and Supports for LGBTQ Adolescents in the United States and Canada. J Homosex 2018;65(8):969–89. https://doi.org/10.1080/00918369.2017.1364944.

94. McDonald K. Social Support and Mental Health in LGBTQ Adolescents: A review of the literature. Issues Ment Health Nurs 2018;39(1):16–29. https://doi.org/10.1080/01612840.2017.1398283.

95. Braveman P, Arkin E, Orleans T, et al. What is health equity? Behavioral Science & Policy 2018;4(1):1–14.

96. Center for Intersectional Justice, Available at: https://www.intersectionaljustice.org/. Accessed 3 October, 2022.

Climate Change and Child Health Equity

Katherine C. Budolfson, MD, MPH[a], Ruth A. Etzel, MD, PhD[b],*

KEYWORDS

- Climate crisis • Advocacy • Health equity • Pediatrics
- Recurrent respiratory disease • Mold • Pulmonary hemorrhage • Stachybotrys
- Flooding • Apnea • Sudden death

KEY POINTS

- The climate crisis poses current and future risks to pediatric health, with disproportionate negative effects on vulnerable children.
- Pediatric clinicians can address and mitigate the health effects of climate change in the clinical encounter.
- Collective action is needed by pediatric clinicians to advocate for eliminating the use of fossil fuels and to enact climate-friendly policies at local, state, national, and global levels.

CASE

A 23-month-old boy lived at home with his parents in public housing in a low-lying area of the city of Manchester. During severe rainstorms, the one-bedroom apartment frequently flooded, and as a result, was chronically damp and moldy. From birth, the boy often had respiratory illnesses and was brought to the urgent care center frequently with a chief complaint of "trouble breathing." The parents were immigrants from Sudan, and the boy's mother spoke very little English. The boy's parents made numerous complaints about the black mold that was visible in the kitchen and bathroom and also made requests to move from the apartment to another apartment because of the black mold. These requests were supported by a visiting nurse but never were addressed by the public housing department. The public housing officials seemed to be dismissive and to place blame on the tenants' lifestyle. The father was told to paint over the mold.

In early December, the boy was taken to the urgent care center due to his flulike symptoms and difficulty breathing and was then transferred to the hospital, where

[a] Baylor College of Medicine, Texas Children's Hospital, Houston, TX, USA; [b] Milken Institute School of Public Health, The George Washington University, 950 New Hampshire Avenue, Northwest, Washington, DC 20052, USA
* Corresponding author.
E-mail address: retzel@gwu.edu

Pediatr Clin N Am 70 (2023) 837–853
https://doi.org/10.1016/j.pcl.2023.03.012
0031-3955/23/© 2023 Elsevier Inc. All rights reserved.

pediatric.theclinics.com

he was given supportive treatment and discharged. The boy's mother showed the doctor photographs on her phone of extensive mold growth in the apartment. Because of her limited English proficiency and the lack of a translator, little discussion took place. At home, the boy continued with difficulties and his breathing became worse, so his parents took him back to the urgent care center 2 days later. On arrival, he was in respiratory failure. He was transferred to the hospital where he was pronounced dead on arrival.

The pathologist who performed the autopsy stated that the boy's throat was swollen to a degree that would compromise his breathing. His windpipe and other airways were also swollen and congested. There was evidence of fungus in his blood and lungs, and the pathologist affirmed that exposure to fungi was the most plausible explanation for the inflammation. An inspection of the apartment found "extensive mold" on the walls and ceilings of the bathroom and kitchen and also found mold in a cupboard in the bedroom. The inspector told the doctor that the apartment would have been contaminated "for some considerable time."

This case illustrates one of the most common problems associated with the climate crisis: severe flooding that leads to chronically moldy home environments. This is an equity issue because low-income families may not have resources to clean up water damage and mold. Such families may be forced to live in water-damaged environments for months or years. The housing department or the landlord may be unwilling to spend the money needed to properly remediate the water damage. Immigrants from other countries, especially those with limited English proficiency, may not fully understand the risks associated with environmental hazards, and they may not know how to navigate the public housing system to get attention. Child health professionals should recognize that children should not live in moldy environments and should take steps to ensure that they are removed from such environments and not return until the water damage is properly repaired.

INTRODUCTION

The climate crisis is the greatest public health threat facing the health and well-being of children and future generations.[1–3] It also is a major driver of health inequity through disproportionate negative effects on historically marginalized populations, including communities of color, those living in poverty, and indigenous and immigrant populations. Pediatric clinicians are uniquely poised to advocate at the personal, professional, community, and national/international levels to raise the alarm and spur positive change.[4] This article summarizes the current science on the health effects of climate change on children and the intersection of climate change and child health equity, describes medicine's contribution to climate change, and provides practical advocacy strategies at the individual, patient-centered, organizational, professional society, and national/international levels.

CLIMATE CHANGE AND PEDIATRIC HEALTH

The climate crisis is a global emergency, declared the greatest public health threat facing the world. Children are uniquely vulnerable to the effects of climate change, with children under the age of 5 suffering greater than 88% of the disease burden from catastrophic changes to the environment.[5–7]

There is consensus among scientists that climate change is due to greenhouse gas emissions generated by human activities, primarily fossil fuel combustion. Carbon dioxide and other greenhouse gases release trapped heat in the atmosphere, causing a greenhouse effect, resulting in an average temperature increase of over 1.5°F

(0.833°C) in the United States over the past century.[8] Increases in global temperature have led to many secondary effects, including heat waves, reduction in ice sheets, rising sea levels, and increased frequency and severity of severe weather events and wildfires. The widespread ecologic devastation resulting from these effects will only worsen if decisive action is not taken promptly. Limiting temperature increases to a total of 2°C will prevent the most catastrophic consequences of climate change.[9] Although the current worsening trajectory of climate change and pediatric health is dire, quick and widespread action by individuals, organizations, communities, and nations will prevent worsening catastrophic effects and ameliorate some current effects.

Climate change's effects are seen in the prenatal period, with numerous studies showing maternal stress during pregnancy from environmental factors, such as heat, nutrition, exposure to infections and toxins, and natural disasters.[7,10] After birth, children are more susceptible to exposures owing to their higher surface area in proportion to body weight. Because children, pound for pound, eat and drink more, breathe more air, and have greater surface area for dermal exposure to toxicants than adults, their exposures are proportionately greater than in adults occupying the same environment. Children also have cumulative exposure across their lifetimes.[11–14] Finally, children are dependent on their adult caregivers and community structures and have less autonomy than adults over the environments in which they live.[15]

Weather Disasters

Globally, the number and severity of weather disasters have increased significantly because of warming from greenhouse gases. These weather events include severe storms, floods, wildfires, heatwaves, and droughts. The immediate health effects of a weather disaster for children may include injuries, infectious diseases, respiratory illnesses, and even death.[16,17] However, the health effects extend far beyond the weather events themselves. Survivors often experience psychological sequelae of trauma, leading to increased mental health care needs.[18] Disruption of local ecosystems can create conditions favorable for disease and increased opportunity for transmission of vector-borne diseases. Destruction of property and subsequent economic effects can lead to housing, food, and economic insecurity for children and families. For patients with high medical needs (particularly those with technology dependence), weather disasters and associated power outages, flooding, and disruption of the water supply can be fatal if appropriate evacuation and preparedness plans are not in place and followed.[19]

Heat Stress

Heat waves already are the leading weather-related cause of death in the United States, and children are particularly susceptible to heat-related morbidity.[20] Increasing temperatures globally threaten the health of children starting in the prenatal period. Maternal heat stress during pregnancy is associated with negative pregnancy outcomes, including preterm birth, low birth weight, stillbirth, and increased rates of postpartum depression.[21] Infant mortality increases by up to 25% on extremely hot days.[22] Heat stress effects continue into childhood and adolescence, with increased numbers of emergency room visits for heat-related illnesses seen for children under 15 years of age.[23] Heat illness is a major cause of morbidity and mortality for teenage athletes.[24]

Air Quality

Increased heat contributes to ground-level ozone pollution.[11] Children experience higher exposure to air pollutants owing to physiologic factors, including increased minute ventilation and continuing lung development.[25] Ozone exposure affects lung development in children over time, leading to a reduction in total lung volume, and is associated with higher rates of chronic lung disease.[26,27]

Asthma is the most prevalent chronic respiratory disease in children, and rates have increased significantly in the United States over the past several decades.[28] Climate change is contributing to increasing asthma rates through several risk factors, including increased ozone exposure, greenhouse gases, and molds.[29] Wildfires and resultant smoke are another major cause of asthma exacerbations in children while also further elevating ozone levels.[30,31] Moreover, prolonged heat has generated longer pollen seasons with higher counts, worsening symptoms for children with allergies and asthma.[32] Climate change also results in increased indoor air pollution and mold growth after flooding, further worsening asthma and allergy symptoms for many children.[33] Infants are uniquely vulnerable to acute and sometimes fatal pulmonary hemorrhage if they live in moldy, water-damaged homes.[34–40]

Infectious Disease

Increases in vector-borne, food-borne, and waterborne disease will continue as the effects of climate change worsen.[41] The most notable vector-borne diseases transmitted by mosquitoes and ticks, such as malaria and Lyme disease, are already increasing as changing climates expand the regions hospitable to these insects and increase exposures.[42] As the climate warms, unusual infections, such as primary amebic encephalitis caused by *Naegleria fowleri* (a thermophilic ameba), which used to be reported only in the southern United States, are now occurring in states in the northern United States.[43] Natural disasters and temperature changes resulting in drought or flooding can increase the transmission of gastrointestinal disease by contamination of clean water and food sources.[44]

Resource Insecurity

Children and families are at high risk of resource insecurity as a direct result of climate change. These resources include food, water, energy, housing, and other economic insecurities (**Fig. 1**). Through a combination of severe weather events, droughts, and heat waves, climate change puts crops at risk and has the potential to disrupt the global food supply chain at any time. This greatly increases the likelihood of families experiencing food insecurity on top of existing structural barriers to accessing high-quality nutrition for children.[45]

Aging infrastructure throughout the United States, with a particular lack of funding for improvements in marginalized communities, puts many at risk of losing access to safe water, electricity, and other necessities. With higher stress placed on this failing infrastructure in the settings of natural disasters and extreme temperatures, these issues are set to become even more frequent. This is particularly concerning for patients with high medical needs who have equipment requiring electricity or clean water for safe operation.[46] However, this risk extends to all families if no access to clean water exists for drinking, for preparing formula, or for other daily needs. Finally, housing insecurity will be magnified even further as flooding, environmental exposures, and other sequelae of climate change result in abrupt loss or damage to housing.[47]

Psychological Sequelae

Natural disasters are known to cause long-term psychological sequelae in children.[48,49] The most commonly seen psychiatric disorders as a result of experiencing traumatic natural disasters are posttraumatic stress disorder, major depressive disorder, and anxiety. Increases in perceived stress, panic attacks, sleep issues, and

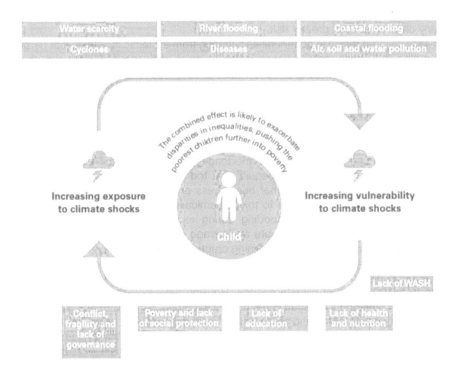

Fig. 1. Mechanism of climate impacts on child health. WASH: water, sanitation, and hygiene. (https://www.unicef.org/reports/climate-crisis-child-rights-crisis. Figure © UNICEF.)

somatic symptoms also are commonly seen. These often are underrecognized and may go untreated for long periods of time, leading to long-term psychological effects and disruption.[18]

Even in the absence of exposure to the acute effects of natural disasters, many children and adolescents are worried about what the future holds, and many suffer from anxiety and depression linked to the climate crisis.[50] A 2021 survey administered to 10,000 children and young people (aged 16–25 years) in 10 countries (Australia, Brazil, Finland, France, India, Nigeria, Philippines, Portugal, the United Kingdom, and the United States) found that respondents across all countries were worried about climate change (59% were very or extremely worried and 84% were at least moderately worried).[51] Many young people perceive that the government has failed to respond to the climate crisis. A new term, solastalgia, has been coined to describe the anxiety among young people that results from concern about the future of the planet.[52]

CLIMATE CHANGE AND HEALTH EQUITY

The climate crisis is a social justice and human rights issue and should be approached with a health equity lens.[53] Climate justice recognizes that those who are least responsible for the factors causing climate change also are the ones whose well-being suffers the most from the effects of climate change.[54] Children are an inherently vulnerable population who disproportionately experience the negative health effects of climate change, but additional socioeconomic, cultural, and environmental factors place many children at even greater risk.

Many children reside in communities suffering from systemic injustices that perpetuate inequity. These include communities of color, indigenous populations, those living in poverty, and immigrant populations. Marginalized groups can experience not only increased exposure to the direct impacts of climate change but also increased sensitivity and reduced adaptive capacity for recovery owing to the social determinants of health inequity.[55]

Children of color suffer from the consequences of redlining, the historical racist practice of perpetuating economic disadvantages to black and immigrant communities by labeling them "high risk" for mortgages and other loans. These policies laid the groundwork for decades of inequity that today result in children living in these neighborhoods experiencing higher heat stress owing to higher temperatures and fewer trees, increased exposure to toxic chemicals owing to proximity to industrial areas, and worsened risk of flooding during extreme weather events.[56] Today, formerly redlined neighborhoods are an average of 2.6°C hotter than non-redlined counterparts, inextricably linking redlining practices with inequities in climate change morbidity in these communities.[57]

People living in marginalized housing communities experience higher rates of exposure to the sequelae of climate change. Housing risks include living in urban heat islands and suffering the negative effects of heat stress, areas with aging and poorly maintained infrastructure, and areas with increased air pollution. Black children in the United States are twice as likely as white children to develop asthma and have significantly higher odds of hospitalization and mortality from asthma exacerbations.[58] Communities of color also are more likely to be living in areas that are high risk for flooding.[59]

Indigenous communities also suffer disproportionate effects of climate change. Indigenous communities across the United States already have experienced drastic ecologic changes, including disruption to food supply, worsened erosion and flooding, threats to water security, and general disruption to traditional ways of life.[60,61] Policies to address climate change must include special consideration for these populations to ensure equitable provision of protective measures (**Fig. 2**).

ADVOCACY AND CLIMATE CHANGE—THE PEDIATRIC CLINICIAN'S ROLE

Pediatric clinicians have the unique ability to address both the upstream causes and the downstream consequences of climate change through advocacy and clinical practice. By screening for and addressing the needs of patients, with a health equity and justice lens, pediatric clinicians can mitigate the morbidity of climate-related illness. Through personal action, organizational quality improvement, community mobilization, professional society actions, and national and international advocacy, pediatric clinicians can exert broad positive change to mitigate the worst climate change's health effects on future generations.

Individual

One of the easiest domains to make quick changes to benefit the environment is in one's own daily life. Making efforts to reduce personal carbon emissions and waste and making educated purchases from companies with positive environmental impacts are good ways to start. Reducing carbon emissions includes actions such as using active transport methods, such as walking or biking, when able. If motorized travel

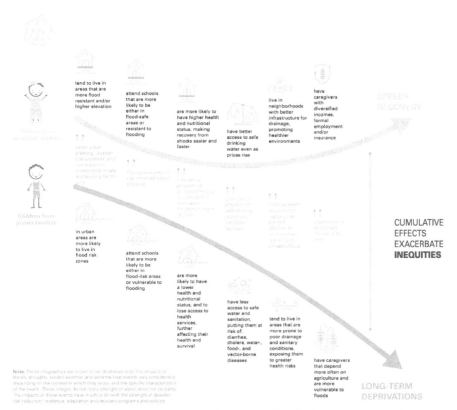

Fig. 2. Floods and severe storms can exacerbate inequities. (Unless we act now: The impact of climate change on children, November 2015. © United NationsChildren's Fund (UNICEF). https://www.unicef.org/reports/unless-we-act-now-impact-climate-change-children.)

is needed, selecting fuel-efficient or electric vehicles and carpooling can minimize the detrimental effects.

One's own carbon footprint extends beyond personal emissions and into the upstream carbon emissions from the production of purchased goods. The products and foods purchased can be made through manufacturing processes that emit carbon and other pollutants. Transportation of these goods, often internationally, also creates significant carbon emissions. Whenever possible, buying locally produced food and goods can limit the carbon produced through transportation. Investigating companies through which purchases are made to ensure appropriate environmental standards are followed is essential.

Finally, reducing, reusing, and recycling are as important as ever. Reduction of waste in our daily lives, and the corresponding reduction of purchases of new goods, not only reduces the amount of landfill waste but also reduces the upstream carbon emissions from production of these wasted goods.

Those working in health care in the United States may not yet feel the effects of climate change, primarily because we live lives of comparative privilege; most of us can afford to purchase air conditioners, for example, if it is too hot. We may encounter colleagues in health care who express doubt that this problem needs immediate attention. It can be helpful to point out that this is an ethical issue—consumption of fossil fuels by people in high-income countries is causing a huge burden of disease among people in low- and middle-income countries, who consume comparatively little fossil fuel. It is also an intergenerational issue—we may not be alive to witness the worst effects of the climate crisis, but our children and grandchildren will be.

Clinical Encounters

Whether in an inpatient or outpatient setting, the effects of climate change on the health of each patient should be considered. Simple environmental health questions, like those for exposure to lead, are already used in pediatric practice. Adding questions about climate risks can guide counseling during the clinic visit. Screening for social determinants of health often includes many questions relevant to risks from

---

Box 1
Key questions for clinicians to ask that address climate risk

1. Are you worried or concerned that in the next 2 months you may not have stable housing that you own, rent, or stay in as a part of a household?
   - ☐ Yes
   - ☐ No

2. Think about the place where you live. Do you have problems with any of the following? (Check all that apply)
   - ☐ Mold
   - ☐ Damp or musty smell
   - ☐ Flooding
   - ☐ Inadequate heat
   - ☐ No air conditioning
   - ☐ No cooling fans
   - ☐ No screens on windows (or screens with holes)
   - ☐ No or not working smoke detectors
   - ☐ Water leaks
   - ☐ Standing water
   - ☐ None of the above

3. Do you use well water?
   - ☐ Yes
   - ☐ No
   - ☐ Don't know

4. Within the past 12 months, were you worried that your food would run out before you got money to buy more?
   - ☐ Often
   - ☐ Sometimes
   - ☐ Never
   - ☐ Don't know/refuse to answer

5. Within the past 12 months, the food you bought just didn't last and you didn't have money to get more.
   - ☐ Often true
   - ☐ Sometimes true
   - ☐ Never true
   - ☐ Don't know/refuse to answer

6. In the past 12 months, has the electric, gas, oil, or water company threatened to shut off services in your home?
   - ☐ Yes
   - ☐ No
   - ☐ Already shut off

climate change.[62] **Box 1** shows core questions that clinicians can ask to assess climate risk; they focus on housing and utilities, use of well water, and food security.

A pediatric clinician also can introduce climate change into the conversation by connecting its effects with a child's symptoms or other effects a family is experiencing. For example, a clinician can say something like, "Burning fossil fuels is affecting health by worsening air pollution; children are breathing polluted air now and in the future. Are you worried about air pollution's effects on your child's lungs?" This kind of message can help parents to make the links between climate change and children's health (**Box 2**).[63]

Anticipatory guidance addressing health threats exacerbated by climate change can help prepare patients and families to avoid or effectively address them. Special care should be taken to ensure any already apparent clinical effects of climate change on the child are addressed during the clinical visit (**Fig. 3**). The American Academy of Pediatrics developed an online toolkit for the pediatric clinician with resources, including handouts, for numerous climate change and pediatric health topics.[64] Resources include tips for approaching the conversation with parents and children, including engagement with adolescents and encouraging individual advocacy efforts.[64]

Practice or Institution

Health care is responsible for 4.4% of global net emissions. The United States is the largest contributor globally to health care–related emissions, generating 27% of that total. Health care emissions constitute 10% of the United States' total emissions of carbon dioxide, methane, and nitrous oxide.[65] These emissions result from a broad array of sources, including health care facilities and equipment, transportation, and supply chain. Although individual and patient-centered changes are important and beneficial, generating larger-scale changes require turning focus to practice and institutional environmental practices. Areas to target, strategies for implementation, and resources are discussed in this section.

In a shared practice or larger institution, creating a climate-friendly environment can be challenging. The first step is assessing the current organizational attitudes toward improving environmental impact. System-wide changes require broad support, which may or may not already exist institutionally. In a large organization, starting this process often requires identification of others currently working in this space to build a collaborative. On the administrative staff, executives who work in facilities or environmental services can be helpful starting points to create partnerships. It also may be

---

Box 2
Selected samples of ways to introduce climate change in clinical visits

For patients with asthma:
"Climate change and air pollution are caused by the same thing—burning fossil fuels. Together they make air quality worse, and that can make lung disease worse. Checking air quality and avoiding busy roadways when you go out for exercise can help protect you."

For patients with lung disease:
"Wildfires are becoming more common because of climate change. The smoke and particles can travel many miles and can be dangerous for everyone, but especially people with lung disease. It is important to check air quality information when there are wildfires. Here are some ways to do that (www.airnow.gov) and tips to reduce exposure."

Based on Senay E, Sarfaty M, Rice MB. Strategies for Clinical Discussions About Climate Change. Ann Intern Med. 2021;174(3):417-418. doi:10.7326/M20-6443.

Screening for Sequlae of Climate Change

Anticipatory Guidance

- Promote plant-based diets, breastfeeding, and reduction of cow's milk and meat intake to improve nutrition and decrease dietary contribution to climate change
- Promote physical activity as a part of a healthy lifestyle, while also promoting the positive effects of active transport methods on the environment and local air quality
- During sports physicals, discuss the effects of heat stress and the importance of hydration, cooling, and avoiding the hottest times of the day to exercise
- Discuss heat safety with families, including avoiding leaving children in hot cars
- Advise sunscreen use with broad-spectrum SPF and other sun safety measures
- Discuss disaster-preparedness, including the development of a family plan, ensuring children know parental contact information, and providing local resources when needed
- Advise DEET-containing insect repellant use in areas with vector-borne disease transmission

Disease Management

- Stay up-to-date on local outbreaks and counsel patients who are at risk
- For children with allergies and asthma, include air quality index and pollen counts in action plans, advising indoor play on days with poor air quality or high pollen counts
- Create a plan with children with complex medical conditions for disaster-preparedness, ensuring access to necessary supplies in an emergency kit
- During the medication reconciliation, ensure patients are storing medications in temperature-controlled areas to ensure no loss of efficacy
- Consider medication contributions to heat sensitivity, dehydration, sun sensitivity when counseling patients about side effects

Fig. 3. Suggested ways to address climate change in clinical visits. (Source: Philipsborn et al.[19])

helpful to ask about what has already been achieved, what was tried but unsuccessful, and if the institution has any outstanding goals.

After identifying allies on both the administrative and the physician sides of the organization, the next step is to identify the most pressing areas of change. These can be organized into "asks" for institutional leadership. Often a first step is for the formal recognition of an environmental committee, with appropriate charters in place to grant formal organizational acknowledgment of the collaboration. This serves to establish structure and communicates institutional support for the effort.

As with any advocacy effort, timing is important. Although environmental impact may not be a current institutional priority, establishing consistent communication with leadership can spur institutional support or simply be available when institutional priorities align. Being ready and organized with a plan when an organization achieves readiness to change can jumpstart efforts and ensure that motivated people are sitting at the table for these discussions.

Developing a readiness plan is best done in collaboration with those who have extensive experience. There are many national and international organizations with the mission to "green" health care and provide guidance to those who want to start the process. Several organizations have generated exceptional resources to assist clinicians with the practical steps to create a more sustainable work environment. The American College of Physicians has a climate change toolkit with practical resources to get started, including specific talking points for each region of the United States.[66] Practice Greenhealth, an organization helping health care institutions improve their environmental impact, identified the target domains of buildings, energy, chemicals, procurement, waste, water, food, the operating room, and transportation.[67] **Fig. 4** summarizes key strategies to improve environmental friendliness in each of these domains. Not every domain will be relevant for every practice or institution, but the items listed can be helpful starting points for the areas applicable to one's setting.

Professional Society Actions

Professional organizations and societies may have a large carbon footprint if they hold national or international in-person meetings to which their members travel over long

Buildings	- Construct using energy-efficient materials
	- Source materials from reputable, climate-friendly companies focused on reduction of environmental impact
	- Avoid construction materials with toxic chemicals
	- Consider disaster-preparedness in building design
Energy	- Purchase electricity from renewable energy sources
	- Prioritize energy efficiency throughout facilities with equipment, lighting, and other electricity-consuming items
	- Automate shut-off of items where possible
Chemicals	- Evaluate current chemical use, including cleaners and disinfectants, for harmful components that may detrimentally affect the health of your staff and patients
	- Avoid products, including construction and furniture, that release toxic chemicals over time
Procurement	- Adopt sustainable procurement standards
	- Consider sustainability in production, shipment, and long-term use of products when selecting what to purchase
	- Avoid purchase of single-use items when able
	- Avoid products that contain hazardous chemicals
Waste	- Assess current waste and identify target areas for waste reduction
	- Implement easily accessible recycling and composting bins
	- Avoid single-use items where possible and evaluate methods for single-use device reprocessing
Water	- Utilize eco-friendly equipment, such as laundry machines and sterilizers, to minimize water use
	- Opt for sustainable landscaping that does not require irrigation
	- Perform regular assessments for leaks in infrastructure
Food	- Promote plant-based food items
	- Analyze and reduce food waste
	- Source sustainable, environmentally friendly ingredients
	- Eliminate plastic and single-use items where able
	- Provide compost and recycling for disposal
Operating Room	- Establish procedures for anesthetic gas reduction and capture
	- Source reusable equipment and utilize reprocessing for medical devices
	- Standardize OR kits where possible to reduce waste
Transportation	- Promote and incentivize active transportation, carpools, and electric vehicles for employees
	- Establish policies to limit idling vehicles on premises

Fig. 4. The key strategies to improve environmental friendliness in selected domains.

distances. Recently, many such organizations have promised to take steps to reduce their footprints by holding more virtual meetings.[68–75] The major pediatric professional organizations in the United States have not yet made such a commitment, and pediatric clinicians can ask them to consider this action.

There also is a growing movement to encourage medical organizations and societies to divest from fossil fuels.[76–79] Pediatric clinicians can contribute by asking their professional organization if they have taken action to divest their portfolio from fossil fuels.

National and International Advocacy

Realizing that the climate crisis is caused by excessive burning of fossil fuels, some pediatric clinicians have opted to move even further upstream with their advocacy efforts.

The United Nations (UN) Framework Convention on Climate Change established an international environmental treaty in 1992 to combat "dangerous human interference with the climate system," in part by stabilizing greenhouse gas concentrations in the atmosphere.[80] The Conference of Parties meets each year to review progress on this treaty. In 2015, an agreement was reached in Paris to try to limit global warming to 1.5°C, or not more than 2°C.[81] The countries that signed this agreement, however, have failed to live up to their promises. To date, health professionals and discussions about the health impact of climate change on human populations have not been a major part of the yearly UN Climate Change Conference negotiations. Pediatric clinicians in pediatric societies and professional organizations around the world can engage in advocacy with their country delegations and missions leading up to the UN Climate Change Conference in 2023, and each year thereafter, in order to urge their leaders to fulfill the promises of the Paris Agreement.[82]

There are multiple roles for health professionals in combating the climate crisis. They can serve as providers, leaders, educators, and advocates. It is imperative that each pediatric clinician engage in order to safeguard the health of today's children and future generations.[83]

SUMMARY

Climate change has profound effects on children that will continue to worsen without drastic global action. The disproportionate effects of climate change on marginalized pediatric populations, particularly children in poverty, further worsen health inequities. Pediatric clinicians can advocate for climate justice through personal, organizational, community, professional society, and national/international actions. Screening, guidance, and treatment for sequelae of climate change can be incorporated into regular pediatric visits. Health care institutions must take responsibility for their contribution to the climate crisis and take action to become climate friendly for the patients, families, and communities they serve. The voice of clinicians who care for children is an important voice to persuade government leaders to immediately reduce the emissions of greenhouse gases.

CLINICS CARE POINTS

- When evaluating an infant with apnea or recurrent respiratory problems, ask about any moldy or musty smells in the home.
- Any home with moldy or musty smells should be evaluated before sending the infant home.
- When requesting an autopsy of an infant with recurrent respiratory problems, a Prussian blue stain of lung tissue should be done to look for hemosiderin.

DISCLOSURE

The authors have nothing to disclose.

REFERENCES

1. Costello A, Abbas M, Allen A, et al. Managing the health effects of climate change: Lancet and University College London Institute for Global. Lancet

2009;373(9676):1693–733.   https://doi.org/10.1016/S0140-6736(09)60935-1. Health Commission [published correction appears in Lancet. 2009 Jun 27;373(9682):2200].

2. Perera F, Nadeau K. Climate change, fossil-fuel pollution, and children's health. N Engl J Med 2022;386(24):2303–14.

3. Nadeau K, Perera F, Salas RN, et al. Climate, pollution, and children's health. N Engl J Med 2022;387(18):e45.

4. Ahdoot S, Pacheco SE. American Academy of Pediatrics Council on Environmental Health. Global climate change and children's health. Pediatrics 2015; 136(5):e1468.

5. Watts N, Amann M, Arnell N, et al. The 2019 report of The Lancet Countdown on health and climate change: ensuring that the health of a child born today is not defined by a changing climate. Lancet 2019;394(10211):1836–78. https://doi. org/10.1016/S0140-6736(19)32596-6.

6. Zhang Y, Bi P, Hiller JE. Climate change and disability-adjusted life years. J Environ Health 2007;70(3):32–6.

7. Sheffield PE, Landrigan PJ. Global climate change and children's health: threats and strategies for prevention. Environ Health Perspect 2011;119(3):291–8. https://doi.org/10.1289/ehp.1002233.

8. Melillo JM, Richmond TC, Yohe GW. Climate Change Impacts in the United States: The Third National Climate Assessment. Washington, DC: US Global Change Research Program; 2014.

9. Swaminathan M, Kesavan P. Agricultural research in an era of climate change. Agric Res 2012;1(1):3–11.

10. Deschenes O, Greenstone M, Guryan J. Climate change and birth weight. Am Econ Rev 2009;99(2):211–7. https://doi.org/10.1257/aer.99.2.211.

11. Kim JJ, American Academy of Pediatrics Committee on Environmental Health. Ambient air pollution: health hazards to children. Pediatrics 2004;114(6): 1699–707. https://doi.org/10.1542/peds.2004-2166.

12. Pronczuk J. Where the child learns. In: Pronczuk-Garbino J, editor. Children's Health and the Environment—A Global Perspective: A Resource Manual for the Health Sector. Geneva: World Health Organization; 2005. p. 40–5.

13. American Academy of Pediatrics Council on Environmental Health, Etzel RA. In: Pediatric Environmental Health. 4th Edition. Itasca, IL: American Academy of Pediatrics; 2019.

14. United Nations Children's Fund (UNICEF). Unless we act now: The impact of climate change on children. UNICEF, New York, NY. https://www.unicef.org/reports/unless-we-act-now-impact-climate-change-children. Published November 1, 2015. Available at: https://www.unicef.org/publications/files/Unless_we_act_now_The_impact_of_climate_change_on_children.pdf.

15. Ebi KL, Paulson JA. Climate change and children. Pediatr Clin North Am 2007; 54(2):213–vii. https://doi.org/10.1016/j.pcl.2007.01.004.

16. Ivers LC, Ryan ET. Infectious diseases of severe weather-related and flood-related natural disasters. Curr Opin Infect Dis 2006;19(5):408–14. https://doi. org/10.1097/01.qco.0000244044.85393.9e.

17. Miranda DS, Choonara I. Hurricanes and child health: lessons from Cuba. Arch Dis Child 2011;96(4):328–9. https://doi.org/10.1136/adc.2009.178145.

18. Goldmann E, Galea S. Mental health consequences of disasters. Annu Rev Public Health 2014;35:169–83. https://doi.org/10.1146/annurev-publhealth-032013-182435.

19. Philipsborn RP, Cowenhoven J, Bole A, et al. A pediatrician's guide to climate change-informed primary care. Curr Probl Pediatr Adolesc Health Care 2021; 51(6):101027. https://doi.org/10.1016/j.cppeds.2021.101027.

20. Centers for Disease Control and Prevention. CDC's Tracking Network in action: Extreme heat. https://www.cdc.gov/nceh/features/trackingheat/index.html.

21. Zhang Y, Yu C, Wang L. Temperature exposure during pregnancy and birth outcomes: an updated systematic review of epidemiological evidence. Environ Pollut 2017;225:700–12.

22. Basagaña X, Sartini C, Barrera-Gómez J, et al. Heat waves and cause-specific mortality at all ages. Epidemiology 2011;22(6):765–72.

23. Sorensen CJ, Salas RN, Rublee C, et al. Clinical implications of climate change on US emergency medicine: Challenges and opportunities. Ann Emerg Med 2020;76(2):168–78. https://doi.org/10.1016/j.annemergmed.2020.03.010.

24. Centers for Disease Control and Prevention (CDC). Nonfatal sports and recreation heat illness treated in hospital emergency departments–United States, 2001-2009. MMWR Morb Mortal Wkly Rep 2011;60(29):977–80.

25. Chance GW, Harmsen E. Children are different: Environmental contaminants and children's health. Can J Public Health 1998;89(Suppl 1):S10–1.

26. To T, Zhu J, Larsen K, et al. Progression from asthma to chronic obstructive pulmonary disease. Is air pollution a risk factor? Am J Respir Crit Care Med 2016; 194(4):429–38. https://doi.org/10.1164/rccm.201510-1932OC.

27. Gauderman WJ, Avol E, Gilliland F, et al. The effect of air pollution on lung development from 10 to 18 years of age [published correction appears in N Engl J Med. 2005 Mar 24;352(12):1276]. N Engl J Med 2004;351(11):1057–67. https://doi.org/10.1056/NEJMoa040610.

28. Serebrisky D, Wiznia A. Pediatric asthma: a global epidemic. Annals of Global Health 2019;85(1).

29. Fuller MG, Cavanaugh N, Green S, et al. Climate change and state of the science for children's health and environmental health equity. J Pediatr Health Care 2022; 36(1):20–6. https://doi.org/10.1016/j.pedhc.2021.08.003.

30. Jaffe D, Chand D, Hafner W, et al. Influence of fires on O_3 concentrations in the western U.S. Environ Sci Technol 2008;42(16):5885–91. https://doi.org/10.1021/es800084k.

31. Dennekamp M, Abramson MJ. The effects of bushfire smoke on respiratory health. Respirology 2011;16(2):198–209. https://doi.org/10.1111/j.1440-1843.2010.01868.x.

32. Poole JA, Barnes CS, Demain JG, et al. Impact of weather and climate change with indoor and outdoor air quality in asthma: A work group report of the AAAAI Environmental Exposure and Respiratory Health Committee. J Allergy Clin Immunol 2019;143(5):1702–10.

33. Mallett LH, Etzel RA. Flooding: what is the impact on pregnancy and child health? Disasters 2018;42(3):432–58.

34. Etzel RA, Montaña E, Sorenson WG, et al. Acute pulmonary hemorrhage in infants associated with exposure to *Stachybotrys atra* and other fungi. Arch Pediatr Adolesc Med 1998;152(8):757–62.

35. Jarvis BB, Sorenson WG, Hintikka EL, et al. Study of toxin production by isolates of *Stachybotrys chartarum* and *Memnoniella echinata* isolated during a study of pulmonary hemosiderosis in infants. Appl Environ Microbiol 1998;64(10):3620–5.

36. Dearborn DG, Yike I, Sorenson WG, et al. Overview of investigations into pulmonary hemorrhage among infants in Cleveland, Ohio. Environ Health Perspect 1999;107(Suppl 3):495–9.

37. Flappan SM, Portnoy J, Jones P, et al. Infant pulmonary hemorrhage in a suburban home with water damage and mold (*Stachybotrys atra*). Environ Health Perspect 1999;107(11):927–30.

38. Novotny WE, Dixit A. Pulmonary hemorrhage in an infant following two weeks of fungal exposure. Arch Pediatr Adolesc Med 2000;154(3):271–5.

39. Weiss A, Chidekel AS. Acute pulmonary hemorrhage in a Delaware infant after exposure to *Stachybotrys atra*. Del Med J 2002;74(9):363–8.

40. Thrasher JD, Hooper DH, Taber J. Family of 6, their health and the death of a 16 month old male from pulmonary hemorrhage: identification of mycotoxins and mold in the home and lungs, liver and brain of deceased infant. J Clin Toxicol 2014;2:1–9. https://doi.org/10.14205/2310-4007.2014.02.01.1.

41. Altizer S, Ostfeld RS, Johnson PT, et al. Climate change and infectious diseases: from evidence to a predictive framework. Science 2013;341(6145):514–9. https://doi.org/10.1126/science.1239401.

42. Caminade C, McIntyre KM, Jones AE. Impact of recent and future climate change on vector-borne diseases. Ann N Y Acad Sci 2019;1436(1):157–73. https://doi.org/10.1111/nyas.13950.

43. Cooper AM, Aouthmany S, Shah K, et al. Killer amoebas: Primary amoebic meningoencephalitis in a changing climate. JAAPA 2019;32(6):30–5.

44. Thomas KM, Charron DF, Waltner-Toews D, et al. A role of high impact weather events in waterborne disease outbreaks in Canada, 1975 - 2001. Int J Environ Health Res 2006;16(3):167–80. https://doi.org/10.1080/09603120600641326.

45. Brown ME, Antle JM, Backlund P, et al. Climate Change, Global Food Security, and the U.S. Food System 2015;146. Available online at. http://www.usda.gov/oce/climate_change/FoodSecurity2015Assessment/FullAssessment.pd.

46. Hipper TJ, Davis R, Massey PM, et al. The disaster information needs of families of children with special healthcare needs: A scoping review. Health Secur 2018;16(3):178–92. https://doi.org/10.1089/hs.2018.0007.

47. Ebi KL, Balbus JM, Luber G. Human health. In: Reidmiller DR, Avery CW, Easterling D, et al, editors. Impacts, Risks, and Adaptation in the United States: Fourth National Climate Assessment, volume II. Washington, DC, USA: U.S. Global Change Research Program; 2018. p. 539–71.

48. Neria Y, Nandi A, Galea S. Post-traumatic stress disorder following disasters: a systematic review. Psychol Med 2008;38(4):467–80. https://doi.org/10.1017/S0033291707001353.

49. Bothe DA, Olness KN, Reyes C. Overview of children and disasters. J Dev Behav Pediatr 2018;39(8):652–62. https://doi.org/10.1097/DBP.0000000000000600.

50. Majeed H, Lee J. The impact of climate change on youth depression and mental health. Lancet Planet Health 2017;1(3):e94–5. https://doi.org/10.1016/S2542-5196(17)30045-1.

51. Hickman C, Marks E, Pihkala P, et al. Climate anxiety in children and young people and their beliefs about government responses to climate change: a global survey. Lancet Planet Health 2021;5(12):e863–73.

52. Albrecht G, Sartore GM, Connor L, et al. Solastalgia: the distress caused by environmental change. Australas Psychiatry 2007;15(Suppl 1):S95–8. https://doi.org/10.1080/10398560701701288.

53. Levy BS, Patz JA. Climate change, human rights, and social justice. Annals of Global Health 2015;81(3):310–22.

54. Preston I, Banks N, Hargreaves K, et al. Climate change and social justice: an evidence review. York, UK: Joseph Rowntree Foundation; 2014.

55. Gamble JL, Balbus J, Berger M, et al. Ch. 9: Populations of concern. The Impacts of Climate Change on Human Health in the United States: A Scientific Assessment. Available at: https://health2016.globalchange.gov/populations-concern. Published April 4, 2016.

56. Gutschow B, Gray B, Ragavan MI, et al. The intersection of pediatrics, climate change, and structural racism: Ensuring health equity through climate justice. Curr Probl Pediatr Adolesc Health Care 2021;51(6):101028. https://doi.org/10.1016/j.cppeds.2021.101028.

57. Hoffman JS, Shandas V, Pendleton N. The effects of historical housing policies on resident exposure to intra-urban heat: a study of 108 US urban areas. Climate 2020 Jan;8(1):12.

58. Volerman A, Chin MH, Press VG. Solutions for asthma disparities. Pediatrics 2017;139(3):e20162546. https://doi.org/10.1542/peds.2016-2546.

59. Keenan MB, Shankar P, Haas P. Assessing disparities of urban flood risk for households of color in Chicago Illinois. Center For Neighborhood Technology (CNT). Municipal Policy Journal 2019;4(1):1–18.

60. Ford JD, Willox AC, Chatwood S, et al. Adapting to the effects of climate change on Inuit health. Am J Public Health 2014;104(Suppl 3):e9–17.

61. U.S. Environmental Protection Agency, Indian Health Service, Department of Agriculture, and Department of Housing and Urban Development, 2008: Meeting the Access Goal: Strategies for Increasing Access to Safe Drinking Water and Wastewater Treatment to American Indian and Alaska Native Homes. Infrastructure Task Force Access Subgroup, U.S. Environmental Protection Agency. 2008; 34. Available at: https://www.epa.gov/sites/default/files/2015-07/documents/meeting-the-access-goal-strategies-for-increasing-access-to-safe-drinking-water-and-wastewater-treatment-american-indian-alaska-native-villages.pdf.

62. American Academy of Family Practice. Social Determinants of Health. Guide to Social Needs Screening. Available at: https://www.aafp.org/dam/AAFP/documents/patient_care/everyone_project/hops19-physician-guide-sdoh.pd.

63. Senay E, Sarfaty M, Rice MB. Strategies for clinical discussions about climate change. Ann Intern Med 2021;174(3):417–8.

64. American Academy of Pediatrics. Connecting the dots: climate solutions for children's health. Available at: https://www.aap.org/en/news-room/campaigns-and-toolkits/connecting-the-dots-climate-solutions-for-childrens-health/.

65. Eckelman MJ, Sherman J. Environmental impacts of the U.S. health care system and effects on public health. PLoS One 2016;11(6):e0157014.

66. Toolkit: Climate change and health. Advocacy in action. Available at: https://www.acponline.org/advocacy/advocacy-in-action/toolkit-climate-change-and-health. Published October 3, 2022.

67. Sustainability solutions for healthcare. Available at: https://practicegreenhealth.org/.

68. Sarabipour S, Khan A, Seah YFS, et al. Changing scientific meetings for the better. Nat Hum Behav 2021;5(3):296–300.

69. Zotova O, trin-Desrosiers CP, Gopfert A, et al. Comment: Carbon-neutral medical conferences should be the norm. Lancet Planet Health 2020;4(2):e48–50.

70. Bousema T, Selvaraj P, Djimde AA, et al. Reducing the carbon footprint of academic conferences: The example of the American Society of Tropical Medicine and Hygiene. Am J Trop Med Hyg 2020;103(5):1758–61.

71. Etzel RA, Ding J, Gil SM, et al. Pediatric societies' declaration on responding to the impact of climate change on children. Journal of Climate Change and Health 2021. https://doi.org/10.1016/j.joclim.2021.100038.

72. Eskenazi B, Etzel RA, Sripada K, et al. The International Society for Children's Health and the Environment commits to reduce its carbon footprint to safeguard children's health. Environ Health Perspect 2020;128(1):14501.

73. Pascal M, Margolis HG, Etzel RA. Greening the International Society for Environmental Epidemiology. Epidemiology 2021;32(4):466–8.

74. World Association of Family Doctors, Planetary Health Alliance, Clinicians for Planetary Health Working Group. Declaration calling for family doctors of the world to act on planetary health. 2019. https://www.wonca.net/site/DefaultSite/filesystem/documents/Groups/Environment/2019%20Planetary%20health.pdf.

75. Kotcher J, Maibach E, Miller J, et al. Views of health professionals on climate change and health: a multinational survey study. Lancet Planet Health 2021; 5(5):e316–23.

76. Lough S. Doctors call for divestment from fossil fuels. CMAJ (Can Med Assoc J) 2015;187(13):E403.

77. Law A, Duff D, Saunders P, et al. Medical organisations must divest from fossil fuels. BMJ 2018;363:k5163.

78. Howard C, Beagley J, Eissa M, et al. Why we need a fossil fuel non-proliferation treaty. Lancet Planet Health 2022;S2542-5196(22):00222–4.

79. Devi S. Health organisations call for non-proliferation of fossil fuels. Lancet 2022; 400(10357):985.

80. United Nations. United Nations Framework Convention on Climate Change, 1992. Available at: https://unfccc.int/files/essential_background/background_publications_htmlpdf/application/pdf/conveng.pdf.

81. United Nations Framework Convention on Climate Change. The Paris Agreement. 2015. Available at: https://unfccc.int/process-and-meetings/the-paris-agreement/the-paris-agreement.

82. Maibach E, Miller J, Armstrong F, et al. Health professionals, the Paris agreement, and the fierce urgency of now. Journal of Climate Change and Health 2021;1: 100002.

83. Duhaime A-C, Futernick M, Alexander M, et al. Healthcare professionals need to be CCLEAR: Climate collaborators, leaders, educators, advocates, and researchers. Journal of Climate Change and Health 2021;4:100078.

Practice and Policy Change

Crossing the Quality Chasm and the Ignored Pillar of Health Care Equity

Tina L. Cheng, MD, MPH[a,b,*], Ndidi I. Unaka, MD, MEd[a,b],
David Nichols, MD, MBA[c]

KEYWORDS

- Child health • Equity • Quality improvement • Social determinants

KEY POINTS

- Health equity is one of the six pillars of health care quality.
- The quality improvement (QI) process provides the framework to drive interventions to address health equity.
- QI inclusive of the pillar of health equity requires ongoing commitment and is an important step to address health care disparities.

Over 20 years ago, the National Academy of Medicine's reports, *To Err is Human*[1] and *Crossing the Quality Chasm*[2] spurred the quality improvement (QI) movement in health care. Although there has been tremendous progress toward the aspiration of delivering quality health care, among the six pillars articulated in the reports (health care should be safe, effective, timely, patient-centered, efficient, and equitable), the last pillar, equity, has been largely ignored. The coronavirus disease 2019 (COVID-19) pandemic and the murder of George Floyd have highlighted persistent and pervasive inequities across all facets of society including health and health care. Learning from the successes of the QI movement, it is past time to address the pillar of health care equity related to race/ethnicity and socioeconomic status.

The Robert Wood Johnson Foundation defines health equity as a state in which "…everyone has a fair and just opportunity to be as healthy as possible. This requires removing obstacles to health such as poverty, discrimination, and their consequences, including powerlessness and lack of access to good jobs with fair pay,

[a] Cincinnati Children's Hospital Medical Center, 3333 Burnet Avenue MLC 3016, Cincinnati, OH 45229, USA; [b] Department of Pediatrics, University of Cincinnati College of Medicine; [c] Emeritus of the American Board of Pediatrics
* Corresponding author. Department of Pediatrics, University of Cincinnati College of Medicine, Cincinnati Children's Hospital Medical Center, 3333 Burnet Avenue MLC 3016, Cincinnati, OH 45229.
E-mail address: Tina.Cheng@cchmc.org

Pediatr Clin N Am 70 (2023) 855–861
https://doi.org/10.1016/j.pcl.2023.03.013
0031-3955/23/© 2023 Elsevier Inc. All rights reserved.

quality education and housing, safe environments, and health care."[3] Thus, achieving health equity requires a multifaceted approach to address upstream societal obstacles outside of health care systems as well as the climate, processes, and systems within health care organizations.

The QI process includes (1) establishing a culture of quality, safety, and continuous improvement that includes equity, (2) collecting and analyzing data to understand the problem, (3) determining and prioritizing process and outcome measures for improvement, (4) identifying key drivers and developing and test interventions, (5) communicating bidirectionally and sharing results transparently, (6) committing to ongoing evaluation, and (7) spreading successes and best practices as outlined in **Fig. 1**.[4] Examples of how these seven steps of the QI process leads to success are numerous and must be applied to the pillar of equity.

1. ESTABLISH A CULTURE OF QUALITY, SAFETY, AND CONTINUOUS IMPROVEMENT THAT INCLUDES EQUITY

The report, *Crossing the Quality Chasm*, called for fundamental change in the health care system to improve health outcomes. The recommendations spurred widespread change in health care organizations from *quality assurance* which concentrates on the flaws of individuals who contribute to medical errors (the "bad apple" theory) to *QI*, which examines the processes and system-level failures that contribute to medical errors.[5] Similarly, a focus on equity within health care will require significant culture change. An institution's mission, organizational structure, processes, and procedures must explicitly support equity and equity must be integrated within QI efforts. The culture of health care organizations' hospital systems, practices, and academic institutions which include attitudes, behaviors, and actions, must reflect excellence and equity. Although we report on serious safety events, serious inequity events must be included. Just like serious safety events must be considered never events, inequities in care must be considered never events. Just as we strive for zero harm, we must strive for zero inequity in care.

Culture change to promote health equity must include leadership support, purposeful discussion of process and systems issues, and safe reporting of concerns. Institutions must cultivate a climate of psychological safety that encourages individuals to speak up if and when they witness inequitable treatment. Some health systems are clear in encouraging reporting and have developed reporting mechanisms aligned with institutional safety and quality efforts.[6,7] Several health care systems have incorporated training on diversity, equity, and inclusion as a means of igniting shifts in organizational culture. Additional methods involve encouraging clinicians to reflect on the

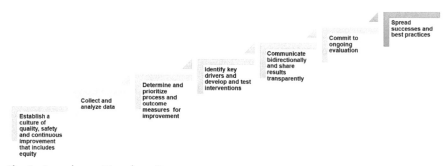

Fig. 1. A roadmap: QI and equity.

ways in which racism in all its forms, discrimination, and poverty contribute to the outcomes of their patients. It is important to consider and discuss these factors during clinical encounters, case presentations as well as during educational activities like morbidity and mortality conferences. Applying learnings about culture change from quality and safety successes is a first step toward ensuring health equity.

2. COLLECT AND ANALYZE DATA

The heart of QI involves data collection and analysis. First, measuring equity requires thorough assessment and optimization of data collection and monitoring systems. At a minimum, data must include accurate collection of demographic information on all patients including insurance status, self-reported race and ethnicity, and language preference. As a result, health care systems should review internal processes for collecting demographic information. Race and ethnicity information in particular should be self-reported and reasons for inaccurate or incomplete information should be mitigated. Population-level measures should reflect relevant structural and social determinants of health domains including economic, geographic, and neighborhood level factors (eg, area deprivation index). Populations with specific needs should receive special consideration (eg, language, immigrant acculturation, birthplace). Analytical approaches must explicitly explore gaps. If differences are found by race and/or ethnicity, stratification by socioeconomic status, and/or insurance type/status is imperative to understand the difference and guide improvement.[8]

Equity measurement can occur on multiple levels including (1) quality metrics stratified by demographic characteristics (eg, race/ethnicity); (2) metrics reflecting population health status; (3) social risk and adversity metrics, (4) organizational climate assessment (eg, patient, family, and provider surveys); and (5) workforce diversity metrics. Traditional health care quality measures must be assessed with regard to these variables to understand the problem and guide intervention.

3. DETERMINE AND PRIORITIZE PROCESS AND OUTCOME MEASURES FOR IMPROVEMENT

Equity-oriented QI work must be prioritized based on data as well as the experiences and needs of patients, families, and communities. Objective measures can quantify the disparities of a defined population and the lived experiences of patients and families must inform interventions for their elimination. QI and equity experts should look at differences in all phases of care within the health care system and at each step in the care process. Then, health system leaders, and clinical teams, in partnership with patients, families, and community members should dig deeper to understand the root causes of the differences. The relevant care steps and processes may involve access, referral patterns, diagnostic and treatment decisions, and transitions of care. Although measuring and addressing services and clinical outcomes related to the first five quality pillars (safety, effectiveness, timeliness, patient-centered, efficiency) have become commonplace in health care, the same must be done for the sixth pillar of equity. Interventions to address disparities may require universal approaches for all patients (eg, lift all boats) whereas other interventions may require a focus on specific neighborhoods or affected groups.

Addressing social determinants of health (SDoH) promotes health equity. Healthy People 2030 defines SDoH as "the conditions in the environments where people are born, live, learn, work, play, worship, and age that affect a wide range of health, functioning, and quality-of-life outcomes and risks."[9] Health care systems are anchor institutions in their communities and have a responsibility to partner with key stakeholders to mitigate the impact of SDoH that confer poor health outcomes on patients by testing and implementing interventions.

4. IDENTIFY KEY DRIVERS, AND DEVELOP AND TEST INTERVENTIONS

Health care organizations must dig deeper to understand the mechanisms that contribute to health inequities—a critical next step to inform interventions. These mechanisms may include racism in all its forms and discrimination that reinforce (1) barriers to health care access, (2) stress and allostatic load, (3) individual-level bias[10–12](eg, a clinician's implicit or explicit assumptions that shape medical decisions), and (4) systems-level bias (eg, clinical practice guidelines that promote raced-based medicine[13]). These mechanisms need to be exposed to appropriately and effectively intervene.

For instance, asthma—which impacts approximately 7 million children and adolescents in the United States—is more prevalent in Black children. Black children and adolescents with asthma have higher rates of urgent care and emergency department visits, are more likely to require hospitalization, and have higher rates of asthma-related mortality.[14,15] Contributing factors for this known health inequity among Black children with asthma may involve multiple factors including[16,17] (1) significant exposure to environmental hazards and neighborhood risk factors due the legacy of redlining and residential segregation,[18,19] (2) clinician bias which negatively impacts the care team's ability to effectively communicate information to families about asthma medications and action plans, and[20] (3) financial and transportation barriers that impact medication adherence and follow-up.[21] Rigorous data analysis and further study move us beyond designing interventions based on downstream and often over-simplified factors that place blame on individual patients and caregivers (eg, nonadherence). Rather, deeper quantitative and qualitative analysis enhances our ability to identify upstream root causes of health inequities at the individual, institutional, and population level and to develop appropriate action plans.

Longstanding efforts in Cincinnati exemplify how clinicians in partnership with community-based organizations used QI approaches to address root causes of disparate pediatric asthma outcomes. Specifically, Cincinnati Children's Hospital Medical Center partnered with the Cincinnati Health Department to establish the Collaboration to Lessen Environmental Asthma Risks (CLEAR) program with the goal of improving pediatric asthma outcomes.[22] Clinicians are able to place CLEAR referrals for hospitalized children with asthma who reside in Hamilton County and screen positive for environmental triggers (eg, mold, mildew, rodents, cockroaches) within the home. The Cincinnati Health Department then reaches out to the family to schedule a home inspection to identify home triggers and facilitate the abatement of environmental hazards.

Another example of the movement from data to intervention is the Vermont Oxford Network's work on health equity for sick newborns.[23,24]

5. COMMUNICATE BIDIRECTIONALLY AND SHARE RESULTS TRANSPARENTLY

Timely, truthful, and transparent communication is critical in uncovering mechanisms that contribute to health inequities and developing action plans. Dashboards that are inclusive of equity metrics are an important means of elevating QI efforts and sharing data within and across health care organizations and with community stakeholders. Health care organizations should convene and support engagement of patients and families as partners through patient and family advisory councils to assist in interpreting data, disseminating results, and co-producing interventions. Health care organizations must ensure advisory councils reflect the community and patient population served and mitigate barriers to participation. The wisdom of all stakeholders is necessary to understand the problem and develop priorities and actions.

6. COMMIT TO ONGOING EVALUATION

QI is an ongoing process. A high-functioning system must collect data, assess, revisit the effectiveness of interventions, and improve on a continual basis to mitigate the risk of degradation of the work. As a result, health care systems must not only prioritize improvement initiatives that aim to narrow equity gaps, they must ensure that these efforts are durable, and that the portfolio of equity-oriented work continues to expand. Equity becomes systemic once it is incorporated into ongoing QI efforts that are tied to organizational priorities and well-supported.

7. SPREAD SUCCESSES AND BEST PRACTICES

Health care transformation and the promotion of equity using improvement science can only occur through large-scale sharing, learning, and implementation. Learning health systems[25] are conducive to rapid knowledge generation, application, and broad spread of successful interventions. The learning collaborative model has proven to be a powerful model to improve outcomes nationwide.[26] A powerful example of the transformative nature of learning health systems is Children's Hospitals' Solutions for Patient Safety Collaborative. This endeavor, which originated with eight children's hospitals in Ohio, was founded on the principles of high-reliability organizations, data transparency, and sharing best practices to promote synergy between improving processes and institutional safety culture across these hospitals.[27] There is no such learning collaborative for health care equity. The time has come. Important core practices for establishing a learning health system where improvement processes and an equity culture converge include (1) leadership by and co-production with individuals with lived experiences and (2) engagement beyond the health care system.

There has been remarkable progress in QI in the past two decades. Incorporating the health equity pillar into the QI playbook offers promise and is long overdue.

CLINICS CARE POINTS

- Use an evidence-based framework (eg, Model for Improvement) when using QI to address equity gaps.
- Start with disaggregating data to identify equity gaps and prioritize QI initiatives.
- Co-design key drivers and interventions with all stakeholders including community partners, patients, and families and avoid being health care centric.

DISCLOSURE

No financial assistance was received to support this article. This work is original, not previously published, and not submitted for publication or consideration elsewhere. T.L. Cheng, N.I. Unaka, D. Nichols: No disclosures of financial ties or potential/perceived conflicts of interest. Each author conceptualized and wrote portions of the article, revised each draft, and approved the final article.

REFERENCES

1. Institute of Medicine (US). In: Kohn LT, Corrigan JM, Donaldson MS, editors. Committee on quality of health care in America. To Err is Human: Building a safer health system. Washington (DC): National Academies Press (US); 2000. PMID: 25077248.
2. Institute of Medicine (US). Committee on quality of health care in America. Crossing the quality Chasm: a New health system for the 21st Century. Washington (DC): National Academies Press (US); 2001. PMID: 25057539.
3. Braveman P, Arkin E, Orleans T, et al. What is health equity? And what difference Does a Definition Make? Princeton, NJ: Robert Wood Johnson Foundation; 2017.
4. Hughes RG. Tools and Strategies for Quality Improvement and Patient Safety. In: Hughes RG, editor. Patient Safety and Quality: An Evidence-Based Handbook for Nurses. Rockville (MD): Agency for Healthcare Research and Quality (US); 2008. Chapter 44. Available at: https://www.ncbi.nlm.nih.gov/books/NBK2682/.
5. Knox L, Brach C. The Practice Facilitation Handbook: Training Modules for New Facilitators and Their Trainers. (Prepared by LA Net through a subcontract with the University of Minnesota under Contract No. HHSA290200710010 TO 3.) Rockville, MD: Agency for Healthcare Research and Quality; June 2013. AHRQ Publication No. 13-0046-EF. Available at: https://www.ahrq.gov/sites/default/files/publications/files/practicefacilitationhandbook.pdf, Accessed October 8, 2022.
6. Yale Children's Hospital. Available at:https://www.ynhh.org/childrens-hospital/medical-professionals/clinical-pathways.aspx. Accessed October 18, 2021.
7. University of Washington. (Available at:https://www.washington.edu/raceequity/updates/bias-reporting-tools/Accessed October 18, 2921.
8. Cheng TL, Goodman E, American Academy of Pediatrics Committee on Pediatric Research. Race, Ethnicity, and Socioeconomic Status in Research on Child Health. Pediatrics 2015;135(1):e225–37.
9. Healthy People 2030, U.S. Department of Health and Human Services, Office of Disease Prevention and Health Promotion. Available at:https://health.gov/healthypeople/objectives-and-data/social-determinants-health. Accessed June 20, 2021.
10. Raphael JL, Oyeku SO. Implicit bias in pediatrics: An emerging focus in health equity research. Pediatrics 2020;145(5).
11. Goyal MK, Kuppermann N, Cleary SD, et al. Racial disparities in pain management of children with appendicitis in emergency departments. JAMA Pediatr 2015;169(11):996–1002.
12. Wakefield EO, Pantaleao A, Popp JM, et al. Describing perceived racial bias among youth with sickle cell disease. J Pediatr Psychol 2018;43(7):779–88.
13. Cerdeña JP, Plaisime MV, Tsai J. From race-based to race-conscious medicine: how anti-racist uprisings call us to act. Lancet 2020;396(10257):1125–8.
14. McQuaid EL. Barriers to medication adherence in asthma. Ann Allergy Asthma Immunol 2018;121(1):37–42.
15. Akinbami LJ, Moorman JE, Simon AE, et al. Trends in racial disparities for asthma outcomes among children 0 to 17 years, 2001-2010. J Allergy Clin Immunol 2014;134(3):547–53.e5.
16. Zahran HS, Bailey CM, Damon SA, et al. Vital Signs: Asthma in Children — United States, 2001–2016. MMWR Morb Mortal Wkly Rep 2018;67(5):149–55.
17. Akinbami LJ, King M. Trends in Asthma Prevalence, Health Care Use, and Mortality in the United States, 2001–2010. NCHS Data Brief 2012;(94):8.

18. Nardone A, Casey JA, Morello-Frosch R, et al. Associations between historical residential redlining and current age-adjusted rates of emergency department visits due to asthma across eight cities in California: an ecological study. Lancet Planet Health 2020;4(1):e24–31.

19. Beck AF, Huang B, Chundur R, et al. Housing Code Violation Density Associated With Emergency Department And Hospital Use By Children With Asthma. Health Aff 2014;33(11):1993–2002.

20. Beck AF, Moncrief T, Huang B, et al. Inequalities in Neighborhood Child Asthma Admission Rates and Underlying Community Characteristics in One US County. J Pediatr 2013;163(2):574–80.e1.

21. McQuaid EL. Barriers to medication adherence in asthma: the importance of culture and context. Ann Allergy Asthma Immunol 2018;121(1):37–42.

22. Beck AF, Simmons JM, Sauers HS, et al. Connecting at-risk inpatient asthmatics to a community-based program to reduce home environmental risks: Care system redesign using quality improvement methods. Hosp Pediatr 2013;3:326–34.

23. Boghossian NS, Geraci M, Lorch SA, et al. Racial and Ethnic Differences Over Time in Outcomes of Infants Born Less Than 30 Weeks' Gestation. Pediatrics 2019;144(3):e20191106.

24. Vermont Oxford Network for Health Equity. Potentially Better Practices for Follow Through https://public.vtoxford.org/health-equity/potentially-better-practices-for-follow-through/Accessed December 4, 2022.

25. Friedman C, Rubin J, Brown J, et al. Toward a science of learning systems: a research agenda for the high-functioning Learning Health System. J Am Med Inform Assoc 2015;22(1):43–50.

26. Lannon CM, Peterson LE. Pediatric Collaborative Networks For Quality Improvement and Research. Acad Pediatrics 2013;13:S69–74.

27. Lyren A, Brilli RJ, Zieker K, et al. Children's hospitals' solutions for patient safety collaborative impact on hospital-acquired harm. Pediatrics 2017;140(3).

Achieving Child Health Equity: Policy Solutions

Benard P. Dreyer, MD

KEYWORDS

- Poverty • Racism • Immigrant • Health care • Early childhood • Family • LGBTQ+
- Environment

KEY POINTS

- Policy solutions for child health equity exist and many are proved to be effective.
- Early childhood is a time where interventions are critically important.
- Direct financial support to families reduces child poverty and improves child outcomes.
- The intersection of poverty with racial-ethnic identity and racism is especially harmful.
- Protection of LGBTQ + children and adolescents, as well as immigrant children and families is necessary.

There are several policy solutions for achieving child health equity at the federal and the state and local level. Many of these policies have been supported by the National Academy of Science, Engineering and Medicine (NASEM) and the American Academy of Pediatrics. **Table 1** lists all the suggested policy solutions.

The theoretic underpinning of these suggested policies is the bioecological model, first proposed by Bronfenbrenner and Ceci in 1994 (**Fig. 1**). The child is situated in the center, surrounded by concentric circles of their environmental influences from proximal to distal (parent and family well-being; school and parental workplace policies; neighborhood and community resources; and finally social, health and economic systems, policies, and values). Although the policy solutions described are part of the outer concentric circle, many of them work through their impact on more proximal environmental influences on the child, from the family to the community.

Individual pediatricians can advocate for these policies and make a difference for children and families. They can make changes in their practice, encourage their hospitals and health systems to act, and advocate at the local, state, and federal level. See **Fig. 2** for suggested actions.

New York University, Grossman School of Medicine, 550 1st Avenue, New York, NY 10016, USA
E-mail address: Benard.Dreyer@nyulangone.org

Pediatr Clin N Am 70 (2023) 863–883
https://doi.org/10.1016/j.pcl.2023.04.003
pediatric.theclinics.com

Table 1
Policy solutions for child health equity

Equity Area	Program	Policy Solutions
Health care	Medicaid/CHIP	Raising eligibility to at least 300% of the FPL (preferably 400%)
		Families above eligibility level should be able to buy into coverage through Medicaid/CHIP
		Medicaid physician payments should match those of Medicare
		All immigrant children should be eligible for Medicaid/CHIP regardless of when they arrived in the United States or their legal status. The LIFT the BAR act should be passed by Congress
		Federal dollars should cover all public health insurance of children who meet eligibility
		Medicaid's menu of services (EPSDT) and cost-sharing rules should be extended to those covered by CHIP
		CHIP should be made a permanent entitlement
		Bureaucratic barriers to continuous enrollment should be removed
		Health care networks should provide access to all pediatric subspecialty services
	VBP Models	State Medicaid VBP models should focus on the specific needs of children including outcomes along the life course and using cross-sector collaborations
		Kindergarten readiness and high school graduation rates should be considered as target outcomes for children
		A bundle of office-based interventions (eg, ROR, VIP, Healthy Steps) should be considered for VBP funding
	IHS	Support for mandatory adequate, equitable, and timely funding for the IHS is necessary to improve the health of AI/AN children and adolescents

Direct financial support to families	Child Allowance/Reformed Child Tax Credit (CTC)	Reinstate the reformed Child Tax Credit in the American Rescue Act of 2021 that provided $3600 per child younger than 5 y and $3000 per child from 6–17 y to low- and middle-income families each year, paid monthly
	EITC	Increase the federal EITC by 40%
	CDCTC	Make the CDCTC completely refundable; raise the percentage of expenses covered to 50%; increase the maximum benefit to $8000 for one child and to $16,000 for 2 or more children
	PFML	Create a national PFML benefit of at least 12 wk per year, paying 60%–70% worker's salary during leave
	Minimum Wage	Raise the federal minimum wage to $15 per hour and index it to inflation after that
	Income limits for federal benefits	Raise the income limit to qualify for federal benefits such as SNAP to at least 200% of the FPL
Nutrition	SNAP	Increase SNAP benefits by 30%
		Make permanent SEBTC of $180 per child
		Extend SNAP benefits to all immigrant households irrespective of time of entry or documentation status
	School Meals	Provide universal free meals in schools to all children
Support for early childhood and brain development	Child Care, Preschool, and Prekindergarten	Increase eligibility for CCDF vouchers to up to 200% of FPL for gross income of families;
		See improvements to CDCTC under Direct Financial support to Families
		States and municipalities should fund universal pre-K for all 4-year-olds and provide funding for 25%–50% of 3-year-olds
	MIECHV	Congress should increase funding to MIECHV by $200 million per year for 5 y and also increase tribal allocations
	Primary Care Literacy and Parenting Interventions	See VBP models under Health Care section
End family homelessness	Housing Choice Voucher Program	Increase the number of housing vouchers available so that 70% of those families that qualify for housing vouchers have access to them
	HPRP	Congress should reinstitute HPRP at a financial level similar to the funding provided for the program from 2009 to 2012 ($1.5 billion over 3 y)

(continued on next page)

Table 1 (*continued*)

Equity Area	Program	Policy Solutions
Make housing and neighborhoods environmentally safe	Low-Income Home Energy Assistance Program (LIHEAP)	Congress should increase annual appropriations for LIHEAP substantially from the present $5 billion to cover all the low-income and tribal families who are eligible for and seek assistance
	Lead service line replacements through EPA	Increase the funding for replacement of lead pipes serving homes, day care centers, and schools to a level that will replace all lead service lines (an additional $30 billion more than the $15 billion allocated as part the Infrastructure and Jobs bill of 2021)
	Air pollution mitigation	The EPA should increase air quality standards and address environmental racism/child health through better regulation and stronger enforcement of existing rules
	Tree canopies in poor city neighborhoods	Cities should modify their tree-planting programs to plant many more trees in those communities that have inadequate tree canopies in order to ameliorate the impact and to reduce the negative health effects of urban heat islands on poor communities and communities of color
Gun Violence Prevention	Federal laws and regulations	Make background checks universal
		Initiate buyer regulations: increase age limits to buy a firearm; require a permit/license; require a waiting period before purchase
		Ban semiautomatic military-style weapons and high-capacity magazines
		Require safety mechanisms such as trigger locks
		Allow the CPSC to regulate guns for safety including the use of "smart" gun technology to prevent access to unauthorized users and decrease unintentional deaths and suicides
	State laws and regulations	Institute strong CAP laws in every state in the United States
		Initiate Safe Storage laws in every state in the United States

LGBTQ + Health Equity	Same-sex marriage and parenting by gay and lesbian parents	Congress must pass the RFMA reintroduced in Congress in 2022
	Support for transgender and gender-diverse children and adolescents	Repeal or prevent passage of state laws that criminalize treatments of transgender youth Advocate for all states to mandate insurance coverage for transgender youth Repeal or prevent passage of state laws that limit participation in high school and college athletics based on biological sex Advocate for the inclusion of gender identity in state hate crime legislation
Protect immigrant children and families	Treatment of children at the southern border	Enforce all the provisions of the Flores agreement, including ending without delay the detention of children and families and discharging them to community Never use the Flores agreement provisions to excuse separating children from their parents
	Deferred Action for Childhood Arrivals (DACA) and the American Dream and Promise Act of 2021 (Dream Act)	Congress should make DACA permanent and open up DACA to new applicants Allow DACA recipients to apply for PELL grants Congress should pass the Dream and Promise Act of 2021 Congress should pass the LIFT the BAR act of 2021–2022

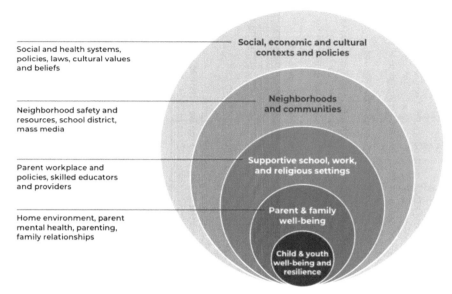

Fig. 1. The bioecological or whole child model of child development. (The Bioecological Model. https://ccfwb.uw.edu/about-us/the-bioecological-model/.)

HEALTH CARE
Medicaid and the Children's Health Insurance Program

Medicaid and the Children's Health Insurance Program (CHIP) insure almost 50% of all children in the United States. However, low provider payments in Medicaid leads to access problems for children. Medicaid's payments to physicians average approximately two-thirds of those paid by Medicare, thus discouraging physician participation. Networks should be broad enough to provide access to all pediatric subspecialty services, including in rural areas and tribal lands and crossing state lines as needed. In addition, the requirement that states fund a significant portion of Medicaid (on average 43%) leads to states limiting enrollment or keeping per child expenses low, especially during times of budget shortfalls. Because states must balance their budgets, allocations to Medicaid by states are part of a "zero sum game."[1,2] Because CHIP is not an entitlement, it must get refunded by congress periodically. In 2017, this led to interruption of coverage for children on CHIP.

Medicaid/CHIP also do not cover all immigrant children. As of 2018, 34 states have chosen to insure all legally residing immigrant children without a 5-year wait but 16 states have chosen not to take that option.[3] In addition, 6 states and the District of Columbia insure all children irrespective of immigrant status. In 2019, compared with an overall prevalence of uninsurance among US children of about 5%, citizen children living with at least one noncitizen parent had a rate of 9% 25% of documented immigrant children and 35% of undocumented immigrant children were uninsured.[4]

Because of the intersection of poverty and race/ethnicity, as well as the added impact of structural racism, almost 60% of African American/Black, Latinx, and American Indian/Alaskan Native children are covered by Medicaid/CHIP. Almost half of Hawaiian native children are similarly insured.[5] Therefore, improving Medicaid and CHIP is a racial health equity issue.

AAP Website: AAP.org/en/advocacy:

> Issues to address, e.g. immigrant child health, health care access, gun violence, climate change, child nutrition

> State Advocacy

> Advocacy Action Center: taking action on individual issues, easily contact your senators and house representatives

AAP Chapter: become active in your chapter to impact state-level issues concerning child poverty and equity

AAP Annual Legislative Conference in Washington DC: attend the conference and visit legislators on "the Hill"

NASEM Roadmap to Reducing Child Poverty:
https://nap.nationalacademies.org/catalog/25246/a-roadmap-to-reducing-child-poverty
Read the entire report and find issues that you are passionate about

Look up individual AAP policies that you are committed to and learn what more can be done by the individual pediatrician

Make an appointment to visit your federal and state legislators when they are in their home office

Join your local school board to advocate for better policies for poor children regarding their education and nutrition

Join AAP sections and councils that focus on issues regarding child poverty and equity and become part of the conversation (e.g. Council on Community Pediatrics [COCP], Section on Minority Equity, Health and Inclusion [SOMHEI], Council on Immigrant Child and Family Health {COICFH])

Advocate that your hospital and/or health system to take on interventions that affect child poverty and equity

Change your practice to include a focus on social determinants of health and institute interventions that are evidenced-based to improve child outcomes for poor and minoritized children and families

Fig. 2. Advocacy actions for the individual pediatrician.

Strengthening Medicaid and CHIP could be done through a series of policy changes. First raising eligibility to 300% of the Federal Poverty Level (FPL) would cover more than 50% of children and reach a sizable number of the uninsured. Raising eligibility to 400% of the FPL would essentially cover all uninsured children. Families above these income eligibility limits should be allowed to buy into coverage through Medicaid/CHIP. Second, Medicaid physician payments should match those of Medicare. Third, coverage should be given to all immigrant children regardless of when they arrived in the United States or their legal status (one bill pending in Congress that partially addresses this problem is the LIFT the BAR act[6]). Fourth, federal dollars should cover all public health insurance for children up to the 300% or 400% of the FPL. Medicaid's complete menu of services for children (EPSDT: Early and Periodic Screening, Diagnostic, and Treatment) and cost-sharing rules should extend to those children covered by CHIP. Fifth, CHIP should become an entitlement (permanent), akin to Medicaid, not requiring periodic refunding.[2] Finally bureaucratic barriers to continuous enrollment should be removed. Waiting periods for CHIP should be abolished. Continuous enrollment in Medicaid/CHIP for at least a year, and possibly from birth to 6 years should be instituted to ensure that early childhood immunizations, screenings, and brain development are enhanced.[7,8]

Value-Based Payment Models to Support Children's Health and Wellness

VBP models that have been pursued by policymakers to improve the quality of care and population health of Medicaid patients, often with an additional goal of cost savings. State-level Medicaid VBP models often are focused on adults and not on children's needs (with outcomes and cost savings much later in the life course and often not in the health sector). Although there have been pilot programs targeting children, even these programs have usually not addressed child health equity issues and the long-term success of poor children beyond the quality of medical care they receive.[9]

Related to state-level VBP models are interventions at the health system level. An example is the Nationwide Children's Hospital Pediatric Vital Signs Project. Partnering with the community, Nationwide chose 8 vital sign goals, including kindergarten readiness, high school graduation, and teenage pregnancy.[10]

Another promising program is the NYC Health and Hospitals 3-2-1 Impact program that is a 2-generational intervention for pregnant and postpartum women and their children. The families get maternal depression screening and services, Reach Out and Read (ROR), Video Interaction Project, and Healthy Steps—all focusing on early brain development, parenting support, and kindergarten readiness.[11] Advocacy is needed to get insurance payers, including Medicaid, to provide payment for these programs, even when these interventions have proven effectiveness.

VBP focused on improving children's outcomes has received recent impetus from the Center for Medicare and Medicaid Innovation Awards for the Integrated Care for Kids (InCK) model. Eight awardees are now experimenting with integrating care across health and social sectors and coming up with alternative VBP models; this is a great opportunity to address kindergarten readiness by supporting a bundle of office-based interventions (eg, ROR) and connections to programs in the early childhood education arena (eg, Early Head Start, prekindergarten [pre-K]). Ultimately, the hope is to mitigate disparities based on poverty and racism.[11] Measures of kindergarten readiness could be based on "Healthy and Ready to Learn" and "Maryland's Ready 4 Kindergarten Measure (R4K)." Although there is ample evidence of the effectiveness of individual interventions and programs, the impact of VBP models on child outcomes is as yet unproved.[12]

Adequate Funding for the Indian Health Service

The Indian Health Service (IHS) is chronically underfunded and at the mercy of federal appropriations, which results in receiving less than 50% of needed support. For example, in 2017 the IHS received about $4000 per capita funding, as compared with almost $11,000 per capita funding in the Veterans Affairs Health system. This grossly inadequate funding leads to stark disparities in all health services including oral and mental health. Policies supporting mandatory adequate, equitable, and timely funding of the IHS are critically important.[13]

DIRECT FINANCIAL SUPPORT TO FAMILIES
Child Allowance/Reformed Child Tax Credit

One of the major recommendations from the NASEM report entitled "Roadmap to Reducing Child Poverty" was for the federal government to institute a child allowance (also known as a reformed Child Tax Credit [CTC]) of at least $3000 per child each year. It would be completely refundable (ie, even those without income would get the full credit) and paid monthly. NASEM estimated that such a child allowance would cut child poverty rates by 40%.[14] When the American Rescue Plan was passed in 2021 (see later discussion), those predictions became reality.

Research shows that in addition to reducing child poverty rates, cash subsidies for families improve child emotional, behavioral, and academic outcomes.[15] Early results from the Baby's First Years study confirm that cash benefits seem to improve early brain development.[16]

The Biden administration passed the American Rescue Plan in March 2021, which included a reformed CTC modeled on the NASEM recommendations. Sadly, it was not reallocated in 2022 and child poverty rates increased back to prior levels. Congress should reinstitute the reformed CTC as quickly as possible. This policy action would increase child health socioeconomic and racial equity.[15]

Earned Income Tax Credit

The Earned Income Tax Credit (EITC) is a refundable federal tax credit for low- and middle-income working families. It was introduced in 1975 and has been expanded under each president beginning with Ronald Reagan. The EITC has been successful at encouraging parents to work (therefore increasing income from work) and further reducing child poverty by providing cash benefits. Furthermore, expansions of the EITC seem to improve the longer term health and academic outcomes of children in families receiving these benefits. NASEM, in its report on reducing child poverty, recommended increasing the EITC by 40%, and this enhancement would likely reduce child poverty rates by 15% to 20%. It is worthy of recommending.[14]

Child and Dependent Care Tax Credit

Child care expenses can be an insurmountable barrier to employment for low-income parents, particularly when their children are too young for school. In the United States, the cost of child care for children younger than 5 years averages approximately $8500 per year. Poor families with a young child often spent about 20% of their income on child care. The federal government helps cover the cost of child care to working families through the Child and Dependent Care Tax Credit (CDCTC). The CDCTC is a nonrefundable tax credit that reimburses a portion of the qualifying child care expenses of working parents with children younger than 13 years. In addition to being nonrefundable, meaning the poorest families are left out of this benefit, it only covers 35% of expenses up to a maximum of $3000 for one child and $6000 for 2 or more children. That means that the maximum benefit is $1050 for one child, nowhere near the $8500 average cost of child care. Research on child care programs suggests that any expansion of child care subsidies would reduce child poverty, both because such subsidies add to family financial resources and because it can make it possible for families to work and increase their earnings.[14]

The American Rescue Plan of 2021 enhanced the CDCTC in several ways, but only for 1 year (2021). It made the CDCTC completely refundable. It also raised the percentage of expenses covered from 35% to 50%, and increased the maximum benefit to $8000 for one child and $16000 for 2 or more children; this means that the maximum benefit for one child is $4000, 4 times greater than the existing CDCTC.[17] This policy should be reinstituted at the level of the 2021 tax credit in order to decrease socioeconomic and racial health inequities.

Paid Family and Medical Leave

The United States is the only high-income country that lacks a national paid family and medical leave program. Federal law affords a little more than half of workers' access to unpaid leave but provides no national paid leave. Nine states and the District of Columbia have paid leave programs that exist or are being implemented, but most workers do not live in those states.[18] States offering Paid Family and Medical Leave (PFML) generally offer up to 12 weeks per year, paying 60% to 70% of the worker's salary during leave and usually financed by payroll deductions.

PFML used for maternity/paternity leave has major benefits for the child and parents. Receipt of PFML increases breastfeeding, decreases infant mortality, increases well-child visits and vaccination rates for children, and decreases maternal depression. Fathers who take paternity leave become more involved fathers and take on household and parenting duties.[19] Especially in low-income families, PFML leads to increased income, decreased poverty, and overall better economic security of young children.[20] There are racial-ethnic disparities in access and use of PFML. Latinx and Black families have less access to these programs and, therefore, cannot use them for maternity, medical reasons, child care, and caring for sick family members.[21] The same is true for the present unpaid Federal family medical leave program.[22] The United States should create a national PFML benefit modeled on those in the states that have implemented them.

Minimum Wage and the Basic Needs Family Budget

The present federal minimum wage is $7.25 per hour. One wage earner working full time (40 h/wk) will earn $15,000 a year. If 2 parents work full time, they will earn $30,000 a year, barely more than the FPL for a family of 4 ($27,750 in 2022). Basic needs budgets include costs for housing, food, child care, health insurance, out-of-pocket medical expenses, transportation to work, other necessities (eg, clothing, broadband), payroll, and income taxes. A basic needs budget for a family of 4 varies by state, from a low of $60,000 to a high of $100,000 or more in 2020.[23] Therefore, increasing the minimum wage to closer to $15 per hour will allow a family of 4 with 2 wage earners to approach the lower end of an adequate basic needs budget.

The size of basic needs budgets also points to revising federal income requirements for benefits based on the FPL to at least 200% of the FPL. Low-income families earning less than 200% of the FLP are not likely to meet their basic needs. Research supports raising these income limits.[24,25]

NUTRITION
SNAP

Food insecurity is related to poverty level and race ethnicity. Thirty-one percent of children living in households with income less than 130% of the FPL (the present gross income requirement to receive SNAP benefits) are food insecure. However, even below 185% of the FPL, 27% of children are food insecure. It is only for children living in househols earning greater than 185% of the FPL that the percent who are food insecure dropts to 5%. Twenty percent of Black households are food insecure, and 16% of Latinx households are food insecure as compared with 7% of White households.[26]

Research documents that food insecurity leads to negative impacts on academic success and social emotional development of children and adolescents.[27–29] In addition, SNAP is a near-cash benefit that reduces child poverty by more than 5%.[14]

NASEM recommended increasing SNAP by 30%. NASEM also recommended adding a Summer Electronic Benefit Transfer for Children of $180 per child to address food gaps for children during the summer when they lack access to school lunch and breakfast programs.[14] Although this program for summer meals was provided during the COVID-19 pandemic, it should now be made permanent. Furthermore, NASEM recommended extending SNAP benefits to all immigrant households, irrespective of time of entry to the United States, and documentation status. Documented child immigrants are already eligible for SNAP without a 5-year waiting period, but their parents, even with green cards, are not eligible.

Universal Free School Meals

Children consume up to 50% of their calories in school, and for many low-income children school meals may be their only meal of the day. Research on the National School Lunch Program, Summer Food Service Program, and Child Care Food Program found that these programs were associated with significantly lower rates of food insecurity in low-income households. Research also found that they led to improved diet quality and academic performance for children in low-income and food-insecure households.[30]

During the COVID-19 pandemic, the United States Department of Agriculture provided universal free meals to all children in school. Congress has not voted to extend that benefit. Reinstating universal free meals in school would eliminate the stigma associated with free and reduced-price school meals; decrease parental burden; decrease the administrative burden on school staff; and ensure that all children in the school get 2 meals a day (breakfast and lunch).

SUPPORT FOR EARLY CHILDHOOD AND BRAIN DEVELOPMENT

Poor and low-income children, including many Black and Latinx children, frequently enter kindergarten significantly behind their higher-income peers in language and math skills. It is hard for children to make up this disparity. By the third grade, these disparities are stable and last into the higher grades.[31,32] By the fourth grade, reading proficiency is associated with higher high school graduation rates and better economic success as adults. Fourth grade reading levels reveal stark disparities for poor- versus higher income children. Only 20% of poor children are proficient readers compared with 50% of those in higher income families. Only 17% of Black children, 19% of Latinx children, and 22% of American Indian/Alaska Native (AI/AN) children are proficient compared with 55% of White children. Immigrant children are also disadvantaged, and only 7% of dual-language learners are proficient readers (in English) compared with 66% of those who are English language learners.[33] Children exposed to adverse childhood experiences causing toxic stress are also more likely to have problems in school, including being less engaged and repeating a grade.[34]

Child Care, Preschool, and Prekindergarten

State and local preschool and pre-K programs improve academic readiness for school and have persistent positive impacts beyond school entry. However, states are only providing pre-K to 33% of 4-year-olds and 5% of 3-year-olds. Higher quality child care programs also lead to better language and cognitive outcomes in the years before kindergarten entry.[34] Research from studies of high-quality early childhood education programs document improved cognitive and social abilities, including better math and language scores, than controls.[35]

Several policies are suggested by these studies.

1. In addition to help from the CDCTC, the Child Care Development Fund (CCDF) provides vouchers to low-income families to offset the cost of child care. At present, CCDF vouchers have federal income limits similar to SNAP. NASEM suggests

increasing the federal income limit (and therefore federal funds) to 150% of the FPL for families to receive vouchers,[14] but 200% of the FPL seems more appropriate. Some states, similar to New York, have higher income limits for families approximating 200% of FPL.

2. Although some states and municipalities offer "universal" pre-K, most do not. Most funding is for pre-K for 4-year-olds, and little attention has been focused on pre-K for 3-year-olds.[36] States should provide universal pre-K to all 4-year-olds and 25% to 50% of 3-year-olds.

Maternal, Infant, and Earl Childhood Home Visiting Program

Home visiting programs create more positive early childhood experiences and lead to children being ready for school and having improved language development.[34] Home visiting also improves parenting, provides early detection and treatment of maternal depression, and decreases child abuse. The Administration for Child and Families (ACF) has conducted an evaluation of many Maternal, Infant, and Earl Childhood Home Visiting Program (MIECHV) programs, called Home Visiting Evidence of Effectiveness or HomeVEE, and found many impactful programs staffed by nurse or community health worker home visitors.[37] However, the program is grossly underfunded, and only 150,000 of a potential 18 million families that could benefit from the program are enrolled because of budget constraints. Congress should increase funding by $200 million per year for 5 years and increase tribal allocations as well.[38]

Primary Care Literacy and Parenting Interventions

As noted earlier, there are interventions as part of primary pediatric care that improve child language, cognitive, and social development that prepare them to learn and succeed in kindergarten.[34,39,40] These interventions should be funded by VBP mechanisms in Medicaid.

END FAMILY HOMELESSNESS

Approximately 1.6 million children experience homelessness in a year, and more than 200,000 are homeless each night. More than 70% of homeless families are Black or Latinx, and therefore, homelessness is an inequity at the intersection of poverty and race. Homeless families often have sustained a long period of housing insecurity or being doubled up before entering a shelter. Homeless children suffer from high rates of food insecurity, poor health, and developmental and academic problems.[41] Homeless children test more poorly on academic subjects at least partially due to multiple school changes and disruptions.[42]

Housing Choice Voucher Program

Low-income renters in the United States spend two-thirds of their income for rent; this has led to high rates of eviction and housing displacement of poor- and low-income families with children. The federal Housing Choice Voucher Program provides financial support to poor families. Unfortunately, there are a finite number of housing vouchers and only 25% or those who qualify are able to get housing vouchers, often spending long times on waiting lists. NASEM suggested increasing the percentage of eligible families who should have access to a housing voucher to 70%.[14]

The Homelessness Prevention and Rapid Rehousing Program

The Homelessness Prevention and Rapid Rehousing Program (HPRP) was a short-lived program that was funded from 2009 to 2012. HUD provided $1.5 billion in

HPRP grants to local and state governments to prevent homelessness and restore housing stability for people who became homeless. Nearly 90% of participants exited HPRP to permanent housing[43]; this was a highly effective program that should be reinstituted by Congress.

MAKE HOUSING AND NEIGHBORHOODS ENVIRONMENTALLY SAFE
Low-Income Home Energy Assistance Program

Home energy is an equity issue for poor families and families of color. Almost 40% of low-income households and 30% of households of color report that they were unable to pay their energy bills and 50% of low-income households report that they had to reduce or forego expenses for food or medicine in order to pay an energy bill. Tribal communities are also at high risk. Those families are likely to experience heating and utility disconnections, which gravely impact health if done during freezing or heat stress times of the year.[44]

The Low-Income Home Energy Assistance Program (LIHEAP), funded through Department of Health and Human Services and administered through the states, is the federal government's support program for utility costs of low-income families. It provides financial support for energy bills, as well as funds for repair or replacement of heating and cooling equipment. It receives yearly appropriations from Congress of about $5 billion. Only about 20% of households that are eligible for LIHEAP receive funds; therefore, advocates suggest increasing the annual appropriations substantially up to as much as $40 billion.[44]

Lead Service Line Replacements Through the Environmental Protection Agency

Poor communities and communities of color are at increased risk of having lead in their drinking and cooking water due to lead pipes in service to their homes, day care centers, and schools. There is no safe level of lead exposure. Lead is especially toxic to children, causing reduced IQ, language development, and attention span and increased aggression and impulsivity, as well as life-long health impacts. According to a Swedish study, an increase in lead levels in the blood from 5 to 10 µg per deciliter is associated with a decrease in nineth grade Grade Point Average of 2.2 percentile points and a 2.3% decrease in the likelihood of graduating high school.[45] Exposure to lead is an equity issue. Poor children, children on public health insurance, and Black and Latinx children are at highest risk for lead intoxication.[46] Because of historic racial disparities in poor housing and lead exposure, Black infants are estimated to experience a 50% higher average loss of IQ points attributable to blood lead than White infants.[47]

The Flint Michigan water crisis brought the problem of lead in water pipes to the nation's attention. The bipartisan Infrastructure and Jobs bill passed in November 2021 includes $15 billion over 5 years to replace lead pipes and service lines across the country; this is a great start and long overdue. But the Environmental Protection Agency (EPA) estimates that the cost to replace all the lead pipes in the United States is closer to $28 to $47 billion. This is a policy that needs further action.[45]

Air Pollution Mitigation

Other areas related to environmental justice are even more complex. Poor communities have historically been riddled with urban highways. Chemical plants, refineries, and other industrial sites that pollute the air and water have been located closer to poor communities and communities of color. A Toxics Release Inventory prepared by the EPA shows that African Americans and other minority groups make up 56%

of those living near toxic sites such as refineries, landfills, and chemical plants. Negative effects include chronic health problems such as asthma in children and adults as well as hypertension and cancer. The American Academy of Pediatrics (AAP) suggests that the EPA should increase air quality standards and better regulate and more strongly enforce existing rules.[48]

Tree Canopies in Poor City Neighborhoods

Inequities in "greening of communities," especially tree canopies, exist for high-poverty neighborhoods and communities of color. Tree canopies are particularly good at reducing health effects associated with urban heat islands. It is estimated that urban heat islands can cause temperatures to be 5° to 7° warmer during the day and 22° warmer at night. Communities of color have 33% less tree canopy on average than majority white communities. Neighborhoods with 90% or more of their residents living in poverty have 41% less tree canopy than communities with only 10% or less of the population in poverty.[49] The policy solution is for cities to modify their tree-planting programs (which exist in most cities) to plant many more trees in those communities that have inadequate tree canopies.

GUN VIOLENCE PREVENTION

Firearms are the leading cause of death in children, adolescents, and young adults 0 to 24 years of age in the United States. Homicides account for 58%, suicides account for 37%, 2% are unintentional, and legal intervention accounts for 1%. There are significant disparities by race and ethnicity as well as gender and sexual orientation. Overall, boys die from firearms 4.5 times as often as girls. Black youth die from homicide at nearly twice as high as the rate for American Indian children, 4 times higher than the rate for Hispanic children, and about 10 times higher than the rate for white and Asian American children. AI/AN male youth have the highest suicide rates. LGBTQ + youth attempt suicide 4.5 times as often as heterosexual youth, but data on completed suicides are limited.[50–52]

The Bipartisan Safer Communities Act, passed and signed into law in June 2022, was the first legislation to seriously address firearm violence since 1994. The Act implements several gun safety laws, including expanded background checks for those purchasing a gun who are younger than 21 years and prohibiting gun purchases for those who committed a qualifying crime when they are younger than 18 years. It clarifies Federal Firearms License requirements, provides funding for state red flag laws (Extreme Risk Protection Orders), further criminalizes arms trafficking and straw purchases, and includes a partial closure of the "boyfriend loophole." It also provides significant funding for children and adolescent mental health services.[53]

Although the Bipartisan Safer Communities Act is ground breaking, there are several other policy solutions not yet promulgated:[54]

Federal Laws and Regulations

1. Make background checks universal. Background checks, using information from federal and local law enforcement sources, should be done before all firearm purchases (including firearms sold at federally licensed dealers and other transactions at gun shows, private sales and transfers, and online).
2. Initiate buyer regulations, including laws that increase age limits, require buyers to obtain a permit or license, and require a waiting period before firearm purchase.
3. Ban semiautomatic military-style weapons and high-capacity magazines.
4. Require safety mechanisms, such as trigger locks, by law.

5. Change the regulation of the Consumer Product Safety Commission (CPSC) to repeal a previous ruling from 1976 that prohibits the CPSC from making a ruling that restricts the manufacture or sale of firearms and firearms ammunition. This ruling has prevented the adoption of "smart" gun technology, which is available but not in use. These "smart" firearms would recognize and allow use by authorized users and prevent use by unauthorized users, thereby preventing many unintentional pediatric deaths and likely greatly reducing youth firearm suicides.

State Laws and Regulations

State legislators should pass Child Access Prevention (CAP) laws and Safe Storage laws to prevent access to guns. CAP laws hold adults (parents) in civil or criminal liability if a child gains access to a gun. Safe storage laws focus on compliance with mandated safe storage of guns. Although CAP laws target prevention of unintentional deaths and injuries in children, there is evidence that they also decrease suicides and homicides. Stronger CAP laws, meaning those with criminal liability for negligent storage of firearms, show greater reductions in both teen suicide and unintentional deaths.[55,56] Strong CAP and Safe Storage laws should be instituted in all US states.

Evidence supports the effectiveness of gun safety laws to prevent firearm deaths.[54–57]

LGBTQ + HEALTH EQUITY
Same-Sex Marriage and Parenting by Gay and Lesbian Parents

The AAP has long strongly supported same-sex marriage and parenting by same-sex couples. In 2013, a policy statement expressed support for marriage equality for all, including those who are of the same sex. This policy additionally called for the repeal of the 1996 Defense of Marriage Act (DOMA) that denies to members of married same-sex households access to benefits equivalent to those afforded to married parents of different genders and forbids the federal government from recognizing same-sex marriages.[58]

On 2015, the Supreme Court ruled in *Obergefell v. Hodges* that the 14th Amendment required all US states to recognize same-sex marriages. This ruling rendered DOMA unenforceable and essentially moot. Although there had been previous efforts to pass a Respect for Marriage Act (RFMA) legalizing same-sex marriages, it seemed that RFMA was now de facto federal law. However, in 2022, a concurring opinion by one of the Supreme Court justices regarding another case suggested that the Supreme Court reconsider the *Obergefell* ruling. In response to that threat, RFMA was reintroduced in Congress, with revisions including protections for interracial marriages.[59] The bill has passed the House but not yet in the Senate. The Senate should pass this important bill.

Support for Transgender and Gender-Diverse Children and Adolescents

The AAP published a policy in 2018 in support of transgender and gender-diverse children and adolescents.[60] That policy stated that children and adolescents who so identify should have access to gender-affirming and developmentally appropriate health care; that insurance plans should offer coverage specific to the needs of transgender youth (including coverage for medical, psychological, and when appropriate, surgical gender affirming interventions); and that pediatricians should advocate for policies and laws that protect transgender youth from discrimination and violence (including at the school and community level).

Lawmakers from several states have introduced bills aimed at restricting medical access or procedures for transgender minors.[61] The bills include proposals to criminalize treatments and surgeries and classify some medical procedures as child abuse. One state has passed a bill to prohibit insurers from covering gender transition procedures for minors. State legislators in many states introduced bills to limit participation in high school or college athletic teams based on "biological sex," and some states have already passed these bills. Although some states with hate crime bills include gender identity or gender expression, many states do not. Policy solutions include repealing or preventing passage of state laws that criminalize treatments for transgender youth or limit participation in high school and college athletics based on biological sex; advocating for all states to mandate insurance coverage for transgender youth; and inclusion of gender identity in state hate crime legislation.

PROTECT IMMIGRANT CHILDREN AND FAMILIES
Treatment of Children at the Southern Border

For the last 2 years, approximately 10,000 to 18,000 unaccompanied minors and 200,000 to 300,000 families with children have been crossing the southwest border each month.[62] Several policies/laws exist that either protect or harm these children. The AAP's policy on the detention of immigrant children addresses many of these regulations.[63]

The 1997 Flores Settlement agreement is the basis of nationwide policy for the detention and treatment of unaccompanied minors in immigration custody. It requires the government to release children from immigration detention without unnecessary delay to their parents, other adult relatives, or licensed programs. It requires recreation, education, and medical care in the least restrictive environment, as well as food, shelter, and clothes. Facilities holding these minors must be licensed by the state to care for children. Frequently these rules are not followed. In 2015, the court ruled that children in family detention centers (accompanied children) must be treated according to Flores as well. The Trump administration planned to terminate the Flores Settlement, but the Biden administration reversed that decision.

Two policies instituted in the Trump administration, the Migrant Protection Protocols (Remain in Mexico or MMP) in 2019 and Title 42 of the public health code at the start of the COVID pandemic, have trapped many children and families on the Mexican side of the border in squalid and dangerous situations. The Biden administration ended MMP in June 2022. Title 42 allows the CDC to prohibit the entry of persons from other countries into the United States to prevent spread of communicable diseases. In the spring of 2022, the CDC thought it was no longer needed, but a court order has kept it in place.[64] Title 42 finally expired in May 2023 with the end of the Covid-19 public health emergency.

Policy solutions include enforcing all the provisions of the Flores agreement, including ending without delay the sheltering or detention of children and families and discharging them to the community; never using the Flores Settlement requirement to release children expeditiously (but not requiring the same for their parents) in order to separate children from their parents; and with the ending of Title 42, expedite alowing children and families to cross the border without expulsion.

Deferred Action for Childhood Arrivals and the American Dream and Promise Act of 2021(Dream Act)

Undocumented youth who were brought to the United States by their parents before the age of 16 years and are in school, or graduated, or in the armed forces may apply for Deferred Action for Childhood Arrivals (DACA). DACA allows recipients to have protection from deportation, get a Social Security card and work, have a driver's license, attend college, and pay in-state tuition rates. The more than 800,000 so-called dreamers cannot apply for PELL grants to defray the costs of college. DACA, promulgated in 2012 during the Obama administration, is under threat of being declared unlawful by the courts. At present, DACA recipients can renew their status, but no new applications are being accepted. Advocates have asked Congress to make it permanent, but there is resistance to addressing DACA without a comprehensive immigration law.

The Dream Act of 2021 would provide an expedited pathway to becoming legal permanent residents (green card) and citizens for DACA recipients and other immigrants, such as immigrants with Temporary Protected Status. It was passed in the House but stalled in the Senate.[6,65]

Policy solutions to help dreamers include making DACA permanent, opening up DACA to new applicants, allowing dreamers to apply for PELL grants, and passing the Dream Act. Congress should also pass the LIFT the BAR act, which would allow all DACA recipients and all other immigrants lawfully present in the United States to access federal benefits. It would also remove the 5-year waiting period for many immigrant children which still is a barrier in many states to accessing CHIP.[6] Both DACA and the Dream Act have been strongly supported by more than 70 medical organizations including the AAP.

CLINICS CARE POINTS

- Help eligible children enroll in Medicaid or CHIP if they are not already enrolled.
- Help your families fill out their tax returns in order to get their EITCs through medical-financial partnerships
- Screen for food insecurity in all low-income families; make sure they are enrolled in WIC, SNAP, and school meals; and refer food insecure families to local pantries.
- Make sure immigrant families know that all pregnant women and children are eligible for WIC benefits unrelated to their immigration status.
- Make sure immigrant families know that SNAP and Medicaid/CHIP benefits for their children are not part of the public charge and they should not deny their children these benefits out of fear of deportation or of never being able to apply for citizenship.
- Make sure that immigrant families know that the Trump era public charge expansions have been rescinded by the Biden administration.
- Start a Reach Out and Read Program if one does not already exist to your practice or clinic.
- Make sure that children at risk for lead poisoning are screened with blood lead tests. Children enrolled in Medicaid are required to get tested for lead at ages 12 and 24 months or age 24 to 72 months if they have no record of ever being tested. All children in low-income households, and who are immigrants from low- or middle-income countries, whether or not enrolled in Medicaid, should be tested for lead.
- Ask about guns in homes of the families you care for and counsel about safe storage and suicide risk.
- Provide a welcoming and sensitive environment and evidence-based health care for transgender children and adolescents.
- Advocate for transgender children and adolescents in your local school districts to be able to participate in school athletics based on their preferred, not biological, gender/sex.

- Assist families with housing and immigration problems through medical-legal partnerships.
- Refer families at higher risk for maternal depression and child neglect to evidence-based home visiting programs

DISCLOSURE

The author has nothing to disclose.

REFERENCES

1. Perrin JA, Kenny GM, Rosenbaum S. Medicaid and child health equity. NEJM 2020;383:2595–8.
2. Alker KC, Kenny GM, Rosenbaum S. Children's health insurance coverage: progress, problems, and priorities for 2021 and beyond. Health Aff 2020;39:1743–51.
3. Available at: https://ccf.georgetown.edu/wp-content/uploads/2018/05/ichia_fact_sheet.pdf. Assessed October 12, 2022.
4. Rosenberg J, Shabanova V, McCollum S, et al. Insurance and health care outcomes in regions where undocumented children are Medicaid-eligible. Pediatrics 2022;150. e2022057034.
5. Available at: https://www.kff.org/racial-equity-and-health-policy/issue-brief/health-coverage-by-race-and-ethnicity/. Assessed October 12, 2022.
6. Available at: https://firstfocus.org/wp-content/uploads/2021/09/FACT-SHEET_LIFT-the-BAR.pdf. Assessed October 12, 2022.
7. Available at: https://firstfocus.org/resources/fact-sheet/fact-sheet-10-ways-to-improve-the-health-coverage-of-americas-children. Assessed October 12, 2022.
8. Available at: https://www.cms.gov/newsroom/fact-sheets/streamlining-eligibility-enrollment-notice-propose-rulemaking-nprm. Assessed October 12, 2022.
9. Available at: https://myasone.org/wp-content/uploads/2021/10/Value-Based-Pmt_Childrens-Health_FINAL.pdf. Assessed October 12, 2022.
10. Kemper AR, Kelleher KJ, Allen S, et al. Improving the health of all children in our community: the Nationwide Children's Hospital and Franklin Count, Ohio, Pediatric Vital Signs Project. J Pediatr 2020;222:227–30.
11. Available at: https://www.nychealthandhospitals.org/pressrelease/system-launches-3-2-1-impact-program-provides-early-intervention-services-to-families/. Assessed October 12, 2022.
12. Sharma A, Flower KB, Wong CA. Incorporating kindergarten readiness as a meaningful measure in pediatric value-based care. JAMA Health Forum 2022; 3:e220616.
13. Bell S, Deen JF, Fuentes M, et al, AAP Committee On Native American Child Health. Caring for American Indian and Alaska Native Children and Adolescents. Pediatrics 2021;147. e2021050498.
14. National Academies of Sciences, Engineering, and Medicine. A roadmap to reducing child poverty. Washington, DC: The National Academies Press; 2019. https://doi.org/10.17226/25246.
15. Dreyer BP. Cash transfers and reducing child poverty in the US. JAMA Pediatr 2022. https://doi.org/10.1001/jamapediatrics.2022.2951.
16. Troller-Renfree SV, Costanzo MA, Duncan GJ, et al. The impact of a poverty reduction intervention on infant brain activity. Proc Natl Acad Sci U S A. 2022; 119(5). e2115649119.

17. Available at: https://www.irs.gov/newsroom/irs-offers-overview-of-tax-provisions-in-american-rescue-plan-retroactive-tax-benefits-help-many-people-now-preparing-2020-returns. Assessed October 12, 2022.
18. Available at: https://www.cbpp.org/research/economy/a-national-paid-leave-program-would-help-workers-families. Assessed October 12, 2022.
19. Available at: https://iwpr.org/wp-content/uploads/2020/09/B334-Paid-Parental-Leave-in-the-United-States.pdf. Assessed October 12, 2022.
20. Stanczyk AD. Does paid family leave improve household economic security following a birth? Evidence from California. Social Service Review 2019;262–304.
21. Available at: access-to-and-use-of-paid-family-and-medical-leave.htm">https://www.bls.gov/opub/mlr/2019/article/racial-and-ethnic-disparities-in-access-to-and-use-of-paid-family-and-medical-leave.htm. Assessed 12 October, 2022.
22. Available at: http://diversitydata.org/sites/default/files/2020-01/ddk_policyequity assessment_fmla_2020_2_0.pdf. Assessed October 12, 2022.
23. Available at: https://www.epi.org/resources/budget/. Assessed October 12, 2022.
24. Duncan GJ, Ziol-Guest KM, Kalil A. Early-childhood poverty and adult attainment, behavior, and health. Child Dev 2010;81(1):306–25.
25. Available at: https://workforce.com/news/minimum-wage-by-state-2022-all-you-need-to-know. Assessed 12 October, 2022.
26. Available at: https://www.ers.usda.gov/topics/food-nutrition-assistance/food-security-in-the-u-s/key-statistics-graphics/#householdtype. Assessed October 12, 2022.
27. Shankar P, Chung R, Frank DA. Association of food insecurity with children's behavioral, emotional and academic outcomes: a systemic review. J Dev Behav Pediatr 2017;38:135–50.
28. Faught EL, Williams PL, Willows ND, et al. The association between food insecurity and academic achievement in Canadian school-aged children. Publ Health Nutr 2017;20:2778–885.
29. Grineski SE, Morales DX, Collins TW, et al. Transitional dynamics of household food insecurity impact children's developmental outcomes. J Dev Behav Pediatr 2018;39:715–25.
30. Ralston K, Treen K, Coleman-Jensen A, et al. *Children's Food Security and USDA Child Nutrition Programs*, EIB-174. U.S. Department of Agriculture, Economic Research Service; 2017.
31. Heckman JJ. Skill formation and the economics of investing in disadvantaged children. Science 2006;312:1900–2.
32. Bradbury B, Corak M, Waldfogel J, et al. Too many children left behind. New York: Russell Sage Foundation; 2015.
33. Available at: https://www.aecf.org/resources/early-reading-proficiency-in-the-united-states. Assessed October 12, 2022.
34. Williams PG, Lerner MA, AAP Council On Early Childhood, AAP Council On School Health. School Readiness. Pediatrics 2019;144(2):e20191766.
35. Donoghue EA, AAP council on early childhood. Quality Early Education and Child Care From Birth to Kindergarten. Pediatrics 2017;140(2):e20171488.
36. Available at: http://www.ecs.org/wp-content/uploads/How-States-Fund-Pre-K_A-Primer-for-Policymakers.pdf. Assessed October 12, 2022.
37. Duffee JH, Mendelsohn AL, Kuo AA, et al. Early Childhood Home Visiting. Pediatrics 2017;140(3):e20172150.
38. https://nationalhomevisitingcoalition.org/. Assessed October 12, 2022.

39. Mendelsohn AL, Mogilner LN, Dreyer BP, et al. The impact of a clinic-based literacy intervention on language development in inner-city preschool children. Pediatrics 2001;107(1):130–4.
40. Mendelsohn AL, Dreyer BP, Flynn V, et al. An RCT of the video interaction project, a low intensity intervention to promote development in at-risk young Latino children: impact on cognitive and language outcomes at 21 months. J Dev Behav Pediatr 2005;26(1):34–41.
41. Council on Community Pediatrics. Providing care for children and adolescents facing homelessness and housing insecurity. Pediatrics 2013;131(6):1206–10.
42. Rubin DH, Erickson CJ, San Augustin M, et al. Cognitive and academic functioning of homeless children compared to housed children. Pediatrics 1996; 97(3):289–94.
43. Available at: http://www.evidenceonhomelessness.com/factsheet/hprp/. Assessed October 12, 2022.
44. Available at: https://www.liheap.org/white-paper#policy-recommendations. Assessed October 12, 2022.
45. Available at: https://www.brookings.edu/blog/up-front/2021/05/13/what-would-it-cost-to-replace-all-the-nations-lead-water-pipes/. Assessed October 12, 2022.
46. Hauptman M, Niles JK, Gudin J, et al. Associated With Detectable and Elevated Blood Lead Levels in US Children: Results From a National Clinical Laboratory. JAMA Pediatr 2021;175(12):1252–60.
47. Boyle J, Yeter D, Aschner M, et al. Estimated IQ points and lifetime earnings lost to early childhood blood lead levels in the United States. Sci Total Environ 2021; 778:146307.
48. Available at: https://www.aap.org/en/advocacy/transition-plan-2020/strong-communities/environmental-health/. Assessed October 12, 2022.
49. Available at: https://www.scientificamerican.com/article/trees-are-missing-in-low-income-neighborhoods/. Assessed October 12, 2022.
50. Available at: www.cdc.gov/injury/WISQARS. Assessed October 12, 2022.
51. Lee LK, Douglas K, Hemenway D. Crossing lines–a change in the leading cause of death among U.S. children. N Engl J Med 2022;386(16):1485–7.
52. Fowler KA, Dahlberg LL, Haileyesus T, et al. Childhood firearm injuries in the United States. Pediatrics 2017;140(1):1–11.
53. Available at: https://www.congress.gov/bill/117th-congress/senate-bill/2938/text?r=5&s=1. Assessed October 12, 2022.
54. Lee LK, Fleegler EW, Goyal MK, et al. AAP Policy Statement: Firearm-Related Injuries and Deaths in Children and Youth: Injury Prevention and Harm Reduction. Pediatrics 2022. https://doi.org/10.1542/peds.2022-060070.
55. Lee LK, Fleegler EW, Goyal MK, et al. AAP Technical Report: Firearm-Related Injuries and Deaths in Children and Youth. Pediatrics 2022. https://doi.org/10.1542/peds.2022-060071.
56. Schell TL, Cefalu M, Griffin BA, et al. Changes in firearm mortality following the implementation of state laws regulating firearm access and use. Proc Natl Acad Sci USA 2020;117(26):14906–10.
57. Galea S, Abdalla SM. State firearm laws and firearm-related mortality and morbidity. JAMA 2022;328(12):1189–90. https://doi.org/10.1001/jama.2022.16648.
58. American Academy of Pediatrics, Committee On Psychosocial Aspects Of Child And Family Health. Promoting the Well-Being of Children Whose Parents Are Gay or Lesbian. Pediatrics 2013;131(4):827–30.
59. Available at: https://www.congress.gov/bill/117th-congress/house-bill/8404/text. Assessed October 12, 2022.

60. Rafferty J, AAP Committee On Psychosocial Aspects Of Child And Family Health, AAP Committee On Adolescence, AAP Section On Lesbian, Gay, Bisexual, And Transgender Health And Wellness. Ensuring Comprehensive Care and Support for Transgender and Gender-Diverse Children and Adolescents. Pediatrics 2018;142(4):e20182162.
61. Available at: https://usafacts.org/articles/state-level-laws-and-statutes-affecting-transgender-americans/. Assessed October 12, 2022.
62. Available at: https://www.cbp.gov/newsroom/stats/southwest-land-border-encounters. Assessed October 12, 2022.
63. Linton JM, Griffin M, Shapiro AJ, AAP council on community pediatrics. Detention of Immigrant Children. Pediatrics 2017;139(5):e20170483.
64. Available at: https://www.govinfo.gov/content/pkg/USCODE-2011-title42/html/USCODE-2011-title42-chap6A-subchapII-partG-sec265.htm. Assessed October 12, 2022.
65. Available at: https://americasvoice.org/blog/immigration-101-what-is-the-dream-and-promise-act/. Assessed October 12, 2022.

Moving?

Make sure your subscription moves with you!

To notify us of your new address, find your **Clinics Account Number** (located on your mailing label above your name), and contact customer service at:

Email: journalscustomerservice-usa@elsevier.com

800-654-2452 (subscribers in the U.S. & Canada)
314-447-8871 (subscribers outside of the U.S. & Canada)

Fax number: 314-447-8029

Elsevier Health Sciences Division
Subscription Customer Service
3251 Riverport Lane
Maryland Heights, MO 63043

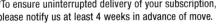